D1567499

SEIZURES

CURRENT CLINICAL NEUROLOGY

Daniel Tarsy, MD, *Series Editor*

Seizures

Medical Causes and Management

Edited by

Norman Delanty, MB, FRCPI

Department of Clinical Neurological Sciences
Royal College of Surgeons in Ireland
Beaumont Hospital, Dublin, Ireland

Foreword by

Marc Dichter, MD, PhD

Professor of Neurology, Director, Penn Epilepsy Center,
Hospital of the University of Pennsylvania, Philadelphia, PA

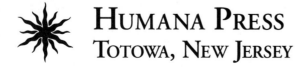

Humana Press
Totowa, New Jersey

© 2002 Humana Press Inc.
999 Riverview Drive, Suite 208
Totowa, New Jersey 07512

www.humanapress.com

The content and opinions expressed in this book are the sole work of the authors and editors, who have warranted due diligence in the creation and issuance of their work. The publisher, editors, and authors are not responsible for errors or omissions or for any consequences arising from the information or opinions presented in this book and make no warranty, express or implied, with respect to its contents.

Due diligence has been taken by the publishers, editors, and authors of this book to assure the accuracy of the information published and to describe generally accepted practices. The contributors herein have carefully checked to ensure that the drug selections and dosages set forth in this text are accurate and in accord with the standards accepted at the time of publication. Notwithstanding, since new research, changes in government regulations, and knowledge from clinical experience relating to drug therapy and drug reactions constantly occur, the reader is advised to check the product information provided by the manufacturer of each drug for any change in dosages or for additional warnings and contraindications. This is of utmost importance when the recommended drug herein is a new or infrequently used drug. It is the responsibility of the treating physician to determine dosages and treatment strategies for individual patients. Further, it is the responsibility of the health care provider to ascertain the Food and Drug Administration status of each drug or device used in their clinical practice. The publishers, editors, and authors are not responsible for errors or omissions or for any consequences from the application of the information presented in this book and make no warranty, express or implied, with respect to the contents in this publication.

This publication is printed on acid-free paper. ∞

ANSI Z39.48-1984 (American National Standards Institute) Permanence of Paper for Printed Library Materials.

Cover design by Patricia F. Cleary.

For additional copies, pricing for bulk purchases, and/or information about other Humana titles, contact Humana at the above address or at any of the following numbers: Tel: 973-256-1699; Fax: 973-256-8341; E-mail: humana@humanapr.com or visit our website at http://humanapress.com

Printed in the United States of America.   10 9 8 7 6 5 4 3 2 1

Library of Congress Cataloging-in-Publication Data

Seizures: medical causes and management / edited by Norman Delanty ; foreword by Marc Dichter.
     p. ; cm. -- (Current clinical neurology)
   Includes bibliographical references and index.
   ISBN 0-89603-827-0 (alk. paper)
   1. Convulsions. I. Delanty, Norman. II. Series
   [DNLM: 1. Seizures--diagnosis. 2. Seizures--therapy. WL 340 S462 2002]
  RC394.C77 S45 2002
  616.8'45--dc21

                                                                          2001039367

Foreword

Seizures are frightening events. They frighten the patients who experience them; they frighten those who witness them; they also frighten many physicians who have to deal with them. Most individuals with seizures present to family physicians or to emergency room physicians. However, despite the fact that seizures are among the most common neurological conditions, most general practitioners, family practice specialists, and internists do not see large numbers of patients with seizures. Given the apoplectic appearance of generalized tonic clonic convulsions, it is not difficult to understand why they arouse such emotional responses in those that experience them, those that witness them, and those whose care is sought for them.

Seizures are symptoms of something wrong with the brain. Many different kinds of perturbations in brain anatomy, chemistry, or physiology can produce seizures. For many individuals, seizures occur in the context of an acute illness and will not recur once that illness is treated. These individuals do not have epilepsy. They have transient disturbances in brain function attributable to systemic medical conditions. It is important to recognize these issues, because, first, the seizure may be the initial, or even only, manifestation of the underlying medical problem and this needs to be recognized. Second, if the underlying medical condition can be diagnosed and effectively treated, the seizures often disappear and the patients do not need to take medication for long periods of time, nor become disabled from their seizures. For other patients, epilepsy will actually present in the context of a systemic illness, either coincident with the illness or directly caused by the illness. These individuals will have multiple problems: their primary illness and their epilepsy, and often both need to be evaluated and treated separately.

What kinds of conditions cause seizures? Almost every variety of disturbance in one's general medical state can result in seizures, including infections, drugs, metabolic disturbances, multiorgan failure, trauma, neoplasms, and so on. In *Seizures: Medical Causes and Management*, Norman Delanty has brought together an impressive panel of experts in various medical conditions that result in seizures, with the admirable goal of bringing order to what, in many cases, is a chaotic, uneven, and widely dispersed literature on the medical causes of seizures and their management. *Seizures: Medical Causes and Management* is designed to elevate the expertise of both generalists (non-neurologists) and neurologists in the area of seizure evaluation and treatment. It addresses issues not generally emphasized in either the general medical literature or in the specialized neurology literature, and does so in sufficient detail to raise the discussion several notches above that generally presented. Most textbooks will focus on a disease and then perhaps mention in passing that seizures may be one of its symptoms. This book focuses on the circumstances under which seizures develop in any given condition, how to recognize this potential life-threatening complication, and how to effectively treat it within the context of that disease. As such it is destined to become a "must have" book for almost anyone practicing medicine—in the office or in the hospital—regardless of one's specialty or the mix of patients in one's practice.

Seizures are *big* events in the life of an individual. Seizures may have *big* consequences. Seizures deserve a *big* treatment. Norman Delanty has recognized this and with this book has filled a significant hole in our medical literature.

Marc A. Dichter, MD, PhD

Preface

Seizures: Medical Causes and Management is intended to present a comprehensive discussion of acute symptomatic seizures. These are common in clinical practice and are encountered by a wide range of clinicians. I believe that a book such as this one is needed as the topic appears to have fallen between the two stools of medicine and neurology. Neurologists and epileptologists are frequently asked to assess and advise on management of individuals with these situation-related seizures. This topic has been given relatively scant treatment in the medical literature and in standard text-books, possibly because it straddles many specialties. The present book is intended at least in part to address this shortfall. It aims to provide in one volume a comprehensive treatment of the causes and management of symptomatic seizures associated with a wide variety of medical disorders. It should prove a valuable resource to those caring for patients who are at risk of seizures in the setting of systemic illness. I hope that neurologists, internists, anesthesiologists, and intensive care unit and emergency physicians will all find it of value.

Chapter 1 serves as a broad introduction, discussing general principles and intro-ducing important terms and definitions. Chapter 2 is an attempt to unify a discussion of the pathophysiology of acute symptomatic seizures, although this is also discussed where appropriate in later chapters. Chapter 3 deals with acute symptomatic seizures caused by underlying primary central nervous system insult. Chapters 4 to 16 are divided into those dealing with specific etiologic areas of acute symptomatic seizures, such as seizures resulting from organ failure, alcohol-related seizures, and seizures in cancer patients. The important topic of the differential diagnosis between seizure and syncope is discussed in Chapter 17. I felt it important to include a specific chapter on seizures in the tropics (Chapter 18). Chapter 19 discusses issues pertaining to the intensive care unit, and Chapter 20 deals with symptomatic status epilepticus. The final chapter (Chapter 21) is a discussion of the use of anticonvulsants in systemically sick patients. Although there is inevitable overlap between chapters, this has been kept to a minimum.

I am grateful to all the authors, for both their excellent contributions and their patience as I worked through this project while moving between continents. I am delighted that Marc Dichter agreed to write the Foreword. I am especially grateful to Paul Dolgert and Craig Adams at Humana Press for their help and understanding. Finally, and most of all, I thank my wife, Breda, and children, Niamh and Saorlaith, for tolerating and supporting me.

Norman Delanty, MB, FRCPI

Contents

Contributors

BRIAN K. ALLDREDGE, PharmD • *Professor of Cinical Pharmacy and Neurology, University of California, San Francisco, San Francisco, CA*

THOMAS P. BLECK, MD, FACP, FCCM, FCCP • *The Louise Nerancy Eminent Scholar in Neurology and Professor of Neurology, Neurological Surgery, and Internal Medicine; Director, Neuroscience Intensive Care Unit; Member, F. E. Dreifuss Comprehensive Epilepsy Center; Department of Neurology, The University of Virginia, Charlottesville, VA*

JANE BOGGS, MD • *Associate Professor of Neurology; Director, Neurophysiology and Epilepsy Services, University of South Alabama, Mobile, AL*

JOHN C. M. BRUST, MD • *Director, Department of Neurology, Harlem Hospital Center; Professor of Clinical Neurology, Columbia University College of Physicians and Surgeons, New York, NY*

RAMEL A. CARLOS, MD • *Department of Neurology, Wake Forest University School of Medicine, Winston-Salem, NC*

FERNANDO CENDES, MD, PhD • *Assistant Professor, Department of Neurology, FCM–UNICAMP, Cidade Universitária, Campinas—SP, Brazil*

PETER B. CRINO, MD, PhD • *Penn Epilepsy Center, Neurological Intensive Care Unit, Department of Neurology, Hospital of the University of Pennsylvania, Philadelphia, PA*

JOSEP DALMAU, MD, PhD • *Department of Neurology, University of Arkansas for Medical Sciences, Little Rock, AR*

NORMAN DELANTY, MB, FRCPI • *Consultant Neurologist, Department of Clinical Neurological Sciences, Royal College of Surgeons of Ireland, Beaumont Hospital, Dublin, Ireland*

MICHELE DEL SIGNORE, DO • *Department of Neurology, Rush-Presbyterian-St. Luke's Medical Center, Chicago, IL*

GAIL D'ONOFRIO, MD • *Section of Emergency Medicine, Yale University School of Medicine, New Haven, CT*

HENRY FRAIMOW, MD • *Associate Professor of Medicine, Division of Infectious Disease, MCP-Hahnemann School of Medicine, Philadelphia, PA*

JACQUELINE A. FRENCH, MD • *Penn Epilepsy Center, Department of Neurology, Hospital of the University of Pennsylvania, Philadelphia, PA*

MICHAEL M. FRUCHT, MD • *Fellow, F. E. Dreifuss Comprehensive Epilepsy Center; Department of Neurology, The University of Virginia, Charlottesville, VA*

PAUL A. GARCIA, MD • *Associate Professor of Clinical Neurology, University of California, San Francisco, San Francisco, CA*

ALVARO R. GUTIERREZ, MD • *Professor of Neurology, West Virginia University School of Medicine, Morgantown, WV*

BRUCE B. LERMAN, MD • *Division of Cardiology, Department of Medicine, Weill Medical College of Cornell University, New York, NY*

SUNEET MITTAL, MD • *Division of Cardiology, Department of Medicine, Weill Medical College of Cornell University, New York, NY*

KEVIN MURPHY, MB, MRCPI • *Department of Clinical Neurological Sciences, Royal College of Surgeons in Ireland; Department of Neurology, Beaumont Hospital, Dublin, Ireland*

CORMAC A. O'DONOVAN, MD • *Department of Neurology, Wake Forest University School of Medicine, Winston-Salem, NC*

NIELS K. RATHLEV, MD • *Department of Emergency Medicine, Boston University School of Medicine, Boston, MA*

MUREDACH REILLY, MB, MRCPI • *Cardiovascular Division, Department of Medicine, University of Pennsylvania Health System, Philadelphia, PA*

JACK E. RIGGS, MD • *Professor of Neurology, Medicine, and Community Medicine, West Virginia University School of Medicine, Morgantown, WV*

COLIN ROBERTS, MD • *Department of Neurology, Hospital of the University of Pennsylvania, Philadelphia, PA*

MYRNA R. ROSENFELD, MD, PhD • *Department of Neurology, University of Arkansas for Medical Sciences, Little Rock, AR*

NIMAL SENANAYAKE, MD, PhD, DSc, FRCP, FRCPE • *Senior Professor of Medicine, Department of Medicine, Faculty of Medicine, University of Peradeniya, Peradeniya, Sri Lanka*

MICHAEL C. SMITH, MD • *Department of Neurology, Rush-Presbyterian-St. Luke's Medical Center, Chicago, IL*

JOERG-PATRICK STÜBGEN, MD, FRCPC • *Associate Professor of Neurology and Neuroscience, Weill Medical College of Cornell University; Associate Attending Neurologist and Neurologist for the Intensive Care Units, New York-Presbyterian Hospital and Hospital for Special Surgery, New York, NY*

ANDREW S. ULRICH, MD • *Department of Emergency Medicine, Boston University School of Medicine, Boston, MA*

CARL J. VAUGHAN, MD, MRCPI • *Division of Cardiology, Department of Medicine, Weill Medical College of Cornell University, New York, NY*

1

Definitions and Epidemiology

Norman Delanty, MB, FRCPI

Introduction and Definitions

An epileptic seizure may be defined as a discrete spontaneous alteration in behavior or a subjective experience occurring due to an abnormal hypersynchronous excessive discharge of a collection of neurons within the brain. Seizures are commonly encountered in hospital practice. Such seizures are often provoked situation-related seizures and occur in patients who do not have epilepsy (defined as recurrent unprovoked seizures) **(Fig. 1)** *(1,2)*. These provoked seizures are also referred to as acute symptomatic seizures and may occur in patients being cared for by general practitioners, internists, surgeons, emergency department physicians, intensivists, anesthesiologists, and other specialists. The evaluation and management of these patients is a significant proportion of the consultative workload of neurologists in hospital practice. Yet, these symptomatic seizures have been relatively ignored in the neurology literature in relation to their importance and frequency in clinical practice. The proper evaluation of acute symptomatic seizures is critical in guiding management, optimizing neurologic outcome, and often avoiding unnecessary long-term treatment with inappropriate and sometimes toxic therapy with anticonvulsant medications.

Acute symptomatic seizures occur in close temporal relationship to a systemic or neurologic insult, and occur as an indirect or direct consequence of this insult **(Table 1)**. These seizures occur in the setting of an initiating illness and are therefore referred to as situation-related seizures. Often the nature of the mechanistic or pathophysiologic relationship between the acute stressor and the seizure is unclear (*see* Chap. 2). Less often, a specific mechanism can be evoked to explain the seizure. Acute symptomatic seizures can be divided arbitrarily into those that are primarily due to *de novo* central nervous system

From: *Seizures: Medical Causes and Management*
Edited by: N. Delanty © Humana Press, Inc., Totowa, NJ

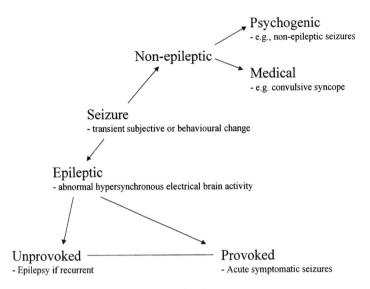

Fig. 1.

(CNS) disease and those due to disease initially arising outside the brain, such as systemic organ failure. It is obvious that such a distinction is artificial and that any failure of homeostasis leading to a seizure in some way affects the nervous system. Meningitis, encephalitis, stroke, and head trauma are all acute disturbances of the brain that are often accompanied by symptomatic seizures. In addition, these disorders may have poorly understood delayed or long-term pathogenetic epileptogenic consequences, which lead to the later development of epilepsy, long after the initial illness. Such epilepsy is often referred to as remote symptomatic epilepsy.

Seizures are categorized into generalized and focal (or partial) types, depending on whether they arise deep within thalamocortical circuits, or whether they arise from a specific site (or focus) within the brain, respectively *(3)*. An absence seizure (petit mal) is an example of a generalized seizure that usually occurs in children and adolescents and is characterized by brief staring, unresponsiveness, and subtle eye blinking, and the immediate return to full awareness at the end of the seizure. A primary generalized tonic-clonic convulsion (a grand-mal seizure) can occur in any of the generalized epilepsies, e.g., in juvenile myoclonic epilepsy. In partial epilepsy, a simple partial seizure arises from one focal part of the brain and occurs without alteration of awareness or consciousness. An aura of a rising epigastric sensation is an example of a simple partial seizure, usually of temporal lobe origin. A complex partial seizure occurs when the seizure arises from one part of the brain and is associated with alteration or loss of awareness. A partial seizure may evolve into a tonic-clonic convulsion, a process referred to as secondary gen-

Table 1
Causes of Acute Symptomatic Seizures

1. Medications (therapeutic, overdose)
2. Alcohol-related
3. Illicit drugs
4. Environmental toxins
5. Electrolyte imbalance
6. Glucose disturbance
7. Organ failure
8. Infection (CNS, systemic)
9. Acute CNS disturbance
10. Multisystem disorders
11. Hypoxic-ischaemic encephalpathy
12. Hypertensive encephalopathy
13. Nonhypertensive posterior leukoencephalopathy
14. Cancer-associated
15. Organ transplant

eralization. Most tonic-clonic convulsions occurring in adults happen as a result of this secondary generalization from an abnormal focus.

Acute symptomatic seizures are related to a provoking illness or circumstance such as illicit drug use. In contrast, epilepsy is clinically defined as recurrent unprovoked seizures. Epilepsy is not one disease; there are many different causes and types. Seizures and epilepsy can be regarded as the clinical manifestation or symptom of underlying brain dysfunction. Any of the provoking factors that cause acute symptomatic seizures in individuals without epilepsy can also aggravate seizures in those with epilepsy. In addition, the distinction between an unprovoked and a provoked seizure is not always clear-cut. For example, the seizures of juvenile myoclonic epilepsy are frequently aggravated by life-style factors such as sleep deprivation and preceding alcohol intake. However, as a general rule, the degree of sleep deprivation and the quantity of prior alcohol consumption provoking seizures in those with epilepsy will not usually cause acute symptomatic seizures in those without epilepsy.

Everyone's brain has the capacity to seize, depending on the interaction between the underlying genetic background, possible past history of brain injury, and the particular nature and magnitude of any acute symptomatic stressors. An individual with epilepsy (i.e., recurrent unprovoked seizures) can be thought of as having a low seizure threshold, whereas an individual who only seizes in the event of being exposed to particularly severe symptomatic insult has a high seizure threshold. Although acute symptomatic seizures are not due to epilepsy, circumstances or conditions causing these seizures are referred to as being epileptogenic, although they could be thought of more correctly as being "seizurogenic."

The management of acute symptomatic seizures involves stabilization of the patient, short-term use of appropriate anticonvulsant drugs such as benzodiazepines and phenytoin, and correction of the underlying cause or causes. If these underlying factors can be corrected, then long-term use of anticonvulsant medication is usually not indicated. It is important that a full explanation of the cause of the seizure be given to the referring physician and to the patients and their families. It is also important to explain that the individual does not have epilepsy. Considerations with regard to driving are guided by laws within the particular jurisdiction. In general, if the underlying cause of the seizure cannot be corrected adequately, the situation should be treated similarly to that pertaining to patients with epilepsy. If the acute symptomatic provocateur can be corrected, it is reasonable practice to advise abstinence from driving for a period of 6 mo.

Nonepileptic Seizures

Some clinical seizures occur unrelated to underlying hypersynchronous discharge of neurons. These are referred to as nonepileptic seizures and may be divided into two categories: medical and psychogenic. As an example of the former, syncope may sometimes cause loss of consciousness with brief tonic-clonic motor activity. This type of convulsive syncope is not an epileptic seizure and does not respond to treatment with anticonvulsant drugs. Underlying psychiatric or psychological processes may also cause seizures that are not due to underlying epileptic phenomena. Examples include nonepileptic seizures occurring due to underlying conversion disorder, dissociative disorder, and panic disorder. These seizures are also referred to as nonorganic or psychogenic seizures, or non-epileptic attack disorder. The term "pseudoseizures" should be avoided because of its confrontational and accusatory connotations. The majority of patients with these nonepileptic seizures are not malingering. These seizures are best seen as a cry for help that needs intervention and treatment in its own right. Nonepileptic seizures are sometimes encountered in hospitalized patients with underlying medical problems and are best managed by epileptologists often using video electroencephalogram (EEG) monitoring to aid in definitive diagnosis *(4)*.

Epidemiology of Acute Symptomatic Seizures

Several studies have examined the epidemiology of acute symptomatic seizures, including those seizures caused by acute neurologic insult. The age-adjusted incidence rate of acute symptomatic seizures was 16.4/100,000 person-years in Martinique, 25.2 in Geneva, 29 in Gironde, France, and 39.0

in Rochester, Minnesota *(5)*. These studies have shown that men are at higher risk than women, and risk is significantly higher at the extremes of age. In the Martinique study, the most common causes were alcohol-related seizures (30.1% of total), seizures due to stroke (20.6%), and those due to head trauma (18.7%) *(6)*. The other main causes were toxins and drugs (11.1%), tumors (9.4%), and metabolic (4.8%) and infectious (4.7%) disease. In the Minnesota study, the leading causes were head trauma (16% of total), cerebrovascular disease (16%), infection (15%), and drug withdrawal (14%) *(7)*. In this study, the risk of experiencing an acute symptomatic seizure in an 80-yr life span was 3.6%, which approaches that of developing epilepsy. In another study of over 13,000 children less than 3 yr of age in Taiwan, the cumulative incidence over a 2-yr period was 460/100,000, with infection being the predominant cause *(8)*. In a hospital study of nearly 2000 consecutive patients admitted to an intensive care unit with a primary non-neurologic diagnosis, acute symptomatic seizures occurred in 61 (or 28%) of 217 patients who developed neurologic complications *(9)*.

It is clear that acute symptomatic seizures are a common problem encountered by many physicians. Specific situations causing these seizures are discussed in detail throughout the remainder of this book. A broad understanding of the principles and definitions outlined in this chapter, as well as correct use of terminology, allows for a greater understanding of these seizures and aids in communication about their etiology and optimum management.

References

1. Boggs J. Seizures in medically complex patients. *Epilepsia* 1997;38(Suppl 4):S55–S59.
2. Delanty N, Vaughan CJ, French JA. Medical causes of seizures. *Lancet* 1998;352:383–390.
3. Murphy K, Delanty N. Primary generalized epilepsies. *Curr. Treatment Options Neurol.* 2000;2:527–541.
4. French J. Pseudoseizures in the era of video-electrocephalogram monitoring. *Curr Opin Neurol* 1995;8:117–120.
5. Jallon P. Epidemiology of acute symptomatic seizures. *Epilepsia* 2000;41(Suppl):127.
6. Jallon P, Smadja D, Cabre P, Le Mab G, Bazin M, EPIMART Group. EPIMART: Prospective incidence study of epileptic seizures in newly referred patients in a French Carribean island (Martinique). *Epilepsia* 1999;40:1103–1109.
7. Annegers JF, Hauser WA, Lee R-J, Rocca WA. Incidence of acute symptomatic seizures in Rochester, Minnesota, 1935–1984. *Epilepsia* 1995;36:327–333.
8. Huang C-C, Chang Y-C, Wang S-T. Acute symptomatic seizure disorders in young children—a population study in southern Taiwan. *Epilepsia* 1998;39:960–964.
9. Bleck TP, Smith MC, Pierre-Louis SJ-C, Jares JJ, Murray J, Hansen CA. Neurologic complications of critical medical illnesses. *Crit Care Med* 1993;21:98–103.

2

Pathophysiology of Acute Symptomatic Seizures

Carl J. Vaughan, MD, MRCPI and Norman Delanty, MB, FRCPI

Introduction

Seizures may arise through the direct or indirect effects of disease on the central nervous system (CNS). Drugs used to treat a variety of systemic illnesses may alter the seizure threshold and cause seizures, and illness may also unmask an underlying tendency to seizures in a stressed patient. In this chapter, we explore the pathogenesis of acute symptomatic seizures in patients who are systemically ill. In some circumstances, much is already known about the mechanisms underlying the development of seizures. However, in many instances these remain speculative and are not completely understood. We will attempt to present putative mechanisms that lead to seizures, based on our current understanding of specific disease processes and their interplay with neuronal excitability. Many of the diseases described in this chapter will be discussed in greater detail in subsequent chapters. This chapter serves to highlight both the general and specific mechanisms responsible for seizure development in a variety of medical illnesses. We have chosen a number of prototypic disorders (i.e., hyponatremia, alcohol withdrawal syndrome, hepatic failure, drug toxicity, and infectious disease) to illustrate particular pathophysiologic processes that orchestrate the development of seizures. We will also focus on the complex and clinically important interplay of discrete pathophysiologic processes, which may aggregate to produce seizures in critically ill patients.

Although seizures may complicate a variety of chronic medical illnesses (**Table 1**), seizures are seen most commonly in patients who are critically ill. In a study of 55 patients with new-onset seizures admitted to an intensive care unit (*1*), seizures were associated with narcotic drug withdrawal in approximately one-third of patients. In a further one-third, the cause was an acute

From: *Seizures: Medical Causes and Management*
Edited by: N. Delanty © Humana Press, Inc., Totowa, NJ

Table 1
Examples of Medical Causes of Seizures

Cerebrovascular disease	Metabolic (*cont.*)
Thombosis	Hypomagnesemia
Embolism	Alkalosis
Hemorrhage	Organ Failure
Vasculitis	Hepatic failure
Cerebral infection	Renal failure
Meningitis	Endocrine
Encephalitis	Hypothyroidism
Abscess	Thyrotoxicosis
Neurosyphilis	Vitamin deficiency
Hypoxic-ischaemic encephalopathy	(e.g., pyridoxine deficiency)
Hypotensive syndromes (shock, Stokes-	Drugs- Therapeutic (e.g., penicillins
Adams attacks, vasodepressor syncope)	imepenem, isoniazid, phenothiazines,
Hypertensive encephalopathy	meperidine, theophylline, cyclosporine
Eclampsia	FK506 [tacrolimus]
Fever	Drugs- Recreational (e.g., cocaine)
Metabolic	Alcohol withdrawal
Hypoglycemia	Sedative drug withdrawal
Hyponatremia/hypernatremia	Environmental toxins (e.g., lead,
Hypocalcemia	mercury, arsenic, strychnine, thallium)

metabolic disorder, predominantly significant hyponatremia (<125 mmol/L serum sodium). In eight patients seizures were attributed to drug toxicity (mainly the use of antiarrhythmic or antibiotic agents). Less than 10% of patients in this study had previously unrecognized structural abnormalities of the CNS that were manifest by focal or generalized tonic-clonic seizures. In 10%, the cause of the seizures remained unknown.

General Mechanisms of Seizure Development

A seizure is produced when neurons within an area of the brain are activated in an unusually synchronous manner. Focal activation of a group of neurons may subsequently spread to involve nearby or distant neurons in an abnormal activation pattern. Any event, or combination of events, that disturbs the delicate balance between neuronal excitation and inhibition can produce a seizure. Many different cellular or biochemical changes such as alterations in ion channel function, neurotransmitter level, neurotransmitter receptor function, or energy metabolism may affect the excitability of neurons and produce seizures. In general, depolarization is mediated by synaptic currents generated by the excitatory neurotransmitters glutamate and aspartate **(Fig. 1)** *(2)*. Neuronal synchronization occurs through local enhancement of excitatory circuits. An increase in synaptic efficacy is thought to be due to recruitment of

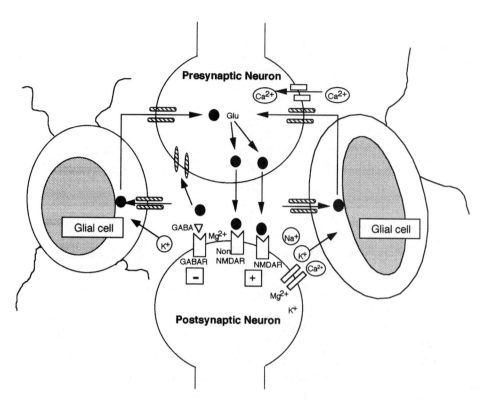

Fig. 1. Neuroexcitability: the presynaptic and postsynaptic neuron. Excitatory amino acids are released from the presynaptic terminal and act on postsynaptic NMDA and non-NMDA receptors (NMDAR) to cause excitation. GABA is an inhibitory neurotransmitter and acts on postsynaptic GABA receptors (GABAR). The glial cells play a central homeostatic role in the control of neuroexcitation by controlling extraneuronal potassium concentration and by removing excitatory neurotransmitters such as glutamate (Glu). Neuronal excitability may also be influenced by ions such as magnesium.

N-methyl-D-aspartate (NMDA) receptors *(3)* **(Fig. 1).** As more NMDA receptors are activated, further depolarization occurs, additional calcium enters the cell, and excitability is enhanced. As these excitatory processes increase, there may be a simultaneous reduction in the activity of inhibitory circuits that are downregulated during high-frequency activation. Neurons can also be synchronized by extracellular currents that may reflect changes in the perineuronal environment, such as local edema, or changes in the extracellular potassium, calcium, or magnesium concentration *(4)*. Finally, neurons may also be synchronized by local ephaptic (nonsynaptic) contacts, which facilitate the development of excitatory circuits *(5,6)*.

In many instances, the precise sequence of events leading to the development of seizures in patients with acute illness remains speculative. However, several pathophysiologic processes appear crucial in the pathogenesis of seizures in the acutely ill **(Table 2).** Changes in the permeability of the

Table 2
Pathophysiologic Mechanisms Producing Seizures in Acutely Ill Patients

Vascular	Changes in the blood brain barrier
	Changes in intracranial pressure
	Hemorrhage
	Cerebral infarction
	Change in cerebral blood flow autoregulation
	Cerebral microhemorrhage and Fe^{2+} liberation
Metabolic	Glucose or electrolyte disturbance (sodium, potassium, calcium, magnesium)
	Endocrine dysfunction (thyroid, adrenal, pituitary)
Neuronal	Neuronal excitotoxicity
	Glial cell dysfunction
	GABA neuronal loss
	Free radical damage
Infection	Central nervous system or systemic infections
	Fever
Drugs and compounds	Drug toxicity
	Drug or alcohol withdrawal
	Recreational drug use
Autoimmune	Systemic inflammatory or autoimmune states i.e. systemic lupus erythematous
Cardiovascular	Arrhythmias
	Loss of blood pressure homeostasis
	Emboli
Hematologic	Thrombotic or hemorrhagic states
Genetic	

blood–brain barrier due to infection, hypoxia, or alterations in cerebral blood flow autoregulation may allow passage of drugs and toxins into the CNS, thus influencing neuronal excitability **(Fig. 2)**. Changes in the integrity of the blood–brain barrier may also influence homeostasis within the neuronal microenvironment that is normally tightly regulated by the glial cell **(Fig. 1).** For example, glial cells normally maintain a low concentration of extracellular potassium *(7)*. Interruption of the blood–brain barrier may directly cause glial cell dysfunction or change the extracellular environment beyond its regulatory capacity. Glial cell dysfunction may lead to seizures by permitting a high ratio of extracellular to intracellular potassium, which depolarizes the neuronal membrane and increases neuronal excitability *(8)*.

Cerebral hemorrhage has been strongly associated with seizure development. For example, this may occur in the setting of spontaneous intracerebral or subarachnoid hemorrhage, which may be associated with hypertension.

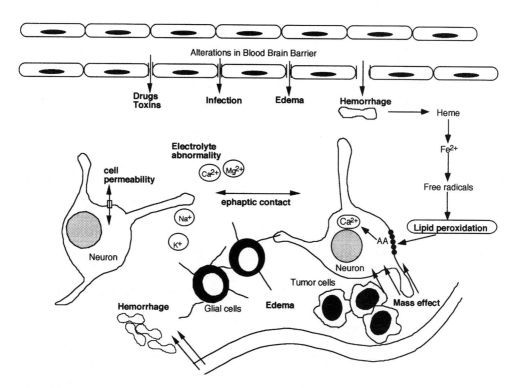

Fig. 2. Pathophysiology of seizures in the systemically ill. A number of pathophysiologic processes may lead to seizures, including alterations in the integrity of the blood–brain barrier, electrolyte abnormalities, changes in neuronal permeability, ephaptic (nonsynaptic) contact between neurons in the setting of edema or infiltrative processes, and hemorrhage or mass effects caused by tumors or infections. The liberation of Fe^{2+} from hemosiderin in areas of hemorrhage may lead to the production of free radicals, lipid peroxidation, and activation of the arachidonic acid cascade. This may elevate intracellular calcium concentration and mediate neuronal excitability, excitotoxicity, and neuronal death.

More subtle alterations in cerebrovascular endothelial cell permeability and integrity as a result of disorders such as hypertensive encephalopathy can lead to the formation of small areas of edema or hemorrhage **(Fig. 2)**. The liberation of iron from hemoglobin may be an important inciting mechanism for seizure development. The presence of free iron within the CNS may lead to the production of free radicals, lipid peroxidation, and activation of the arachidonic acid cascade *(9,10)*. These processes may promote the formation of inositol triphosphate and diacylglycerol, which elevate intracellular calcium concentration; this, in turn, may mediate neuronal excitability, excitotoxicity, and ultimately neuronal death.

In critically ill patients, glucose and/or electrolyte abnormalities are important in the pathophysiology of seizures **(Fig. 2)**. Hypoglycemia is a common cause of both coma and seizures and should be excluded in any patient presenting with a seizure. Disturbances of electrolyte homeostasis are common and may arise in the setting of intravenous fluid therapy, diuretic use, or activation of the hypothalamic/pituitary/adrenal axis. Of particular importance is abnormal central potassium homeostasis. In animal models of epilepsy, increased extracellular potassium decreases neuronal hyperpolarization and promotes seizure activity *(4,7,8)*. Similarly, low extraneuronal concentrations of calcium or magnesium may increase synaptic excitability predisposing to seizures *(11,12,13)*. Low magnesium concentration leads to activation of NMDA receptors, which are normally inhibited by voltage-dependent magnesium blockade. Moreover, changes in the concentration of other ions within the neuronal extracellular environment may also have important influences on the activity of voltage-gated ion channels.

Structural changes in the brain parenchyma that accompany systemic illnesses may produce seizures. A variety of vascular disease processes may produce seizures, and stroke is a common cause of seizures in older people. Seizures may accompany an acute stroke or occur later as a result of a scar formation in brain tissue. This occurs when neurons in the affected area die, and glial cells, mainly astrocytes, cause a glial reaction, which may produce a seizure focus. Altered blood flow may affect neurotransmitter concentration by causing ischemic damage to neurons responsible for production and release of neurotransmitters; γ-aminobutyric acid (GABA) neurons are particularly susceptible to ischemic damage due to their high intrinsic metabolic rate *(14)*. GABA is an inhibitory neurotransmitter that acts on populations of GABA receptors to reduce synaptic excitability (**Fig. 1**). Factors that compromise neurons that produce GABA may increase the likelihood of seizures.

Cardiac disease may also lead to seizures. Patients with structural heart disease and/or atrial fibrillation have an increased tendency to develop thromboembolic stroke that may present with or cause seizures. Patients with a variety of different congenital heart defects have a propensity to develop cerebral emboli or infarction that may also present with a seizure. A patent foramen ovale may present in this manner with emboli arising in the venous circulation, which cross to the left heart through the patent foramen. Although exceptionally rare, cardiac myxomas have been reported to present with a seizure *(15)*.

Abscesses or tumors may have a number of direct and indirect seizure-provoking effects (**Fig. 2**). Mass lesions may disturb cerebral blood flow *(16)* or cerebrospinal fluid (CSF) production/flow and alter the integrity of the blood–brain barrier. In addition, tumors or foci of infection produce local inflammation and lead to the production of pro-inflammatory cytokines. Tumors have a propensity to cause cerebral edema and hemorrhage. Brain edema associated with these pathophysiologic processes may cause neuronal and neuroglial swelling and reduce the relative space between cells. This may increase neuronal excitation because of ephaptic interactions between different groups of neurons *(5,6)* (**Fig. 2**).

An imbalance of neurotransmitters may predispose to seizure activity. Depletion of inhibitory neurotransmitters or accumulation of excitatory neurotransmitters in ailing patients may cause seizures (**Fig. 1**). Increased amounts of excitatory amino acids such as glutamate and aspartate, formed during hypoxic–ischemic injury, may increase neuronal excitability *(17)*. Conversely, depletion of the inhibitory neurotransmitter GABA may also trigger seizures *(18)*. In addition, the formation of free radicals during acute illness may putatively predispose to both seizures and exacerbate neuronal injury *(19)* (**Fig. 2**).

Genetic alterations affecting ion channel or receptor function may predispose to seizures. It is being increasingly recognized that many idiopathic types of epilepsy have a genetic basis *(20)*. Similarly, individuals without a history of epilepsy may have molecular genetic defects that make seizures more likely when homeostasis is disturbed. Subclinical defects in mitochondrial DNA could also predispose to seizures in critically ill patients *(21)*.

A seizure may directly promote further seizure activity through its effects on the brain. Increased excitability may also independently lead to neuronal damage (excitotoxicity). Resting neurons depend on continuously synthesized adenosine triphosphate (ATP) to maintain an electrochemical gradient across the neuronal membrane. During seizures, ATP requirements increase *(22)*, and this may exceed the capacity of cerebral blood flow to deliver additional substrate. Convulsive seizures are also often associated with hypoxia and acidosis that may further exacerbate the energy-depleted state *(23)*.

Sleep deprivation is common in hospitalized critically ill patients, and this may further predispose to the occurrence of acute symptomatic seizures. Sleep deprivation itself is well recognized as a precipitant of seizures in those with and without epilepsy *(24)*. It is thus not uncommon for a student doing frequent "all-nighters" prior to examination time to present to the Emergency Room following a convulsion. In addition, the seizures of the genetic idiopathic epilepsies (e.g., juvenile myoclonic epilepsy) are particularly vulnerable to sleep deprivation. The causes of sleep deprivation in hospitalized patients are many and include undertreated pain and discomfort, environmental noise pollution, frequent disruption by staff during intensive physiologic monitoring, and disease or medication-induced alteration in sleep architecture *(25)*. In one survey of patients' perceptions of intensive care, 46 of 76 patients (61%) reported subjective complaints of sleep deprivation *(26)*. In another study of environmental noise in an intensive care unit, noise levels above 80 decibels were most likely to cause sleep deprivation, and patients identified staff noise as the most disturbing *(27)*. Television and talking accounted for half of sound peaks and were amenable to behavior modification. Further study of this problem is warranted, and in the future, improved engineering design of hospital critical care units may help to alleviate some aspects of noise pollution and thus reduce sleep deprivation and risk of seizures.

Specific Disease Processes and Seizure Pathogenesis

Hyponatremia and Electrolyte Disturbances

Acute hyponatremia (<48-h duration) is generally hospital-acquired and occurs mainly in the postoperative state and/or after excessive fluid administration. Chronic hyponatremia (>48-h duration) usually develops outside the hospital and is generally better tolerated. Some factors appear to aggravate hyponatremic encephalopathy, including female gender (menstruating women) *(28)*, and young age. Hyponatremia produces brain edema, and increased intracranial pressure that may lead to seizures and other neuropathological sequelae, including death *(29,30)*. Hyponatremia is compounded by the tendency of neuronal tissue to undergo demyelination during rapid correction of hyponatremia (central pontine or extrapontine myelinolysis) *(31)*. The mechanisms through which hyponatremia produce neurologic dysfunction and seizures have been studied extensively. Normally, when serum sodium decreases, the brain is protected from edema by actively extruding electrolytes and organic osmolytes. Conversely, during a subsequent increase in serum sodium, re-establishment of intracerebral electrolyte balance occurs but in a delayed manner (often requiring 5 d). In both circumstances the protective mechanisms that normally prevent the development of cerebral edema can be overwhelmed *(29,30)*. The concurrence of both hyponatremia and hypoxia can be particularly problematic and frequently leads to refractory seizures. Hyponatremia aggravates hypoxic brain injury by further reducing the pH after a hypoxic insult. This occurs through a reduction in the availability of sodium for use in the proton exchange pump. As protons build up in the cytoplasm the limited amount of sodium renders the cell unable to restore normal pH *(32)*.

Alcohol Withdrawal Seizure

Alcohol withdrawal seizure (AWS) refers to the seizures that occur secondary to the withdrawal of alcohol after a period of chronic alcohol administration *(33)*. A growing body of evidence indicates that ethanol increases the effect of GABA at $GABA_A$ receptors and contemporaneously blocks the NMDA receptor *(34)*. These events lead to a down-regulation of the GABA system and up-regulation of the NMDA receptor system, which promotes increases in neuronal excitability when ethanol withdrawal occurs. Another mechanism that has been proposed to explain the pathogenesis of AWS is the modified lipid-protein interaction *(35)*. This hypothesis proposes that acute ethanol ingestion modulates the neuronal cell membrane phospholipid that leads to altered protein handling or insertion within the membrane. It is proposed that this alters the relative contribution of $GABA_A$ receptors, NMDA receptors, and voltage-gated Ca^{2+} channels in a manner that promotes neuronal excitability upon withdrawal of alcohol. Low-dose alcohol has been shown to inhibit calcium influx through the NMDA receptor/ionophore, and alcohol has also been shown experimentally to increase the expression of NMDA receptors in the hippocampus. These data suggest that upregulation of the NMDA receptor/ionophore complex plays a role in AWS *(36)*. Other possible mechanisms may relate to the direct effects of unopposed metabolites of alcohol such as aldehydes on nervous tissue, which predominate during the withdrawal period.

Hepatic Encephalopathy

Hepatic encephalopathy is complex neurologic syndrome associated with acute or chronic liver failure. The pathophysiologic basis of hepatic encephalopathy has been investigated extensively *(37)*. Ammonia is considered to play an important role in the onset of hepatic encephalopathy. Seizures in fulminant hepatic failure may be caused by acute ammonia neurotoxicity. Ammonia is directly excitotoxic and is associated with increased synaptic release of glutamate, activation of NMDA receptors, and increased neuroexcitability *(38)*. In contrast, hepatic encephalopathy complicating chronic liver failure is associated with a shift toward a net increase of inhibitory neurotransmitters owing to downregulation of NMDA receptors and inactivation of the glutamate transporter GLT-1 in astrocytes *(37)*. In addition, chronic liver failure is associated with increased inhibitory GABA activity caused by elevated brain levels of GABA, and the direct interaction of increased levels of ammonia with the $GABA_A$ receptor complex. Patients with liver failure are particularly prone to develop drug toxicity, as many drugs undergo extensive hepatic metabolism. Additionally, reduced hepatic synthetic function may reduce serum plasma protein concentration and increase free levels of drugs that are normally highly protein-bound. These changes in drug metabolism and handling may predispose to drug toxicity and seizures.

Febrile Seizures and the Genetic Milieu

Febrile convulsions affect 2–5% of children under age 5. Although these seizures have a variety of causes, it is increasingly recognized that many have a familial component. Genetic linkage analysis in families with febrile seizures inherited as an autosomal dominant trait have revealed that the disease genes responsible for these disorders are located on chromosome

8q13-21 and chromosome 19p13.3 *(39,40)*. To date, the genes responsible for febrile convulsions in these families have not been isolated. These genes are of great interest, as they may have a pivotal role in neuronal responses to fever and other neurologic insults. Febrile convulsions are age-related acute symptomatic seizures in which there is a large genetic background, but one that depend on the occurrence of an additional stressor (i.e., fever) before seizures are manifest. This disorder may therefore be a prototype of many other acute symptomatic seizures that occur in the setting of systemic illness.

Recently, molecular studies in animals have uncovered a number of genetic abnormalities that predispose to seizure activity. Mice harboring a mutation in the gene encoding the α_{1A}-subunit of the voltage-dependent calcium channel are seizure prone *(41)*. Similarly, a mutation in the *Nhe-1* gene, which encodes a sodium–hydrogen exchanger, is responsible for seizures in the slow-wave epilepsy mutant mouse *(42)*. The *Nhe-1* exchanger has a prominent homeostatic role in virtually all cells of the CNS by extruding a hydrogen ion in exchange for sodium, thereby maintaining intracellular pH and cell volume. Molecular genetic studies of human epilepsy have unveiled a number of inherited defects, predominantly in genes coding ion channel subunits *(20)*. In the absence of epilepsy, mutations or polymorphisms in these or other human genes that regulate neuronal homeostasis may produce a subclinical predisposition to seizures that may only become manifest during the stress of an acute illness.

Infectious Agents and AIDS

Many bacterial, viral, fungal, and parasitic infections produce seizures. A spectrum of pathophysiologic processes accompany different infections to produce CNS dysfunction that leads to seizures. Cortical damage may accompany infection with a number of viruses, including herpes, rubella, measles, and human immunodeficiency virus (HIV) *(43)*. Conspicuous cerebral edema and inflammation occurs in varicella-zoster virus infection. Cerebral malaria is very frequently accompanied by seizures. The pathogenesis of cerebral malaria is characterized by capillary thrombosis caused by intravascular aggregation of parasitized red cells, predominantly within the cerebral white matter. Aspergillosis, tuberculosis, hydatosis, cysticercosis, and trypanosomiasis generally produce CNS disease and seizures through the formation of vasculitis, infarction, necrosis, and granuloma or abscess formation. Infection with *Candida* species often leads to meningitis, whereas infection with *Aspergillus* generally leads to hyphal vasculitis, infarction, or abscess formation *(44)*.

Although a seizure may be the presenting symptom in a patient with AIDS, seizures are more common in advanced stages of the disease *(45,46)*. Seizures are usually generalized; however, partial seizures may also occur. Intracranial mass lesions are responsible for over 50% of neurologic disorders in AIDS patients, and seizures are a common presentation of such lesions *(47)*. Mass lesions promote seizure development through local irritation of the brain parenchyma, enhanced ephaptic contact between neurons facilitated by invading inflammatory or neoplastic cells, compression of brain structures, or disruption of blood flow. Venous drainage or CSF circulation in the brain adjacent to a space-occupying lesion may also be disrupted. Toxoplasmosis and primary CNS lymphoma are the most common mass lesions encountered among patients with AIDS *(47)*. Other causes of intracranial lesions that may precipitate seizures include tuberculomas, tuberculous abscesses, and cryptococcal abscesses. Meningitis and encephalitis are also common and may present with seizures. Cryptococcal meningitis is the most frequent meningitis provoking seizures in AIDS *(46,48)*. Meningoencephalitis may lead to the development of seizures through a variety of pathophysiologic processes such as focal irritation and inflammation of the brain parenchyma, disruption of the blood–brain barrier, and through alterations in intracranial pressure and CSF production or flow. Progressive multifocal leukoencephalopathy (PML) may also cause new-onset seizures among patients with AIDS *(49)*. This process does not produce an intracranial mass effect, but it has been postulated that PML precipitates seizures by producing demyelinating foci near the cerebral cortex, which lead to cortical irritability, and/or by interrupting axonal conduction.

Although mass lesions and infections may have a florid presentation with new-onset seizures, the etiology of seizures remains unknown in over 50% of cases. In these patients a number of pathophysiologic processes have been proposed to contribute to the development of seizures. These putative factors include HIV- or immune-mediated neuronal cell death and the production of neurotoxic substances such as eicosanoids, cytokines, or free radicals, which enhance glutamate availability and lead to the activation of voltage-gated calcium channels and NMDA receptors. Patients with AIDS may have a variety of other electrolyte, endocrine, or metabolic abnormalities that may contribute to the development of seizures, including hyponatremia, hypomagnesemia, hypoadrenalism, and renal failure *(50,51)*. Finally, the milieu in patients with AIDS is further complicated by the increasing use of multiple drugs (i.e., antimicrobial drugs and protease inhibitors) with many side effects and the potential for a myriad of drug interactions.

Drugs and Toxins

A variety of drugs and toxins are known to cause seizures. The list of drugs outlined in **Table 1** is a representative sample of a much larger list of compounds that have been associated with the development of seizures *(52,53)*. The most common causes of drug- or toxin-induced seizures are medications, such as the tricyclic antidepressants, theophylline, and isoniazid, or the recreational abuse of drugs such as cocaine, phenylcyclidine, and amphetamines

(54). Cocaine-induced seizures have been documented after a single dose and are often generalized tonic-clonic, and self-limiting *(55).* However, cocaine may be associated with other serious pathologies including severe hypertension, intracranial hemorrhage, stroke, aortic dissection, and spinal cord injuries. Administration of large doses of penicillin may cause seizures, including status epilepticus, through disinhibition of the $GABA_A$ receptor by allosteric modulation of the receptor by the penicillin molecule *(56).* The mechanisms of isoniazid-induced seizures appears to be through depletion of pyridoxine (vitamin B_6) through the formation of isoniazid–pyridoxal hydrazones *(57).* These hydrazones inhibit the enzyme pyridoxal phosphate, leading to additional depletion of pyridoxine. Depletion of pyridoxine in the CNS depletes GABA. It has been shown that in this setting seizures can be prevented by administering large doses of pyridoxine. Theophylline is commonly used in the management of patients with a variety of pulmonary disorders, and theophylline toxicity is frequently associated with the development of seizures *(58).* Recent data from an animal model suggest that theophylline-induced seizures are mediated by $GABA_A$ and NMDA receptors *(59).* The pathophysiologic mechanisms of seizures accompanying salicylate overdose are unclear. A high concentration of salicylate in the CNS is associated with low CNS glucose levels and enhanced CNS oxygen consumption *(60,61).* The high anion-gap metabolic acidosis seen in salicylate poisoning may also contribute to the development of seizures. Seizures may occur after deliberate or accidental exposure to carbon monoxide (CO). This gas binds to hemoglobin to form carboxyhemoglobin, resulting in a reduced tissue oxygen content and cellular hypoxia *(62).* The brain is particularly sensitive to hypoxia, leading to cerebral dysfunction and injury *(63).* Putative mechanisms of neuronal injury accompanying CO poisoning include direct cellular toxicity, hypoxia, lipid peroxidation *(64),* free radical damage *(54),* altered neurotransmitter release, acidosis, and hypotension.

The accidental ingestion of toxins is associated with seizure development. For example, mussels contaminated with the neurotoxin domoic acid, a structural analog of glutamate and kainate, has been reported to cause encephalopathy and prolonged seizures in some patients *(65,66).* Although a large number of other exogenous drugs and toxins may cause seizures (**Table 1**), the molecular and biochemical bases through which these compounds induce seizures are not completely understood.

Interplay Between Different Pathophysiologic Factors and the Genesis of Seizures

In many acutely ill patients who seize, no specific single cause can be found. In these circumstances, it is likely that a number of synergistic subcritical insults aggregate to promote seizure development *(67).* **Figure 3** rep-

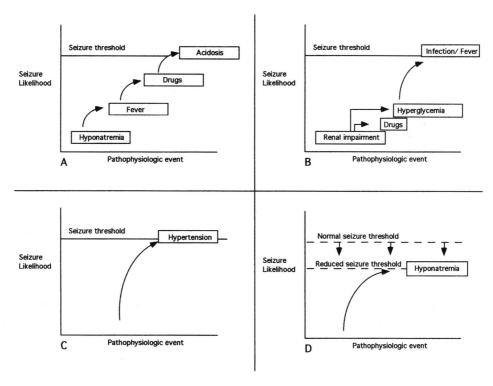

Fig. 3. Putative models of initiating factors and seizure development. (**A**) The acute disease model: A number of cumulative insults are required before seizures develop. (**B**) The chronic disease model: Seizures develop as a consequence of a single insult superimposed on a background of chronic disease. (**C**) The single insult model: A single insult of sufficient magnitude produces seizures in the absence of other precipitants. (**D**) The genetic predisposition model: The genetic constitution of the individual is such that seizures occur in the setting of a relatively minor insult that would not normally cause a seizure.

resents this concept schematically. In **Figure 3A** a number of cumulative insults are required before seizures develop. This is an acute disease model and is common among critically ill patients who develop progressive organ dysfunction and multiorgan failure. The case illustrated in **Figure 3B** is a chronic disease model; and in contrast to the acute disease model, seizures develop as a consequence of a single insult superimposed on a background of chronic disease. Examples of chronic disease models in which seizures occur with an increased frequency are chronic renal failure and in patients with cerebrovascular disease. The single insult model is represented in **Figure 3C;** an example of this model is eclampsia. In eclampsia the rate of blood pressure rise is usually sufficient to produce seizures in the absence of other pathologies. Finally, the genetic predisposition model (**Fig. 3D**) conceptualizes the occurrence of seizures in a subject with a latent seizure tendency but one who does not have epilepsy. This is similar to the single insult model, but in this model the genetic constitution of the individual is such that seizures occur in the setting of a relatively minor insult that would not normally cause a seizure. This model best explains interindividual differences in seizure tendency.

The concept of cumulative synergistic insults **(Fig. 3A)** and seizure development has important therapeutic implications. The therapy of symptomatic seizures in the acutely ill often requires antiepileptic drug therapy. However, it is important to pay close attention to the patient's physiologic milieu at the time of seizure development to determine the presence of one or more reversible factors that perturb CNS homeostasis. Reversal of one or more homeostatic abnormalities in a critically ill patient may prevent seizures from occurring by interrupting the cumulative insults as depicted in **Figure 3A.**

Conclusion

Systemic illnesses often cause seizures. A seizure is produced when neurons are activated in a synchronous manner. The mechanisms causing seizures in the systemically ill patient are incompletely understood. Seizures often reflect an imbalance between neuronal excitation and inhibition and may be due to a variety of cellular or biochemical changes that affect neuronal excitability. The neurotransmitters glutamate and aspartate mediate excitation, and inhibition is mediated by the prominent GABA system. Neurons can be synchronized by changes in the neuronal environment due to alterations in the blood–brain barrier, brain edema, electrolyte disturbance, or through non-synaptic neuronal contact. Seizures are a prominent feature in a number of diseases, including disorders of electrolyte homeostasis, particularly in hyponatremia, and AWS. Seizures are also a conspicuous and important manifestation of many infectious diseases, including HIV. In many patients who seize, there may be no single etiologic factor that accounts for seizure development. Seizures in this setting may be caused by cumulative synergistic insults. Pre-emptive reversal of one or more discrete homeostatic abnormalities in a critically ill patient may prevent their synergism and their culmination in a seizure.

References

1. Wijdicks EF, Sharbrough FW. New-onset seizures in critically ill patients. *Neurology* 1993;43:1042–1044.
2. Greenamyre JT, Porter RH. Anatomy and physiology of glutamate in the CNS. *Neurology* 1994;44:S7–S13.
3. Rogawski MA. Excitatory amino acids and seizures. In: Stone TW (ed.), *CNS Neurotransmitters and Neuromodulators;* vol 2, Glutamate. Boca Raton, FL: CRC, 1995;219–237.
4. Traynelis SF, Dingledine R. Potassium-induced spontaneous electrographic seizures in the rat hippocampal slice. *J Neurophysiol* 1988;59:259–276.

5. Jefferys JG. Nonsynaptic modulation of neuronal activity in the brain: electric currents and extracellular ions. *Physiol Rev* 1995;75:689–723.
6. Jefferys JG, Haas HL. Synchronized bursting of CA1 hippocampal pyramidal cells in the absence of synaptic transmission. *Nature* 1982;300:448–450.
7. Amedee T, Robert A, Coles JA. Potassium homeostasis and glial energy metabolism. *Glia* 1997;21:46–55.
8. Sypert GW, Ward AA Jr. Changes in extracellular potassium activity during neocortical propagated seizures. *Exp Neurol* 1974;45:19–41.
9. Ciuffi M, Gentilini G, Franchi-Micheli S, Zilletti L. Lipid peroxidation induced "in vivo" by iron-carbohydrate complex in the rat brain cortex. *Neurochem Res* 1991;16:43–49.
10. Lamb RG, Harper CC, McKinney JS, Rzigalinski BA, Ellis EF. Alterations in phosphatidylcholine metabolism of stretch-injured cultured rat astrocytes. *J Neurochem* 1997;68:1904–1910.
11. Anderson WW, Lewis DV, Swartzwelder HS, Wilson WA. Magnesium-free medium activates seizure-like events in the rat hippocampal slice. *Brain Res* 1986;398:215–219.
12. Haas HL, Jeffreys JGR. Low-calcium field burst discharges of CA1 pyramidal neurons in at hippocampal slices. *J Physiol* 1984;354:185–201.
13. Avoli M, Drapeau C, Louvel J, Pumain R, Olivier A, Villemure J-G. Epileptiform activity induced by low extracellular magnesium in the human cortex maintained in vitro. *Ann Neurol* 1991;30:589–596.
14. Sloper JJ, Johnson P, Powell TPS. Selective degeneration of interneurons in the motor cortex of infant monkeys following controlled hypoxia: a possible cause of epilepsy. *Brain Res* 1980;198:204–209.
15. Tonz M, Laske A, Carrel T, da Silva V, Real F, Turina M. Convulsions, hemiparesis and central retinal artery occlusion due to left atrial myxoma in child. *Eur J Pediatr* 1992;151:652–654.
16. Hossman KA, Niebuhr I, Tamura M. Local cerebral flow and glucose consumption of rats with experimental gliomas. *J Cereb Blood Flow Metab* 1982;2:25–32.
17. Castillo J, Davalos A, Noya M. Progression of ischaemic stroke and excitotoxic aminoacids. *Lancet* 1997;349:79–83.
18. Olsen RW, Avoli M. GABA and epileptogenesis. *Epilepsia* 1997;38:399–407.
19. Ueda Y, Yokoyama H, Niwa R, Konaka R, Ohya-Nishiguchi H, Kamada H. Generation of lipid radicals in the hippocampal extracellular space during kainic acid-induced seizures in rats. *Epilepsy Res* 1997;26:329–333.
20. Berkovic SF, Scheffer IE. Genetics of human partial epilepsy. *Curr Opin Neurol* 1997;10:110–114.
21. Chinnery PF, Turnbull DM. Clinical features, investigation, and management of patients with defects of mitochondrial DNA. *J Neurol Neurosurg Psychiatry* 1997;63:559–563.
22. Duffy TE, Howse DC, Plum F. Cerebral energy metabolism during experimental status epilepticus. *J Neurochem* 1975;24:925–934.
23. Howse DC, Caronna JJ, Duffy TE, Plum F. Cerebral energy metabolism, pH, and blood flow during seizures in the cat. *Am J Physiol* 1974;227:1444–1451.
24. Shouse MN, da Silva AM, Sammaritano M. Circadian rhythm, sleep, and epilepsy. *J Clin Neurophysiol* 1996;13:32–50.
25. Rosenberg-Adamsen S, Kehlet H, Dodds C, Rosenberg J. Postoperatiive sleep disturbances: mechanisms and clinical implications. *Br J Anaesthesiol* 1996; 76:552–559.

26. Simini B. Patients' perceptions of intensive care. *Lancet* 1999;354:571–572.
27. Kahn DM, Cook TE, Carlisle CC, Nelson DL, Kramer NR, Millman RP. Identification and modification of environmental noise in an ICU setting. *Chest* 1998; 114:535–540.
28. Ayus JC, Wheeler JM, Arieff AI. Postoperative hyponatremic encephalopathy in menstruant women. *Ann Intern Med* 1992;117:891–897.
29. Soupart A, Decaux G. Therapeutic recommendations for management of severe hyponatremia: current concepts on pathogenesis and prevention of neurologic complications. *Clin Nephrol* 1996;46:149–169.
30. Fraser CL, Arieff AI. Epidemiology, pathophysiology, and management of hyponatremic encephalopathy. *Am J Med* 1997;102:67–77.
31. Sterns RH, Riggs JE, Schochet SS Jr. Osmotic demyelination syndrome following correction of hyponatremia. *N Engl J Med* 1986;314:1535–1542.
32. Adler S, Simplaceanu V. Effect of acute hyponatremia on rat brain pH and rat brain buffering. *Am J Physiol* 1989;256:F113–F119.
33. McMicken DB, Freedland ES. Alcohol-related seizures. Pathophysiology, differential diagnosis, evaluation, and treatment. *Emerg Med Clin North Am* 1994; 12:1057–1079.
34. Faingold CL, N'Gouemo P, Riaz A. Ethanol and neurotransmitter interactions: from molecular to integrative effects. *Prog Neurobiol* 1998;55:509–535.
35. Tan CY, Weaver DF. Molecular pathogenesis of alcohol withdrawal seizures: the modified lipid-protein interaction mechanism. *Seizure* 1997;6:255–274.
36. Grant KA, Valverius P, Hudspith M, Tabakoff B. Ethanol withdrawal seizures and the NMDA receptor complex. *Eur J Pharmacol* 1990;176:289–296.
37. Albrecht J, Jones EA. Hepatic encephalopathy: molecular mechanisms underlying the clinical syndrome. *J Neurol Sci* 1999;170:138–146.
38. Albrecht J. Roles of neuroactive amino acids in ammonia neurotoxicity. *J Neurosci Res* 1998;51:133–138.
39. Wallace RH, Berkovic SF, Howell RA, Sutherland GR, Mulley JC. Suggestion of a major gene for familial febrile convulsions mapping to 8q13-21. *J Med Genet* 1996;33:308–312.
40. Johnson EW, Dubovsky J, Rich SS, et al. Evidence for a novel gene for familial febrile convulsions, FEB2, linked to chromosome 19p in an extended family from the midwest. *Hum Mol Genet* 1998;7:63–67.
41. Fletcher CF, Lutz CM, O'Sullivan N, Shaughnessy J, Hawkes R, Frankel WN, Copeland NG, Jenkins NA. Absence epilepsy in tottering mutant mice is associated with calcium channel defects. *Cell* 1996;87:607–617.
42. Cox GA, Lutz CM, Yang CL, et al. Sodium/hydrogen exchanger gene defect in slow-wave epilepsy mutant mice. *Cell* 1997;91:139–148.
43. Schlitt M, Chronister RB, Whitley RJ. Pathogenesis and pathophysiology of viral infections of the central nervous system. In: Scheld WM, Whitley RJ, Durak DT (eds.), *Infections of the Central Nervous System.* New York: Raven, 1991, pp 69–80.
44. Sepkowitz K, Armstrong D. Space-occupying fungal lesions of the central nervous system. In: Scheld WM, Whitley RJ, Durak DT (eds.), *Infections of the Central Nervous System.* New York: Raven, 1991, pp 741–764.
45. Aronow HA, Feraru ER, Lipton RB. New-onset seizures in AIDS patients: etiology, prognosis, and treatment. *Neurology* 1989;39:(Suppl I)428.
46. Wong MC, Suite NDA, Labar DR. Seizures in human immunodeficiency virus infection. *Arch Neurol* 1990;47:640–642.

47. Report of the Quality Standards Subcommittee of the American Academy of Neurology. Evaluation and management of intracranial mass lesions in AIDS. *Neurology* 1998;50:21–26.
48. Labar DR. Seizures and HIV infection. In: Pedley TA, Meldrum BS (eds.), *Recent Advances in Epilepsy.* Edinburgh: Churchill Livingston, 1992, pp 119–126.
49. Moulignier A, Mikol J, Pialoux G, Fenelon G, Gray F, Thiebaut JB. AIDS-associated progressive multifocal leukoencephalopathy revealed by new-onset seizures. *Am J Med* 1995;99:64–68.
50. Lipton SA. AIDS-related dementia and calcium homeostasis. *Ann NY Acad Sci* 1994;747:205–224.
51. Van Paesschen W, Bodian C, Maker H. Metabolic abnormalities and new-onset seizures in human immunodeficiency virus—seropositive patients. *Epilepsia* 1995;36:146–150.
52. Kunisaki TA, Augenstein WL. Drug- and toxin-induced seizures. *Emerg Med Clin North Am* 1994;12:1027–1056.
53. Murphy K, Delanty N. Drug-induced seizures. General principles in assessment, management and prevention. *CNS Drugs* 2000;14:135–146.
54. Messing RO, Closson RG, Simon RP. Drug-induced seizures: a ten-year experience. *Neurology* 1984;34:1582–1586.
55. Pascual-Leone A, Dhuna A, Altafulla I, Anderson DC. Cocaine-induced seizures. *Neurology* 1990;40:404–407.
56. Alldredge BK, Lowenstein DH. Status epilepticus: new concepts. *Curr Opin Neurol* 1999;12:183–190.
57. Miller J, Robinson A, Percy AK. Acute isoniazid poisoning in childhood. *Am J Dis Child* 1980;134:290–292.
58. Shannon M, Lovejoy FH. The influence of age vs serum concentration on life-threatening events after chronic theophylline intoxication. *Arch Internal Med* 1990; 150:2045–2048.
59. Amabeoku GJ. Gamma-aminobutyric acid and glutamic acid receptors may mediate theophylline-induced seizures in mice. *Gen Pharmacol* 1999;32:365–372.
60. Thurston JH, Pollock PG, Warren SK, Jones EM. Reduced brain glucose with normal plasma glucose in salicylate poisoning. *J Clin Invest* 1970;49:2139–2145.
61. Hill JB. Salicylate intoxication. *N Engl J Med* 1973;288:1110–1113.
62. Norkool DM, Kirkpatrick JN. Treatment of acute carbon monoxide poisoning: a review of 115 cases. *Ann Emerg Med* 1985;14:1168–1171.
63. Chance B, Erecinska M, Washer M. Mitochondrial responses to carbon monoxide toxicity. *Ann NY Acad Sci* 1970;174:193–204.
64. Thom SR. Carbon monoxide poisoning-mediated brain lipid peroxidation in the rat. *J Appl Physiol* 1990;68:997–1003.
65. Perl TM, Bedard L, Kosatsky T, Hockin JC, Todd EC, Remis RS. An outbreak of toxic encephalopathy caused by eating mussels contaminated with domoic acid. *N Engl J Med* 1990;322:1775–1780.
66. Teitelbaum JS, Zatorre RJ, Carpenter S, et al. Neurologic sequelae of domoic acid intoxication due to ingestion of contaminated mussels. *N Engl J Med* 1990: 322:1781–1787.
67. Delanty N, Vaughan CJ, French JA. Medical causes of seizures. *Lancet* 1998; 352:383–390.

3

Seizures in Acute Neurological Disorders

Peter B. Crino, MD, PhD

Introduction

Seizures may herald, complicate, or become persistent sequellae of acute neurologic disorders such as acute cerebrovascular insult (stroke or hemorrhage), bacterial or viral meningoencephalitis, and head trauma. The occurrence of seizures in patients with primary neurological insults invariably adds an additional layer of complexity to patient management. For example, diminished arousal after generalized tonic-clonic seizures or status epilepticus (SE) may put a patient at risk for aspiration or hypoxia and may warrant airway protection via intubation and mechanical ventilation. Many patients will develop aspiration pneumonia. Phasic and substantial increases in intracranial pressure (ICP) during generalized tonic clonic seizures may lead to brain herniation in the setting of an existing mass lesion such as an acute stroke, hemorrhage, or brain tumor. Increased mean arterial blood pressure (MAP), hypoxemia, and metabolic or respiratory acidosis may accompany generalized tonic-clonic seizures and complicate the management of patients with acute stroke, sepsis, cardiac ischemia, or pulmonary edema. Finally, systemic toxicity of antiepileptic drugs (AEDs) may be encountered and cause medical complications such as cardiac dysrhythmia, hypotension, the Stevens–Johnson syndrome, other hypersensitivity reactions, and hepatic failure. Some of these complications may be life threatening even if the underlying neurologic event is not. It is important for the clinician, whether in the outpatient, hospital ward, or Emergency Department setting, to remember that a first-time seizure may herald a potentially significant and even disastrous neurologic event. This chapter will focus on the etiologic, diagnostic, and treatment implications of seizures in several acute neurologic disorders such as arterial

From: *Seizures: Medical Causes and Management*
Edited by: N. Delanty © Humana Press, Inc., Totowa, NJ

and venous cerebral infarcts, intracerebral hemorrhage, including hypertensive, subdural, and subarachnoid hemorrhage, meningoencephalitis, and brain trauma.

Seizures in Cerebrovascular Disease

Acute Stroke

Cerebrovascular disease is a common cause of epilepsy in the elderly. Up to 10–15% of patients with acute stroke or transient ischemic attack (TIA) will present with a seizure, and in some studies, twice that number will suffer a seizure within the first 24–48 h after their initial infarct *(1)*. For example, in 71 young patients (aged 15–45 years) affected by a cerebral infarct, post-stroke seizures occurred in 7 patients (10.8%) *(2)*. Seizures in the first 24–48 h are more common than later seizures or epilepsy and tend to be focal motor, brief, and isolated. Epilepsy usually does not follow early seizures, but the risk of subsequent poststroke epilepsy is increased. Late seizures occur months to years after a stroke and are probably the result of structural brain abnormalities leading to the development of an epileptic focus. Of course, the risk of seizures is increased markedly when the cerebrovascular event involves the cerebral cortex, and deep-seated hemispheric or infratentorial lesions rarely produce seizures or epilepsy. There may be a higher incidence of seizures in hemorrhagic stroke, although this remains to be proved. The risk is also increased in patients with other medical problems known to lower seizure threshold, such as renal failure. Venous thrombosis, e.g., cortical vein thrombosis and sagittal sinus thrombosis, carries an increased risk of seizure that may be higher than cerebral arterial thrombosis.

The most common types of seizures associated with cerebrovascular disease include focal motor and generalized tonic-clonic seizures. Focal motor seizures typically emanate from the cortical region that has sustained an ischemic insult. Complex partial seizures may present in the setting of acute stroke and, like focal seizures, typically are believed to emanate from the ischemic region. Whereas single seizures are the most common, recurrent seizures and SE may occur. Surprisingly, convulsive SE is relatively rare in acute stroke. These results have been reported in a large number of retrospective and prospective analyses worldwide. It has also been suggested that embolic infarction has a higher incidence of seizures than does thrombotic infarction, but definitive evidence is again lacking. Interestingly, the presence of seizures in an acute stroke does not seem to correlate with the size of the lesion, functional outcome, or mortality *(3)*.

Several studies have assessed the incidence and course of poststroke seizures. Ninety patients with seizures following acute stroke were studied retrospectively to investigate the common clinical features, prognosis, and electroencephalographic findings *(4)*. Of 90 seizures, 33% appeared early (within 2 wk after the infarction), and 90% of the 30 early seizures appeared within 24 h after the infarction. Of 90 seizures, 56% were single, and SE occured in only 8%. Early-onset seizures were more likely to be partial (57% of 30 patients). Of 90 initial seizures, 39% recurred, and there was no significant difference in recurrence rate between early- or late-onset initial seizures. Seizures in 88% of the 90 patients were managed with monotherapy.

The incidence of early seizures in 1000 consecutive patients with stroke and transient ischemic attacks was evaluated propectively to determine whether seizure occurrence correlates with stroke type, pathogenesis, or outcome *(3)*. Seizures occurred in 44 patients (4.4%), including 24 patients (6.5%) of 370 patients with cortical infarction, and 4 (3.7%) of 109 with hemispheric transient ischemic attacks. Lobar or extensive hemorrhage, or subarachnoid hemorrhage, was also associated with seizures. Lacunar infarcts and deep hemorrhages were not associated with seizures in this series. Interestingly, in patients with cortical infarcts, there was no association between seizure occurrence and stroke pathogenesis. Seizures generally occurred within 48 h of stroke onset and were usually single, partial, and readily controlled. Seizures were not associated with a higher mortality or worse functional outcome.

The development of seizures was evaluated in 219 consecutive patients who had ischemic or hemorrhagic stroke *(5)*. Seizures developed in 13 of 183 patients with ischemic stroke and 9 of 36 patients with hemorrhagic stroke. Seizures were more common in those with cortical lesions and in a lesion occupying more than one lobe. The occurrence of seizures within 15 days of a first stroke or transient ischemic episode was evaluated prospectively in 1640 patients to study relation between seizures and type of stroke *(6)*. Seizures occurred in 90 patients (5.4%), with the most common setting being cardiogenic embolus followed by large vessel atheroma, TIA, subcortical infarcts, and lacunar infarcts. Other causes included supratentorial hematoma and subarachnoid hemorrhage. Seizures were the initial sign of stroke in 80 (89%) of 90 cases and were usually single and partial. Seizure symptoms were most often motor, sensory, or visual. The number and type of seizures, initial stroke severity, infarct size, mortality, and outcome were studied recently in 1197 patients with acute stroke *(7)*. Fifty patients (4.2%) had seizures within 14 days of a stroke. Using a multivariate analyses, only initial stroke severity was related to early seizure, whereas stroke type and lesion localization were not related. The occurrence of an early seizure did not influence the risk of death during hospital stay.

In a recent hospital-based study from South India, up to 40% of seizures presenting to the Emergency Department were related to cerebrovascular disease such as stroke and superior sagittal sinus thrombosis *(8)*. Similarly, in a study of the north–central region of Saskatchewan, seizures were caused by stroke in 19 of 84 (23%) cases analyzed *(9)*. EEGs were abnormal in 61 of 84 (73%) cases, with epileptiform discharge in 33 of 84 (39%). Another study determined the profile of late-onset epileptic seizures following cerebral infarcts, as well as the predictive clinical and radiological factors associated with their development *(10)*. In this analysis 86 patients were evaluated who developed late seizures after cerebral infarction and 285 patients were evaluated who did not develop seizures for at least 1 y after their strokes. Simple partial (motor) seizures, with or without secondary generalization, accounted for 80% of the classifiable seizures. Factors that appeared to be predictive of seizure development were the presence of large cortical infarcts and the presence of apparently preserved cerebral tissue within the infarcted area. Seizures were rare in patients with lacunar infarction, but the presence of associated leukoaraiosis increased the risk. Motor and cognitive deficit, as well as epilepsy, are common in patients with periventricular leukomalacia (PVLM).

Interestingly, SE is an infrequent complication of acute stroke. Several studies have demonstrated an incidence of convulsive SE in acute stroke of approx. 3–5%. Both complex partial SE (*see* ref. 11) and convulsive SE may occur in the acute setting or will arise within the first 24–72 h. Clinically, nonconvulsive SE is heralded by persistant alteration in mental status or subtle motor manifestations. Continuous focal motor seizures (focal motor SE or epilepsia partialis continua) can be an especially disabling complication of acute stroke. A recent study demonstrated that the most common cause of focal SE was acute brain ischemia, which was especially difficult to control *(12)*. Of these patients, many had electrographic evidence of seizures with only subtle clinical manifestations. These investigators suggest that controlling focal SE may be especially problematic despite multiple anticonvulsant agents.

The rising use of cocaine in the 1980s and 1990s has been associated with a well-documented and significant risk of stroke or cerebral hemorrhage and concomitant seizures. Cocaine can provoke seizures, exacerbate preexisting epilepsy, or cause an ischemic or hemorrhagic stroke that leads to seizures *(13)*. Mitochondrial DNA mutations resulting in mitochondrial myopathy, encephalopathy, lactic acidosis, and stroke-like episodes (MELAS) have been linked to seizures (for review, *see* ref. *14*). Silent infarcts have been reported in 17% of young patients with sickle cell disease and are associated with impaired performance on standardized psychometric tests as well as with epilepsy *(15)*. One interesting report suggested that stroke and seizure may be the initial presentation of HIV infection in children *(10)*. Sturge–Weber syndrome is characterized by the presence of a port-wine nevus, epilepsy, stroke-like episodes, headache, and developmental delay.

Evidence obtained using fluorodeoxyglucose (FDG)—positron emission tomography (PET) suggests that progressive hypo-perfusion and glucose hypometabolism are associated with neurologic deterioration in Sturge–Weber syndrome *(17)*. The family of vasculitides that affect the CNS, including giant cell arteritis, primary angiitis of the CNS, Takayasu's disease, periarteritis nodosa, Churg–Strauss syndrome, Wegener's granulomatosis, Behçet's disease, other collagen vascular diseases, and vasculitis secondary to the use of illicit drugs may present with symptoms and signs such as headache, encephalopathy, seizures, and stroke *(18)*. Cerebral autosomal dominant arteriopathy with subcortical infarcts and leukoencephalopathy (CADASIL) is an increasingly recognized autosomal dominant disorder leading to cerebrovascular manifestations in early adulthood that may be associated with seizures in as many as 10–20% of cases *(19)*. Arteriovenous malformations may be complicated by acute stroke or hemorrhage and, therefore, can induce single and recurrent seizures. Patients with small arteriovenous malformations (AVMs) (<3 cm) were more likely to present with hemorrhage, whereas those with large AVMs were more likely to present with seizures *(20)*. In pregnant females, an especially disabling cause of seizures is eclampsia (for review, *see* ref. *21*). Eclampsia is a complex multisystem disorder with potentially severe, irreversible sequelae, including a progressive and often relentless arteriopathy that can result in acute stroke and vasospasm.

Acute Intracerebral Hemorrhage

Seizures may complicate intracerebral hemorrhage (ICH) in as many as 15–25% of cases. In one series *(22)*, seizures occurred in 15% of patients with ICH (early in 12% and delayed in 3%). Seizures were most frequent with lobar hemorrhages and uncommon with deep subcortical hemorrhages. Lobar hemorrhages in the frontal, parietal, or temporal, but not occipital, regions were more commonly associated with seizures. Seizures were most common if the hemorrhage was the result of an aneurysm, angioma, or neoplasm and less common if hypertensive or spontaneous. AVM may be a common cause of lobar hemorrhage with early seizures.

Among 1402 patients with ICH, early seizures occurred in 64 (4.6%) *(23)*. Seizure was the first manifestation of ICH in 19 patients (30%), and SE occurred in 11 patients (17%). SE was the initial presentation of ICH in 6 individuals (9%). The majority of seizures were simple partial (motor) seizures. Fifty-five cases of epileptic seizures associated with spontaneous ICH were reported *(24)*. Seizures appeared as the first symptom in 23 of 55 patients with ICH. Seizures occurred early (within 2 wk) in 18 patients and late (after 2 wk) in 14. Partial seizures were the most frequent type (63%) especially in the setting of lobar hemorrhage. In a retrospective study in 1200 Chinese veterans with cerebrovascular disease, 32% experienced ICH; of these patients, 2.8% developed seizures *(25)*. A prospective analysis of 123 patients with hypertensive ICH revealed that 12% of these patients had seizures within the first 24 h of the ICH ictus *(26)*. The majority of seizure types were partial with fewer being generalized. SE occurred in only 10% of patients following ICH. Another study demonstrated that seizures occurred in 19 of 112 patients (17%) with nontraumatic, supratentorial ICH *(27)*. All seizures occurred at ICH onset. Seizures were significantly associated with extension of blood into the cerebral cortex. These investigators concluded that seizures in ICH occur most commonly at hemorrhage onset, patients without seizures at hemorrhage onset are at very low risk for subsequent seizures during their hospitalization, and hemorrhage involving the cerebral cortex, regardless of site of origin, predisposes to seizures. Cerebral amyloid angiopathy is a well-known cause of cerebral lobar hemorrhage and may be associated with subacute dementia, seizures, or an acute encephalopathy without lobar hemorrhage *(28)*.

The incidence of seizures in subarachnoid hemorrhage is approx. 10%. Seizures may also herald symptomatic but unruptured aneurysm *(29)*. An early retrospective series of 100 consecutive patients with subarachnoid hemorrhage caused by a ruptured aneurysm was performed to determine the incidence and the prognostic implications of seizures during the acute phase *(30)*. Seizures occurred in 26% of the patients, and the majority of seizures occurred near the onset of the initial hemorrhage. The occurrence of early seizures did not correlate with the location of the aneurysm or the prognosis. A proportion of seizures occurred immediately after rebleeding, with no greater morbidity or mortality compared to all patients who rebled. The occurrence of seizures was analyzed retrospectively in 131 consecutive cases of spontaneous subarachnoid hemorrhage *(31)*. Convulsions occurred in 31 patients (24%) and most often within 24 h of bleeding. Motor manifestations of partial seizures had no clear lateralizing value to aneurysm site. Early mortality, rebleeding, and intracerebral hematoma were similar in both seizure and nonseizure groups. Interestingly, late seizures were infrequent in survivors who had suffered seizures in the acute stage. In a prospective study of 253 patients with subarachnoid hemorrhage, 16 (6.3%) had seizures at the onset of bleeding *(32)*. None had a previous history of seizures or evidence of other metabolic derangement. Hemiparesis, Hunt's grade >3, a large amount of subarachnoid blood, and the presence of an aneurysm were significantly more frequent in patients with seizures at the onset of subarachnoid hemorrhage. Although rebleeding, mortality, or severe disability at discharge was more frequent in these patients, seizures were not a significant predictor of long-term prognosis.

Seizures in patients with acute epidural or subdural hematoma occur between 5% and 20% of cases *(33)*. In one study, the incidence of epilepsy in infants with extradural hematoma was 7.5% *(34)*. A large-scale analysis of seizures in acute epidural or subdural hematoma remains to be performed.

Seizures in CNS Infections

Seizures may occur in the setting of any CNS infection, including bacterial or viral meningitis, viral encephalitis, especially resulting from herpes simplex virus (HSV) infection, bacterial abscess, parasitic infection, e.g., toxoplasmosis, cysticercosis, or opportunistic infection, e.g., mucormycosis, and cryptococcosis. For example, the etiological spectrum of symptomatic localization-related epilepsies was generated from a study in South India *(35)*. Seizure occurred in close temporal association with an acute CNS insult in 53% of 991 patients. Infections of the CNS accounted for 77% of patients with symptomatic epilepsy.

In patients with HSV1 encephalitis (HSVE), the most common long-term symptoms are memory impairment (69%), personality and behavioral abnormalities (45%), and epilepsy (24%) *(36)*. Children and adults with HSVE may present with focal or complex partial seizures, can be initially afebrile, and can have a normal brain computerized tomography (CT) scan despite an abnormal EEG *(37)*. Rarely are acute encephalopathy and SE associated with human herpesvirus 6 infection *(38)*. Seizures are present frequently during acute La Crosse encephalitis, and recurrent seizures may occur in 6–13% of patients 1–8 y after infection *(39)*.

Seizures are the presenting sign in the majority of patients with neurocysticercosis (*see* ref. *40*). In one series *(41)*, seizures were present in 48 of 54 patients, representing the most common clinical presenting manifestation. CT scan of the brain revealed parenchymal brain cysticerci in 52 patients. In this report, all patients with seizures were treated with antiepileptic drugs with an excellent rate of seizure control.

Neurologic complications occur in approx. 30% of patients with infective endocarditis and represent a major factor associated with an increased mortality rate. Cerebral embolism is the most common complication and may account for all other sequellae, such as mycotic aneurysm, meningoencephalitis, and brain abscess, that may develop. Emboli are more common in patients with mitral valve infection and in those infected with more virulent organisms such as *Staphylococcus aureus*. Seizures are common in patients with infective endocarditis as well as in those who develop brain abscess. Focal seizures are associated more commonly with acute emboli, whereas generalized seizures are associated more commonly with systemic metabolic factors such as sepsis.

New-onset seizures are frequent manifestations of central nervous system (CNS) disorders in patients infected with HIV (ref. *42*). Seizures are more common in advanced stages of the disease, although they may occur early in the course of illness. In the majority of patients, seizures are of the generalized type. SE is also frequent. Associated metabolic abnormalities increase the risk for SE. Cerebral mass lesions, cryptococcal meningitis, and HIV encephalopathy are common causes of seizures. The prognosis of seizures in HIV-infected patients depends on the underlying cause, and seizures related to focal lesions may be more difficult to control.

Seizures in Acute Head Trauma

Seizures occur in the setting of acute head trauma and may persist as post-traumatic epilepsy. The risk of seizures is increased after traumatic brain injury, but the extent and duration of the increase in risk are unknown. One study examined the ictal phenomenology and outcome of convulsions occurring within seconds of impact following violent collision while playing rugby *(43)*. These investigators evaluated 22 cases of concussive convulsions documented on television videotape. Convulsions began within 2 s of impact and comprised an initial period of tonic stiffening followed by myoclonic jerks of all limbs lasting up to 150 s. Some asymmetry in the convulsive manifestations was common, and recovery of consciousness was rapid. No structural or permanent brain injury was present on clinical assessment, neuropsychological testing, or neuroimaging studies. Epilepsy did not develop in any player during the 3.5 y of follow-up.

Young children are more prone to early seizures, and adolescents and adults, to late seizures following brain trauma. The main risk factors for late seizures are early seizures and depressed skull fracture *(44)*. Severity of brain injury, as measured by a low Glasgow Coma Scale (GCS) score, prolonged unconsciousness, and posttraumatic amnesia (PTA) without local brain lesion, should not be considered risk factors for late post-traumatic seizures. Low GCS and a longer period of unconsciousness after head trauma, especially >12 h, have a higher likelihood of suffering convulsions after head injury *(45)*. A recent study identified the characteristics of brain injuries that are associated with the development of seizures in 4541 children and adults using a multivariate analysis. Significant risk factors for later seizures were brain contusion with subdural hematoma, skull fracture, loss of consciousness, or amnesia for more than 1 day, and an age of 65 years or older *(46)*.

One series reviewed the seizure incidence in 4232 adult patients with mild closed head injury who did not receive prophylactic anticonvulsant agents *(33)*. One hundred patients (2%) experienced seizures within 1 wk after head injury, whereas 43 of these (1% of the series) had seizures within 24 h after trauma. Most of the seizures (84%) that developed during the first week after injury were generalized tonic-clonic. The incidence of generalized tonic-clonic seizures was higher than that of partial seizures within the first 24 h and within the first week following the trauma. No definite intracranial pathological findings were detected by CT in 53% of patients with early posttraumatic seizures. However, six patients had intracranial hemorrhage without intracranial parenchymal damage (three with epidural hematoma and three with subarachnoid hemorrhage). The most common positive CT scan findings in the early posttraumatic-seizure group were ICH (24%), followed by acute subdural hematoma with ICH (17%). Intracerebral parenchymal damage could be identified on CT scans in 41 (48.8%) of 84 patients with generalized tonic-clonic seizures and 5 (31%) of 16 patients with partial seizures with motor symptoms. The intracerebral parenchymal damage was detected most commonly in the frontal lobe (21%) and the temporal lobe (19%). Seven patients with early posttraumatic seizures received emergency craniotomy to remove an intracranial hematoma. This review suggested that early posttraumatic seizures after mild closed head injury have a high incidence (53%) in patients with normal CT scan findings. In another series, the incidence and clinical significance of early post-traumatic seizures after severe closed head injury were assessed prospectively in 3340 adult patients with severe closed head injuries, each of them having a GCS of 3–8 after trauma (*47*). Anticonvulsant agents were not given to these patients unless there was evidence of seizure. One hundred twenty-one patients (3.6%) experienced seizures within 1 wk after head injury, and 42 of these were within 24 h after trauma. The incidence of intracerebral parenchymal damage was higher among those patients who developed seizures in the first week (66.1%) than in those who did not (62.7%). Interestingly, the patients with early seizures had a lower mortality rate. In patients who survived the initial injury, the occurrence of early posttraumatic seizures did not appear to influence the neurological recovery at 6 mo after injury. These investigators concluded that the presence of intracerebral parenchymal damage on CT scan after severe closed head injury did not increase the risk of early posttraumatic seizures and that the occurrence of early seizures did not influence the neurological recovery in patients who survived the initial severe closed head injury.

Several studies have documented the incidence of convulsive and nonconvulsive SE (NCSE) by using continuous EEG monitoring in patients in the Neurointensive Care Unit (NICU) during the initial 14 days following brain trauma. NCSE occurs commonly in the setting of an acute brain injury (*see* ref. *48*). It may persist following cessation of generalized convulsive SE, and it is not uncommonly associated with acute cerebral ischemia. In the absence of EEG testing, NCSE is likely to be missed or delayed. Increasing evidence suggests that brain trauma and NCSE are synergistically detrimental and increase brain injury. In one series of 94 patients with moderate-to-severe brain injuries, convulsive and nonconvulsive seizures occurred in 21 (22%), with many displaying SE *(49)*. In 52% of patients, the seizures were nonconvulsive and were diagnosed on the basis of EEG studies alone.

Mechanisims of Epileptogenesis

In most cases, seizures occurring in the setting of acute neurological disorders result from structural brain injury that affects the cerebral cortex. The degree to which there is overlap between the cellular and molecular pathogenesis of seizure genesis in acute ischemia versus acute hemorrhage remains to be defined. Current wisdom is that there is a disruption of the complex and delicate balance between neural excitation and inhibition in the cerebral cortex as a result of the acute insult. These changes likely affect the excitatory glutamatergic system as well as the inhibitory GABA-ergic system.

The rapid progress in recent years in the molecular and cellular pharmacology of excitatory amino acid receptors has shed light on the pathogenesis of hypoxic–ischemic (HI) injury to the brain. It has become clear that excitotoxic injury also complicates prolonged seizure activity in the brain and that the glutamate family of receptors contributes to epileptogenesis in humans. In experimental animals, ischemia potentiates seizures induced by a variety of measures, including picrotoxin and pentylenetetrazol *(50)*. Excessive activation of glutamate receptors may contribute to neuronal loss after a traumatic or ischemic CNS insult. Such injuries are often associated with hemorrhage and extravasation of hemoglobin, a pro-oxidant and putative neurotoxin. Hemoglobin potentiates the neurotoxicity of low concentrations of α-amino-3-hydroxy-5-methyl-4-isoxazole-propionate (AMPA) and kainate *(51)*.

After transient cerebral ischemia in fetal sheep, cortical seizures are accompanied by a progressive decrease in the concentration of oxidized cytochrome oxidase as measured by near-infrared (IR) spectroscopy *(52)*. These investigators suggest that nitric oxide and nitric oxide synthetase are important mediators of ischemia and epileptogenesis. Brain areas damaged by stroke and seizures express high levels of heat shock protein (HSP72). Overexpression of HSP72 improves neuron survival against focal cerebral ischemia and systemic kainic acid (KA) administration *(53)*. In recent study the effect of chemically induced seizures on cerebral HI damage in immature animals *(54)*. Cerebral HI injury was produced in 7- and 13-d postnatal rats by combined unilateral common carotid artery ligation and hypoxia. Seizures were induced chemically by the subcutaneous injection of KA or inhalation of flurothyl vapor. Histologic examination of brains of animals subjected to seizures prior to HI injury and their HI-only controls showed that seizures occurring before HI injury conferred protection against cerebral damage. These investigators concluded that there was no evidence that seizures in early postnatal development aggravate pre-existing cerebral HI damage.

Changes in gene transcription underscore the molecular pathogenesis of seizure initiation following brain ischemia. For example, differential alterations in expression of c-*fos*, nerve growth factor (NGF), brain-derived neurotrophic factor (BDNF), neurotrophin-3 (NT-3), TrkB, and TrkC mRNAs have been reported at different reperfusion times following unilateral middle cerebral artery occlusion *(55)*. These and other data suggest that HI injury can induce long-lasting changes in gene transcription that affect cell death and survival pathways. Altered expression of the immediate early genes c-*fos*, c-*jun*, and *jun B* and their cognate proteins has been demonstrated by immunocytochemistry following unilateral entorhinal cortex lesion in experimental animals *(56)*. Within the denervated fascia dentata, some of these changes may be linked to the reorganization processes following traumatic brain lesion. Alternatively, the alterations in immediate early gene expression reported in this study may be the result of changes in synaptic activity or postlesional seizures that occur in this lesioning paradigm. An increase in extracellular glutamate has been demonstrated after human traumatic brain injury, which may be secondary to reduced cerebral perfusion pressure and early posttraumatic seizures *(49)*.

The presence of an intracranial hematoma has a robust association with the development of posttraumatic epilepsy. Extravasation of blood is followed by hemolysis and deposition of heme-containing compounds into the neuropil, initiating a sequence of univalent redox reactions and generating various free radical species, including superoxides, hydroxyl radicals, peroxides, and perferryl ions. Free radicals initiate peroxidation reactions by hydrogen abstraction from methylene groups adjacent to double bonds of fatty acids and lipids within cellular membranes. Intrinsic enzymatic mechanisms for control of free radical reactions include activation of catalase, peroxidase, and superoxide dismutase. Steroids, proteins, and tocopherol also terminate peroxidative reactions. Tocopherol and selenium are effective in preventing tissue injury initiated by ferrous chloride and heme compounds. Treatment strategies for prevention or prophylaxis of post-traumatic epilepsy must await absolute knowledge of mechanisms. Antioxidants and chelators may be useful, given the speculation that peroxidative reactions may be an important component of brain injury responses. In addition, potential treatment strategies involving GABA agonists, NMDA receptor antagonists, and barbiturates need further scientific assessment.

Head trauma initiates a sequence of responses that includes altered blood flow and vasoregulation, disruption of the blood–brain barrier, increases in intracranial pressure, focal or diffuse ischemia, hemorrhage, inflammation, necrosis, and disruption of fiber tracts (*see* ref. 57). Head trauma with cerebral contusion or primary ICH causes extravasation of red blood cells, followed by hemolysis and deposition of iron-containing blood products within the neuropil. Liberation of heme compounds is associated with deposition of hemosiderin and, with gliosis, neuronal loss and occasionally the development of seizures. Free radical reactions initiated by iron or heme deposited within the neuropil may be a fundamental reaction associated with brain injury responses, and possibly with posttraumatic epileptogenesis. Hemoglobin has been demonstrated to be neurotoxic when injected into the cerebral cortex in vivo. Exposure of neuronal cultures to hemoglobin for 24–28 h produced widespread and concentration-dependent neuronal death *(51)* that was blocked by the ferric iron chelator deferoxamine. Thus, hemoglobin may be neurotoxic, and its neurotoxicity may contribute to neuronal injury processes after trauma and ICH.

An increase in leukotriene-like immunoreactivity was identified by radioimmunoassay in the gerbil forebrain following ischemia and reperfusion, subarachnoid hemorrhage, or nonlethal concussive brain injury *(58)*. Cerebral vessels and circulating blood are capable of producing leukotrienes, which may have a role in the pathophysiology of cerebral edema formation, cerebral vasospasm, and seizure activity following ICH.

Epileptogenesis following neocortical trauma may result from two sources of disinhibition, including the physical removal of important superficial inhibitory circuits and glutamate-triggered increases in intracellular calcium *(59)*. Using a fluid percussion injury (FPI) model and patch-clamp recordings from hippocampal slices, D'Ambrosio et al. *(60)* found impaired glial physiology 2 d after FPI. A reduction in transient outward and inward K^+ currents was observed that resulted in an abnormal extracellular K^+ accumulation in the post-traumatic hippocampal slices, accompanied by the appearance of CA3 after-discharges. Traumatic brain injury (TBI) causes loss of K^+ conductance in hippocampal glia that results in the failure of glial K^+ homeostasis. Enhanced self-sustaining epileptogenic activity and disinhibition were observed in hippocampal slices from rats exposed to lateral FPI *(61)*.

One study evaluated the incidence of seizure activity following acute traumatic brain injury to the right parietal cortex in artificially ventilated rats *(62)*. Generalized seizure activity occurred within 1 min and was accompanied by a transient increase of aspartate, taurine, glutamate, and glycine. These investigators concluded that elevated levels of aspartate and glutamate may have a role in post-traumatic seizure activity. Following FPI, two typical responses to TBI were recorded *(63)*. Some animals developed seizures at various stages after TBI. When severe injury was induced, ischemic depolarization (ID) developed, whereas mild or moderate injury led to repetitive spreading depression (SD) cycles. Intracranial pressure (ICP) before injury was between 2 and 6 mmHg and increased to 20–22 mmHg 2–3 min after ID. Following severe head injury, ICP remained high and in some cases increased to critical values, causing death of these animals.

Complications of Seizures in Acute Neurological Disturbances

Seizures in the setting of acute neurological disorders such as acute stroke or hemorrhage can lead to numerous medical and neurologic complications. For example, increased ICP, hypoxemia, acidosis, and hypercarbia may contribute to worsening brain ischemia in stroke or subarachnoid hemorrhage. Hypoxia during a generalized tonic clonic seizure can in theory extend neuronal HI injury.

Patients may develop high ICP in the setting of prolonged seizures or SE. Increased ICP can occur during both complex partial and generalized tonic-clonic seizures. Previous work has demonstrated loss of vasomotor regulatory tone in the cerebrovascular bed in the setting of generalized tonic-clonic seizures. As such, the normal mechanisms that protect against increased ICP in the setting of rising MAP are lost. Changes in the pressure–volume compliance curve during generalized tonic-clonic seizures result in large and potentially life-threatening increases in ICP. These considerations are especially important in the setting of large cerebral infarctions or hemorrhages in which ICP is already precariously close to generating an incipient herniation syndrome. Experimental results in cats examined the relationship between prolonged convulsions and ICP *(64)*. Pentylenetetrazole- or bicuculline-induced convulsions resulted in a three- to fivefold increase in ICP attaining maximal pressures of 20–94 mmHg after 20–420 s of seizure activity. Interestingly, the ICP remained high for between 47 s and 10 min but then began to fall gradually, reaching pre-ictal levels after 2–30 min despite the continuation of convulsions. Changes in ICP were independent of changes in blood pressure. In one report, ICP and electroencephalographic activity were monitored in a patient with viral encephalitis and frequent partial motor seizures. Each ictal episode was associated with stable blood pressure and an increase in ICP *(65)*. The average seizure duration was approx. 1 min, and the average maximum increase of ICP above baseline during the seizures was 6.5 mmHg. These investigators used a simple mathematical model to predict the rate of ICP increase, the peak ICP, the phase difference between maximum spike frequency and maximum ICP, and the rate at which ICP returned to pre-ictal values after termination of the seizure. They concluded that the time course of the ICP appears to be determined by the frequency of spikes and the CSF pressure–volume dynamics existing at the time of the seizure.

Metabolic consequences of seizures are more likely to accompany SE and include hypoxia, hypercarbia, respiratory and metabolic (lactic) acidosis, rhabdomyolysis, and cardiac ischemia. In addition to absent respiratory effort during a convulsion, airway obstruction in even a single generalized tonic-clonic seizure can lead to diminished tissue oxygenation. Aspiration pneumonia remains an important risk following either single or prolonged seizures and, if missed, can lead to sepsis, the acute respiratory distress syndrome (ARDS), and the need for prolonged mechanical ventilation. Rarely, neurogenic pulmonary edema may develop in the setting of SE. The syndrome of inappropriate antidiuretic hormone (SIADH) secretion or neurogenic diabetes insipidus can follow convulsive SE. Elevated creatine kinase levels may herald rhabdomyolysis, which can lead to acute renal insufficiency.

Several side effects of AEDs may complicate the clinical picture in patients with seizures and acute neurological disorders. Hypotension in patients receiving intravenous phenytoin can exacerbate poor cerebral perfusion in the setting of acute stroke. Similarly, cardiac dysrhythmia following phenytoin (PHT) *(66)* may diminish cerebral perfusion and worsen brain ischemia. Significant sedation can accompany phenytoin, phenobarbital (PB), and carbamazepine (CBZ) administration, which can cloud interpretation of the mental status exam.

The incidence of head injuries and intracranial hematomas owing to falls caused by seizures is increased in epilepsy patients. In one series of 1760 adult head-injured patients, 582 head injuries (33.1%) were caused by falls and 22 (3.8%) of these were caused by seizures *(67)*. Based on the prevalence rates for epilepsy in the general population of 0.5–2%, the investigators concluded that epilepsy patients are several times more likely to suffer a head injury as the result of a fall.

Diagnostic Considerations

A first-time seizure may in fact be a manifestation of a new and potentially life-threatening neurologic event such as stroke, ICH, subarachnoid hemorrhage, or encephalitis. Seizures in the setting of acute TBI may herald substantial CNS injury. It is also important to remember that concomitant medical illnesses such as hypoxemia, hypoglycemia, hyponatremia, hypocalcemia, hepatic or renal failure, urinary tract infections, pneumonia, sepsis, and iatrogenic or illicit drug use may lower seizure threshold in any individual and especially those with CNS structural injury. In addition, recent expert opinion has suggested that seizures persisting for >5 min should be viewed as SE and treated as such *(68,69)*.

On first assessment of a patient with seizures and known or suspected neurologic disease, a calm and methodical approach is best adopted. If possible, a thorough history should be obtained from patient family members or friends regarding recent symptoms or complaints such as change in mental status, history of TIA or stroke, loss of vision, focal weakness or sensory loss, or change in gait. Use of prescription or illicit drugs should be determined. Initial assessment of vital signs and maintenance of airway, breathing, and circulatory stability ("ABCs") is paramount. Special attention should be given to the presence of cardiac dysrhythmias such as atrial fibrillation, which may predispose to embolic stroke. Once these parameters are ascertained, a rapid but complete neurologic exam should be performed. Salient features of the exam should include determination of mental status and, if indicated, gradation using the GCS. Evidence of localizing signs such as pupillary or eye movement abnormalities, hemiparesis, reflex asymmetry, or extensor plantar reflexes should be sought. If feasible, funduscopic exam may be revealing especially in the setting of increased intracranial pressure (papilledema), acute stroke (Hollenhorst plaques), or septic cardiac emboli (Roth spots). Evidence of CNS infection such as meningismus, headache, fever or supportive evidence such as rash should also be sought and an early decision regarding lumbar puncture should be made. Initial laboratory studies should include electrolytes, serum glucose, O_2 saturation and/or arterial blood gas, complete blood count with differential, toxicology profile, AED levels if detected in toxicology screen, and β-HCG (human chorionic gonadotropin) in female patients.

If there is strong suspicion of acute CNS lesion, a neuroimaging study such as CT or magnetic resonance imagery (MRI) is indicated. If infection is suspected, an initial dose of antibiotics or antiviral medications such as acyclovir may be given prior to imaging and CSF examination. As a general rule, it is better to control a patient's seizures with intravenous medications such as lorazepam or diazepam prior to initiation of a neuroimaging study. Patients who experience seizures in the MR or CT scanner are at risk for injury from fall, aspiration, asphyxiation, and post-ictal confusion or aggression. Additionally, in the absence of known hypersensitivity to benzodiazepines, there are currently no neurologic disorders including potentially life-threatening conditions such as SAH, epidural hemorrhage, meningitis, stroke, or increased ICP, in which rapid treatment of seizures with benzodiazepines is contraindicated. In short, cessation of seizures, even if only for a brief period while more clinical data are obtained, is the goal in the setting of acute neurologic disorders.

EEG Monitoring

A recent review outlines the role of continuous EEG (CEEG) monitoring in the NICU and Emergency Department *(70)*. CEEG may serve as a neurophysiologic monitor that can detect brain abnormalities at a reversible stage and therefore guide timely and physiologically sound interventions *(71)*. CEEG monitoring is of benefit in the early diagnosis and management of cerebral ischemia, acute cerebral infarction, and post-SAH vasospasm. In comatose patients, it can provide important diagnostic and prognostic information. More recently, it has been found advantageous for targeting management of acute severe head trauma patients.

EEG Findings in Acute Stroke

Evidence of focal slow activity may suggest an underlying structural brain lesion such as a cerebral infarct or hemorrhage. Periodic lateralized epileptiform discharges (PLEDs) are most commonly associated with acute vascular lesions and may persist for several months following a stroke. Focal high-voltage delta waves with polyspikes (FHDPS) may correlate with ictal events including focal clonic or myoclonic seizures in patients with MELAS *(72)*. In the subacute and chronic stages, focal spikes or sharp waves and 14- and 6-Hz positive bursts were recorded frequently in MELAS patients. Intracranial EEG in one reported patient with PVLM demonstrated multifocal epileptic discharges *(73)*. In one series, the most common electroencephalographic abnormality in patients with seizures and acute stroke was focal slowing *(4)*. Recurrent seizures occurred in all of the 4 patients with PLEDs and in 75% of the 8 patients with diffuse slowing.

EEG Findings in ICH

The EEG changes associated with ICH are typically focal and more pronounced than those seen in ischemic stroke. More overt EEG changes occur in the setting of lobar hemorrhage than thalamic or basal ganglia hemorrhage. Whereas spikes or sharp waves may develop, they are often not seen in the setting of acute ICH. In contrast, focal ipsilateral delta activity (intermittent or continuous) and loss of normal background cerebral activity, i.e., alpha and sleep spindles, may be observed in regions adjacent and ipsilateral to the ICH. ICH involving the third ventricle or those with extension into the ventricular system or thalamus bilaterally may cause clinical coma. In these patients, the EEG may reveal diffuse bilateral theta and delta with minimal spontaneous reactivity. Finally, cerebellar hemorrhage may occur with little change in the EEG as long as the patient remains awake. If brainstem compression occurs, loss of consciousness will be followed by diffuse delta and theta activity on the EEG. In the setting of subarachnoid hemorrhage, more diffuse abnormalities may be detected such as diffuse theta or delta. Marked suppression of the background amplitudes may also occur. If there is extension of the hemorrhage into the brain parenchyma, focal delta may be seen in this region.

EEG Findings in CNS Infection

In virtually all forms of viral encephalitis, the EEG is abnormal to some extent. Diffuse delta is seen most commonly but intermittent rhythmic delta may also be observed. The EEG in the acute stage of HSVE can show a variety of abnormalities, including unilateral or bilateral periodic sharp waves or attenuation of amplitude, focal or generalized slow waves or epileptiform discharges, or electrographic seizures (for comprehensive review, *see* ref. *74*). No specific EEG patterns are pathognomonic for HSVE, but a focal or lateralized EEG abnormality in the presence of encephalitis is highly indicative of HSV infection. In the acute stage, EEG appears to be more sensitive than CT imaging or radioisotope brain scanning. The EEG findings tend to differ during the course of illness, and the periodic discharges occur only during the acute stage. The EEG findings in either the acute stage or on long-term follow-up do not predict the chance of survival or severity of disability, and EEG changes appear to lag behind the clinical changes. EEG results can become normal in both adults and neonates when the acute stage is over. In one study, the EEG abnormalities included frontotemporal delta slowing in five patients, periodic lateralized epileptiform discharge in three, and runs of spike and periodic activity in one patient each *(75)*. Periodic discharges are considered by many as a sine qua non of HSVE, although PLEDs may be seen in a variety of other disorders. The periodicity of PLEDs in HSVE and other viral encephalidities tends to be more rhythmic and montonous *(76)*.

In one series of 32 patients with tuberculous meningitis, the EEG was abnormal in 24 patients *(77)*. The EEG abnormalities included diffuse theta or delta slowing in 22 patients, frontal intermittent rhythmic delta activity (FIRDA) in 15, asymmetry in 5, and epileptiform discharges in 4 patients. The EEG findings correlated with the severity of meningitis, the degree of coma, and outcome at 3 mo as assessed by the Barthel index score.

EEG Findings in Brain Trauma

After initial loss of consciousness following brain injury, background EEG may show diffuse slowing. Epileptiform abnormalities such as sharp waves and spikes may be seen immediately and may be either focal or widespread. In the setting of mild brain trauma, the EEG may be normal or exhibit subtle slowing. Following severe brain trauma there may be a dramatic cessation of EEG activity. In one series of 76 patients, spontaneous EEG activity was initially absent from 33 patients who were subsequently shown to have no cerebral perfusion by angiography. EEG activity was recorded in 32 patients, but 20 of these died within the ensuing 2–4 d *(78)*. EEG and CT scans of 280 cases of minor head injury in children under 15 yr of age were studied *(79)*. Abnormality on initial EEG was shown in 42.5% patients. Those who lost consciousness had a higher incidence of abnormality than those who did not, and incidence was also higher between 4 and 13 yr of age. The most frequent abnormality was slow waves, seen predominantly in the occipital regions. The EEGs became or remained normal in 95% of patients.

Therapeutic Considerations

Recent evidence suggests that prophylactic AEDs are effective in reducing early seizures following brain trauma, but there is no evidence that treatment with such drugs reduces the occurrence of late seizures (i.e., epilepsy), or has any effect on death and neurological disability *(80)*. Whereas AED prophylaxis for posttraumatic seizures (PTS) is common, results of clinical trials raise questions regarding the benefits of such treatment. A subcommittee of the Brain Injury Special Interest Group of the American Academy of Physical Medicine and Rehabilitation reviewed published literature (1998) regarding AED prophylaxis of PTS and suggested recommendations in the form of a practice parameter *(81)*. The treatment standard is that prophylactic use of PHT, CBZ, sodium valproate (VPA), or PB is not recommended for preventing late PTS, defined as seizures that occur after 1 wk of injury, in the patient in whom there has been no history of seizures following a nonpenetrating traumatic brain injury. However, it is recommended as a treatment option that PHT, PB, and CBZ may be used to prevent early PTS in patients at high risk for seizures following TBI. Finally, prophylactic use of PHT, CBZ, VPA, or PB is not recommended for preventing late PTS following penetrating TBI.

The long-term use of AEDs to prevent postoperative seizures in patients with cerebral aneurysms is common. However, in recent case series of aneurysm patients, there has been a low incidence of seizures. To investigate the incidence of seizures following aneurysm surgery, Baker et al. *(82)* categorized 387 of the 420 craniotomies for aneurysm surgery over a 4-yr period into those deemed to have low risk of seizure. Postoperative anticonvulsant medication in this group was restricted to an average of 3 d. A retrospective analysis of the incidence of early postoperative seizures and late postoperative seizures was performed in the populations of patients with ruptured and unruptured aneurysms with an average follow-up of 2.4 yr. The overall seizure rate in the study group was 5.4%. Patients with ruptured aneurysms had an early postoperative seizure rate of 1.5% and a long-term seizure rate of 3.0%. Early and long-term seizure rates for unruptured aneurysms were 2.6% and 4.4%, respectively. No patients who had early seizures went on to develop epilepsy, and all seizures were well controlled once AEDs were begun. These data support the idea that anticonvulsant medication may be safely restricted to the immediate perioperative period for most patients with aneurysms.

The prevalence of perioperative seizures following subdural hematoma was reviewed in 98 patients *(83)*. The onset of new seizures was found in 17 (18.5%) of 98 patients and was associated with increases in morbidity and mortality. Patients who received prophylactic AED demonstrated a significant decrease in the occurrence of seizures, and these investigators concluded that PHT prophylaxis in patients treated surgically for chronic subdural hematoma was beneficial.

Prophylactic treatment with AEDs is not clearly indicated for most types of strokes. In a study of ICH, Berger et al. *(27)* concluded that the prophylactic use of anticonvulsants in the acute management of ICH patients is unwarranted, especially in those patients in whom the ICH does not involve cortex. In patients with lobar ICH that affects cerebral cortex, AEDs may afford some prophylactic benefit especially in the setting of increased ICP.

In pre-eclampsia or eclampsia, recent multicenter studies show a benefit of magnesium sulfate over either PHT or diazepam in the prevention of seizures. In a prospective study of over 200 female patients, Lucas et al. *(84)* demonstrated that magnesium sulfate was superior to PHT for the prevention of eclampsia in hypertensive pregnant women. In a recent series of 50 eclamptic females randomized to either PHT or magnesium sulfate *(85),* women treated with PHT had a higher incidence of recurrent seizures (10 of 25–40%) than those treated with magnesium sulfate (2 of 25–8%). The majority of the women treated with PHT (6 of 10–60%) had single convulsion after initiation of anticonvulsant therapy and 1 woman in each group had recurrent convulsions. There was no significant difference in perinatal outcome in either group. Maternal morbidity was comparable in both groups, and there was no maternal death in either group. In addition to its anticonvulsant properties, magnesium sulfate may offer additional prophylaxis against stroke in eclampsia.

Summary

Seizures may herald an acute neurologic disturbance and therefore must be fully investigated. The assiduous clinician can glean from a thorough history and careful neurologic exam a rapid assessment of potentially life-threatening disorders and be able to institute appropriate diagnostic tests and therapeutic maneuvers.

References

1. Asconape JJ, Penry JK. Poststroke seizures in the elderly. *Clin Geriatr Med* 1991;7:483–492.
2. Neau JP, Ingrand P, Mouille-Brachet C, Rosier MP, Couderq C, Alvarez A, Gil R. Functional recovery and social outcome after cerebral infarction in young adults. *Cerebrovasc Dis* 1998;8:296–302.
3. Kilpatrick CJ, Davis SM, Tress BM, Rossiter SC, Hopper JL, Vandendriesen ML. Epileptic seizures in acute stroke. *Arch Neurol* 1990;47:157–160.
4. Gupta SR, Naheedy MH, Elias D, Rubino FA. Postinfarction seizures. A clinical study. *Stroke* 1988;19:1477–1481.
5. Lancman ME, Golimstok A, Norscini J, Granillo R. Risk factors for developing seizures after a stroke. *Epilepsia* 1993;34:141–143.
6. Giroud M, Gras P, Fayolle H, Andre N, Soichot P, Dumas R. Early seizures after acute stroke: a study of 1,640 cases. *Epilepsia* 1994;35:959–964.

7. Reith J, Jorgensen HS, Nakayama H, Raaschou HO, Olsen TS. Seizures in acute stroke: predictors and prognostic significance. The Copenhagen Stroke Study. *Stroke* 1997;28:1585–1589.

8. Murthy JM, Yangala R. Acute symptomatic seizures—incidence and etiological spectrum: a hospital-based study from South India. *Seizure* 1999;8:162–165.

9. Holt-Seitz A, Wirrell EC, Sundaram MB. Seizures in the elderly: etiology and prognosis. *Can J Neurol Sci* 1999;26:110–114.

10. Awada A, Omojola MF, Obeid T. Late epileptic seizures after cerebral infarction. *Acta Neurol Scand* 1999;99:265–268.

11. Krumholz A. Epidemiology and evidence for morbidity of nonconvulsive status epilepticus. *Clin Neurophysiol* 1999;16:314–322; discussion 353.

12. Drislane FW, Blum AS, Schomer DL. Focal status epilepticus: clinical features and significance of different EEG patterns. *Epilepsia* 1999;40:1254–1260.

13. Koppel BS, Samkoff L, Daras M Relation of cocaine use to seizures and epilepsy. *Epilepsia* 1996;37:875–878.

14. Simon DK, Johns DR. Mitochondrial disorders: clinical and genetic features. *Annu Rev Med* 1999;50:111–127.

15. Kinney TR, Sleeper LA, Wang WC, Zimmerman RA, Pegelow CH, Ohene-Frempong K, Wethers DL, Bello JA, Vichinsky EP, Moser FG, Gallagher DM, DeBaun MR, Platt OS, Miller ST. Silent cerebral infarcts in sickle cell anemia: a risk factor analysis. The Cooperative Study of Sickle Cell Disease. *Pediatrics* 1999; 103:640–645.

16. Visudtibhan A, Visudhiphan P, Chiemchanya S. Stroke and seizures as the presenting signs of pediatric HIV infection. *Pediatr Neurol* 1999;20:53–56.

17. Maria BL, Neufeld JA, Rosainz LC, Drane WE, Quisling RG, Ben-David K, Hamed LM. Central nervous system structure and function in Sturge-Weber syndrome: evidence of neurologic and radiologic progression. *J Child Neurol* 1998; 13:606–618.

18. Ferro JM. Vasculitis of the central nervous system. *J Neurol* 1998;245:766–776.

19. Dichgans M, Mayer M, Uttner I, Bruning R, Muller-Hocker J, Rungger G, Ebke M, Klockgether T, Gasser T. The phenotypic spectrum of CADASIL: clinical findings in 102 cases. *Ann Neurol* 1998;44:731–739.

20. Piepgras DG, Sundt TM Jr, Ragoowansi AT, Stevens L. Seizure outcome in patients with surgically treated cerebral arteriovenous malformations. *J Neurosurg* 1993; 78:5–11.

21. Kaplan PW. Neurologic issues in eclampsia. *Rev Neurol* (Paris) 1999;155:335–341.

22. Weisberg LA, Shamsnia M, Elliott D. Seizures caused by nontraumatic parenchymal brain hemorrhages. *Neurology* 1991;41:1197–1199.

23. Sung CY, Chu NS. Epileptic seizures in intracerebral haemorrhage. *J Neurol Neurosurg Psychiatry* 1989;52:1273–1276.

24. Cervoni L, Artico M, Salvati M, Bristot R, Franco C, Delfini R. Epileptic seizures in intracerebral hemorrhage: a clinical and prognostic study of 55 cases. *Neurosurg Rev* 1994;17:185–188.

25. Lo YK, Yiu CH, Hu HH, Su MS, Laeuchli SC. Frequency and characteristics of early seizures in Chinese acute stroke. *Acta Neurol Scand* 1994;90:83–85.

26. Faught E, Peters D, Bartolucci A, Moore L, Miller PC. Seizures after primary intracerebral hemorrhage. *Neurology* 1989;39:1089–1093.

27. Berger AR, Lipton RB, Lesser ML, Lantos G, Portenoy RK. Early seizures following intracerebral hemorrhage: implications for therapy. *Neurology* 1988;38:1363–1365.

28. Silbert PL, Bartleson JD, Miller GM, Parisi JE, Goldman MS, Meyer FB. Cortical petechial hemorrhage, leukoencephalopathy, and subacute dementia associated with seizures due to cerebral amyloid angiopathy. *Mayo Clin Proc* 1995; 70:477–480.
29. Raps EC, Rogers JD, Galetta SL, Solomon RA, Lennihan L, Klebanoff LM, Fink ME. The clinical spectrum of unruptured intracranial aneurysms. *Arch Neurol* 1993;50:265–268.
30. Hart RG, Byer JA, Slaughter JR, Hewett JE, Easton JD. Occurrence and implications of seizures in subarachnoid hemorrhage due to ruptured intracranial aneurysms. *Neurosurgery* 1981;8:417–421.
31. Sundaram MB, Chow F. Seizures associated with spontaneous subarachnoid hemorrhage. *Can J Neurol Sci* 1986;13:229–231.
32. Pinto AN, Canhao P, Ferro JM. Seizures at the onset of subarachnoid haemorrhage. *J Neurol* 1996;243:161–164.
33. Lee ST, Lui TN. Early seizures after mild closed head injury. *J Neurosurg* 1992;76:435–439.
34. Leggate JR, Lopez-Ramos N, Genitori L, Lena G, Choux M. Extradural haematoma in infants. *Br J Neurosurg* 1989;3:533–539.
35. Murthy JM, Yangala R. Etiological spectrum of symptomatic localization related epilepsies: a study from South India. *J Neurol Sci* 1998;158:65–70.
36. McGrath N, Anderson NE, Croxson MC, Powell KF. Herpes simplex encephalitis treated with acyclovir: diagnosis and long term outcome. *J Neurol Neurosurg Psychiatry* 1997;63:321–326.
37. Cameron PD, Wallace SJ, Munro J. Herpes simplex virus encephalitis: problems in diagnosis. *Dev Med Child Neurol* 1992;34:134–140.
38. Jones CM, Dunn HG, Thomas EE, Cone RW, Weber JM. Acute encephalopathy and status epilepticus associated with human herpes virus 6 infection. *Dev Med Child Neurol* 1994;36:646–650.
39. Chun RW. Clinical aspects of La Crosse encephalitis: neurological and psychological sequellae. *Prog Clin Biol Res* 1983;123:193–201.
40. Davis LE, Kornfeld M. Neurocysticercosis: neurologic, pathogenic, diagnostic and therapeutic aspects. *Eur Neurol* 1991;31:229–240.
41. del Brutto OH. Neurocysticercosis in children: clinical and radiological analysis and prognostic factors in 54 patients. *Rev Neurol* 1997;25:1681–1684.
42. Garg RK. HIV infection and seizures. *Postgrad Med J* 1999;75:387–390.
43. McCrory PR, Bladin PF, Berkovic SF. Retrospective study of concussive convulsions in elite Australian rules and rugby league footballers: phenomenology, aetiology, and outcome. *Br Med J* 1997;314:171–174.
44. Asikainen I, Kaste M, Sarna S. Early and late posttraumatic seizures in traumatic brain injury rehabilitation patients: brain injury factors causing late seizures and influence of seizures on long-term outcome. *Epilepsia* 1999;40:584–589.
45. Ratan SK, Kulshreshtha R, Pandey RM. Predictors of posttraumatic convulsions in head-injured children. *Pediatr Neurosurg* 1999;30:127–131.
46. Annegers JF, Hauser WA, Coan SP, Rocca WA. A. population-based study of seizures after traumatic brain injuries. *N Engl J Med* 1998;338:20–24.
47. Lee ST, Lui TN, Wong CW, Yeh YS, Izuan WC, Chen T, Hung S, Wu C. Early seizures after severe closed head injury. *Can J Neurosci* 1997;24:359–360.
48. Jordan KG. Nonconvulsive status epilepticus in acute brain injury. *J Clin Neurophysiol* 1999;16:332–340; discussion 353.

49. Vespa PM, Nuwer MR, Nenov V, Ronne-Engstrom E, Hovda DA, Bergsneider M, Kelly DF, Martin NA, Becker DP. Increased incidence and impact of nonconvulsive and convulsive seizures after traumatic brain injury as detected by continuous electroencephalographic monitoring. *J Neurosurg* 1999;91:750–760.

50. Kim DC, Todd MM. Forebrain ischemia: effect on pharmacologically induced seizure thresholds in the rat. *Brain Res* 1999;831:131–139.

51. Regan RF, Panter SS. Neurotoxicity of hemoglobin in cortical cell culture. *Neurosci Lett* 1993;153:219–222.

52. Marks KA, Mallard CE, Roberts I, Williams CE, Gluckman PD, Edwards AD. Nitric oxide synthase inhibition and delayed cerebral injury after severe cerebral ischemia in fetal sheep. *Pediatr Res* 1999;46:8–13.

53. Yenari MA, Fink SL, Sun GH, Chang LK, Patel MK, Kunis DM, Onley D, Ho DY, Sapolsky RM, Steinberg GK. Gene therapy with HSP72 is neuroprotective in rat models of stroke and epilepsy. *Ann Neurol* 1998;44:584–591.

54. Towfighi J, Housman C, Mauger D, Vannucci RC. Effect of seizures on cerebral hypoxic-ischemic lesions in immature rats. *Brain Res Dev Brain Res* 1999; 113:83–95.

55. Kokaia Z, Zhao Q, Kokaia M, Elmer E, Metsis M, Smith ML, Siesjo BK, Lindvall O. Regulation of brain-derived neurotrophic factor gene expression after transient middle cerebral artery occlusion with and without brain damage. *Exp Neurol* 1995;136:73–88.

56. Haas CA, Frotscher M, Deller T. Differential induction of c-Fos, c-Jun and Jun B in the rat central nervous system following unilateral entorhinal cortex lesion. *Neuroscience* 1999;90:41–51.

57. Willmore LJ. Post-traumatic epilepsy: cellular mechanisms and implications for treatment. *Epilepsia* 1990;31(Suppl 3):S67–S73.

58. Kiwak KJ, Moskowitz MA, Levine L. Leukotriene production in gerbil brain after ischemic insult, subarachnoid hemorrhage, and concussive injury. *J Neurosurg* 1985;62:865–869.

59. Yang L, Benardo LS. Epileptogenesis following neocortical trauma from two sources of disinhibition. *J Neurophysiol* 1997;78:2804–2810.

60. D'Ambrosio R, Maris DO, Grady MS, Winn HR, Janigro D. Impaired K(+) homeostasis and altered electrophysiological properties of post-traumatic hippocampal glia. *J Neurosci* 1999;19:8152–8162.

61. Coulter DA, Rafiq A, Shumate M, Gong QZ, DeLorenzo RJ, Lyeth BG. Brain injury-induced enhanced limbic epileptogenesis: anatomical and physiological parallels to an animal model of temporal lobe epilepsy. *Epilepsy Res* 1996;26:81–91.

62. Nilsson P, Ronne-Engstrom E, Flink R, Ungerstedt U, Carlson H, Hillered L. Epileptic seizure activity in the acute phase following cortical impact trauma in rat. *Brain Res* 1994;637:227–232.

63. Rogatsky G, Mayevsky A, Zarchin N, Doron A. Continuous multiparametric monitoring of brain activities following fluid-percussion injury in rats: preliminary results. *J Basic Clin Physiol Pharmacol* 1996;7:23–43.

64. Goitein KJ, Shohami E. Intracranial pressure during prolonged experimental convulsions in cats. J Neurol 1983;230:259–266.

65. Gabor AJ, Brooks AG, Scobey RP, Parsons GH. Intracranial pressure during epileptic seizures. *Electroencephalogr Clin Neurophysiol* 1984;57:497–506.

66. Earnest MP, Marx JA, Drury LR. Complications of intravenous phenytoin for acute treatment of seizures. Recommendations for usage. *JAMA* 1983;249:762–765.

67. Zwimpfer TJ, Brown J, Sullivan I, Moulton RJ. Head injuries due to falls caused by seizures: a group at high risk for traumatic intracranial hematomas. *J Neurosurg* 1997;86:433–437.
68. Lowenstein DH, Alldredge BK. Status epilepticus. *N Engl J Med* 1998; 2;338:970–976.
69. Lowenstein DH, Bleck T, Macdonald RL. It's time to revise the definition of status epilepticus. *Epilepsia* 1999;40:120–122.
70. Jordan KG. Continuous EEG monitoring in the neuroscience intensive care unit and emergency department. *J Clin Neurophysiol* 1999;16:14–39.
71. Vespa P, Prins M, Ronne-Engstrom E, Caron M, Shalmon E, Hovda DA, Martin NA, Becker DP. Increase in extracellular glutamate caused by reduced cerebral perfusion pressure and seizures after human traumatic brain injury: a microdialysis. *J Neurosurg* 1998;89:971–982.
72. Fujimoto S, Mizuno K, Shibata H, Kanayama M, Kobayashi M, Sugiyama N, Ban K, Ishikawa T, Itoh T, Togari H, Wada Y. Serial electroencephalographic findings in patients with MELAS. *Pediatr Neurol* 1999;20:43–48.
73. Gurses C, Gross DW, Andermann F, Bastos A, Dubeau F, Calay M, Eraksoy M, Bezci S, Andermann E, Melanson D. Periventricular leukomalacia and epilepsy: incidence and seizure pattern. Neurology 1999;52:341–345.
74. Lai CW, Gragasin ME. Electroencephalography in herpes simplex encephalitis. *J Clin Neurophysiol* 1988;5:87–103.
75. Misra UK, Kalita J. Neurophysiological studies in herpes simplex encephalitis. *Electromyogr Clin Neurophysiol* 1998;38:177–182.
76. Gross DW, Wiebe S, Blume WT. The periodicity of lateralized epileptiform discharges. *Clin Neurophysiol* 1999;110:1516–1520.
77. Kalita J, Misra UK. EEG changes in tuberculous meningitis: a clinicoradiological correlation. *Electroencephalogr Clin Neurophysiol* 1998;107:39–43.
78. Ganes T, Lundar T. EEG and evoked potentials in comatose patients with severe brain damage. *Electroencephalogr Clin Neurophysiol* 1988;69:6–13.
79. Enomoto T, Ono Y, Nose T, Maki Y, Tsukada K. Electroencephalography in minor head injury in children. *Child Nerv Syst* 1986;2:72–79.
80. Schierhout G, Roberts I. Prophylactic antiepileptic agents after head injury: a systematic review. *J Neurol Neurosurg Psychiatry* 1998;64:108–112.
81. Brain Injury Special Interest Group of the American Academy of Physical Medicine and Rehabilitation. Practice parameter: antiepileptic drug treatment of posttraumatic seizures. *Arch Phys Med Rehabil* 1998;79:594–597.
82. Baker CJ, Prestigiacoma CJ, Solomon RA. Short-term perioperative anticonvulsant prophylaxis for the surgical treatment of low-risk patients with intracranial aneurysms. *Neurosurgery* 1995;37:863–870; discussion 870–871.
83. Sabo RA, Hanigan WC, Aldag JC. Chronic subdural hematomas and seizures: the role of prophylactic anticonvulsive medication. *Surg Neurol* 1995;43:579–582.
84. Lucas MJ, Leveno KJ, Cunningham FG. A comparison of magnesium sulfate with phenytoin for the prevention of eclampsia. *N Engl J Med* 1995;333:201–205.
85. Sawhney H, Sawhney IM, Mandal R, Subramanyam, Vasishta K. Efficacy of magnesium sulphate and phenytoin in the management of eclampsia. *J Obstet Gynaecol Res* 1999;25:333–338.

4

Seizures in Multisystem Disease Affecting the Nervous System

Joerg-Patrick Stübgen, MD, FRCPC

Introduction

This chapter discusses a heterogeneous group of disorders that involve the central nervous system (CNS) and cause seizures (**Table 1**). Nervous system involvement is part of the disease definition or is a complication of the systemic disease process. Neurologic manifestations, including seizures, can present before the systemic illness becomes manifest but more commonly occur in the setting of established disease. Seizures can also be a complication of end-organ damage caused by the underlying illness, or of medications used to treat the illness. The incidence of neurologic complications and seizures varies widely. The etiopathogenesis of seizures is mostly unknown in this diverse group of diseases.

Systemic Immunologic Diseases

Systemic (non-organ-specific) autoimmune diseases, including the systemic vasculitides, occur as a result of disordered immunoregulation. The etiology of these diseases is mostly unknown. Both humeral and cell-mediated immune responses are implicated. More than one type of immune mechanism may be involved in a particular disease. The nervous system is commonly involved in these disorders. CNS involvement may be a presenting manifestation and is a major cause of morbidity. Seizures occur as a complication of the primary process or as a result of systemic complications and treatment.

From: *Seizures: Medical Causes and Management*
Edited by: N. Delanty © Humana Press, Inc., Totowa, NJ

Table 1
Multisystem Disease Associated with Seizures

Systemic immunologic diseases
Systemic lupus erythematosus/Antiphospholipid antibody syndrome
Polyarteritis nodosa
Wegener's granulomatosus
Behcét's disease
Sydenham's chorea
Sarcoidosis
Stiff-man syndrome
Other: Giant cell arteritis
      Sjøgren's syndrome
      Rheumatoid arthritis
      Systemic sclerosis

Mitochondrial disorders
MELAS
MERRF
Leigh syndrome
NARP
Kearns–Sayre syndrome
Reye's syndrome

Inherited metabolic disease
Acute porphyria

Hematologic diseases
Fat embolism syndrome
Dysbarism
Thrombotic thrombocytopenic purpura
Sickle cell disease

Infectious disease
Whipple's disease

Systemic Lupus Erythematosis/Antiphospholipid Antibody Syndrome

Systemic lupus erythematosis (SLE) is a chronic inflammatory connective tissue disorder of unknown cause that can involve joints, kidneys, serous surfaces, and vessel walls. It occurs predominantly in young women. The sera of most patients contain antinuclear antibodies (ANA), often including anti-DNA antibodies. The prevalence of CNS involvement is variable and depends on clinical definition, with estimates between 18% and 70%. The clinical features cover a wide range of symptoms, from mild depression and cognitive behavioral abnormalities to stroke, epilepsy, and severe psychiatric disorders. Systemic disease may be inactive at the onset of CNS manifestations. Seizures are one of the most common neuropsychiatric complications of SLE, second only to organic brain syndrome and psychiatric disorders *(1)*. Secondary generalized tonic-clonic seizures are more common than complex partial seizures. Seizures may infrequently be the initial presentation of SLE or may precede the diagnosis by several years. Seizures mostly occur during an exacerbation and do not subsequently recur, although epilepsy may develop in a minority of patients. The reported prevalence of seizures in SLE patients ranges from 7% to 74%, but a reasonable estimate is around 15% *(2,3)*. Differentiation of seizures caused by the direct effect of active SLE on the CNS from seizures as a secondary event during severe disease (e.g., hypertension, uremia, electrolyte disturbance, infection, or corticosteroid treatment) may be difficult *(4)*. Seizures occur with increased frequency terminally, probably because death in SLE is often related to either renal failure or fulminant CNS disease. Anticonvulsants such as hydantoins and primidone may unmask SLE or induce a lupus-like syndrome, but these clinical disorders usually regress following withdrawal of the drug.

The pathogenesis of seizures in SLE remains unclear. Both secondary generalized and focal seizures are likely to occur as a result of ischemic vascular disease or possibly from antibodies that bind to cerebral tissue. Antineuronal antibodies have been associated with seizures *(3)*. However, those antibodies also occur in non-lupus patients with seizures and in SLE patients without seizures; perhaps seizures induce antibody production. Cerebrospinal fluid (CSF) antineuronal antibodies are present only when serum antineuronal antibodies are detectable and indices of blood–brain barrier damage are elevated; thus blood–brain barrier damage may be required before antibody-mediated neuropsychiatric disease and seizures become manifest. The causal role of a variety of other autoantibodies (anti-ribosomal-P, anti-synaptosomal, and anti-ganglioside) in neuropsychiatric lupus is an area of active research *(5–7)*.

Seizures in SLE are also correlated with a high prevalence of serum antiphospholipid antibodies (APAs) *(4,8)*. There was a statistically significant increase in the prevalence of APAs in SLE patients with seizures compared to control SLE patients *(4)*. The APAs, specifically anticardiolipin (aCL) antibodies and lupus anticoagulant (LAC), have been studied in SLE. Studies suggest a relationship between seizures and aCL antibodies, even in patients without SLE *(9)*. Moderate-to-high titers of immunoglobulin G (IgG) aCL antibodies are most strongly implicated in relation to seizures, whereas the IgM isotype appears to be less specific *(4)*. These findings suggest that the IgG isotype may have a pathogenetic role in SLE-associated seizures. The mechanism through which aCL antibodies cause seizures in SLE patients is unclear *(10,11)*. Epileptogenic cerebral ischemic lesions are not detected in all patients. The coexistence of vascular lesions in a high percentage (43%) of SLE patients with seizures and positive aCL antibodies provides evidence that this association may be significant *(4)*. Alternatively, the aCL antibodies could also reflect a common, perhaps genetically determined, predisposition both to develop seizures and to produce autoantibodies, as seems to be the case for aCL antibodies and schizophrenia. Another possible mechanism may be an immune reaction to antigens expressed specifically by neurons that have epileptic activity, as has been demonstrated for several types of seizure-induced genes or cell products. However, the absence of CSF aCL antibodies in patients with positive serum aCL antibodies, acute CNS SLE, and seizures mitigates against a role for aCL antibodies as a direct antineuronal antibody. Finally, LAC was not statistically more prevalent in SLE patients with seizures compared to patients without seizures, but this too requires further research *(4)*.

Polyarteritis Nodosa

Polyarteritis nodosa (PAN) is a disease characterized by segmental inflammation and necrosis of medium-sized muscular arteries, with secondary ischemia of tissue supplied by affected arteries. PAN is a clinicopathologic syndrome caused by a particular qualitative and quantitative relationship between antibodies and any of a variety of antigens that participate in the formation of immune complexes. These complexes are not cleared by the reticuloendothelial system but are deposited in the vessel walls where they initiate an inflammatory reaction. The common denominator of the various types of neurologic abnormalities is tissue ischemia, resulting in a variety of functional and structural alterations in neural tissue. CNS manifestations have been reported in 3–41% of patients in clinical series and generally have been given little attention *(12–14)*. For unclear reasons, CNS disease occurs later and has a lower incidence, compared to peripheral neuropathy. In a series of 114 PAN patients (possibly including some with Wegener's granulomatosus [WG]), 13 patients suffered seizures: 6 secondary generalized tonic-clonic, 4 focal, and 3 both *(12)*. In another series of 25 patients, 5 suffered a diffuse process characterized by encephalopathy with secondary generalized or focal seizures *(13)*. The encephalopathy proved to be rapidly reversible with definitive treatment, suggesting that it was related to functional rather than structural abnormalities secondary to diffuse cerebral ischemia. Seizures always occurred in the setting of acute illness and were never a long-term sequela, despite follow-up periods as long as 12 yr. CNS involvement does not worsen the outlook of PAN when appropriately treated with corticosteroids and/or cyclophosphamide.

Wegener's Granulomatosis

WG begins as a localized granulomatous inflammation of upper and lower respiratory tract mucosa and may progress into a generalized necrotizing granulomatous vasculitis and glomerulonephritis. Neurological involvement occurs in 22–54% of patients with WG *(15–17)*. Seizures were reported in 10 of 324 consecutive patients in a large series *(17)*. All patients had secondary generalized tonic-clonic seizures. Seizures occurred as a result of a systemic vasculitis, cerebral granulomatous involvement, progressive renal or pulmonary failure or terminally in association with sepsis, or disseminated intravascular coagulation. Rarely has WG presented with a seizure prior to the diagnosis of the disorder. In one reported case, seizure was clinically attributed to cerebral vasculitis remote from the granulomatous involvement of the sinuses *(18)*. The pathogenesis of this disorder is unknown, and the favored hypothesis is an immune-mediated vasculitis triggered by a nasopharyngeal infection. Serum antineutrophil cytoplasmic antibody (ANCA) is a highly sensitive and specific test for WG. Effective treatment is with corticosteroids and cyclophosphamide.

Behçet's Disease

Behçet's disease is a polysymptomatic, recurrent systemic vasculitis with a chronic course and an unknown cause. Infectious agents, immune mechanisms, and genetic factors are invoked in the etiology. The prevalence of CNS involvement ranges from 3% to 44% *(18–20)*. Neurological manifestations can be the presenting feature (<3%). Seizures are regarded as an important clue to CNS involvement and are reported to occur in 4–8% of patients in large series of Behçet's disease *(21)*. These seizures can be either focal or generalized, and usually respond well to anticonvulsant medication. Magnetic resonance imagery (MRI) demonstrates lesions predominantly of the brainstem and the deep cerebral structures at different stages of illness. The most important pathologic changes in the nervous system in Behçet's disease are diffuse perivascular inflammatory cell infiltration of the leptomeninges, small multifocal necrotic lesions in gray and white matter of the brain, brainstem, and spinal cord, and, thrombosis of the dural sinuses. Immunosuppressive treatment includes boluses of intravenous (IV) methylprednisolone for several days and 2.5 mg/kg cyclophosphamide per day, especially with severe vasculitis. Favorable results are reported with 0.1 mg/kg chlorambucil per day for several months.

Sydenham's Chorea

Sydenham's chorea (SC) is a movement disorder of young people (mostly 5–15 yr), manifested predominantly by involuntary movement and infrequently by other neurologic symptoms. The etiology is unknown, but there is a strong association with rheumatic fever and antecedent group A streptococcal infection. Pathophysiological mechanisms remain obscure, and the role of detected antibodies to striatal and subthalamic neurons must still be determined. Perhaps genetically vulnerable children, when exposed to a group A streptococcal infection, produce antibodies that mistakenly recognize cells within the basal ganglia and cause an inflammatory response. The neuropathology of SC consists of neuronal degeneration and vascular abnormalities, including inflammatory lesions, vasodilation, and petechial hemorrhages. The pathologic substrate for chorea has not been identified. The association of SC with seizures has not been well documented, and the incidence is unclear *(22)*. Seizures may occur during SC; however, if subtle, they may be masked by frequent choreic movements and thus not recognized *(23,24)*. Secondary generalized tonic-clonic convulsions and complex partial seizures have been described. Electroencephalogram (EEG) abnormalities (irregular posterior slowing, epileptic spikes, high voltage sharp waves) are more frequent than overt clinical seizures, and have been reported in 30–70% of patients with or without an acute brain syndrome. EEG changes are transient and return to normal within 1–4 wk. Seizures are confined to the acute attack of SC. Permanent EEG slowing and focal epilepsy have been reported separately.

Sarcoidosis

Sarcoidosis is a multisystem granulomatous disorder of unknown etiology, characterized histologically by noncaseating epithelioid granulomas involving various organs or tissues, with symptoms dependent on the site and degree of involvement. A single provoking agent or disordered defense reactions triggered by various insults may be responsible, and genetic factors may be important *(25)*. Neurosarcoidosis (NS) affects 5% of patients with systemic sarcoidosis *(26)*. Half of the patients with NS will present with neurologic symptoms. The CNS can be the only site involved. Manifestations of meningeal, parameningeal, cranial nerve, hypothalamic, and pituitary involvement are most common *(27)*. Parenchymal disease, especially periventricular, and involvment of the ependymal lining (leading to hydrocephalus) are also common. Intracranial mass lesions are infrequent. In leptomeningitis or focal pachymeningitis, inflammatory cells infiltrate the brain parenchyma after invading the subarachnoid and Virchow-Robin spaces. Collections of granulomata may coalesce to form a mass lesion; invasion of the cortex may act as a seizure focus. Epilepsy may continue as a sign of previous granuloma involvement and scarring even thought the process is no longer active. Seizures occur in up to 21% of patients with NS *(28,29)*. Seizures may be the first manifestation (up to 10%) of NS. Generalized tonic-clonic seizures are most common (up to 92%), and partial seizures occur in up to 31% of patients. Seizures are unrelated to electrolyte or calcium imbalance, anoxia, trauma, infection, or end-organ failure. Granulomatous meningoencephalitis is a feature of nearly all reported cases, and a minority of patients show evidence of space occupying granulomata. Patients with NS and seizures are more likely to have a progressive or relapsing clinical course. The presence of seizure disorder in association with NS is correlated with a worse prognosis *(30)*. Increased morbidity and mortality (75%) is the result of the extent of intracranial involvement rather than the seizures *per se*. Seizures in this group of patients are easily controlled with combinations of steroids and antiseizure medication. Patients may follow a fulminant course and die within months after seizure onset. A group of patients may survive with a chronic seizure disorder *(31)*. No clinical or laboratory features distinguish between these two groups. The EEG and CSF findings correlate poorly with the clinical picture. Only patients with solitary space-occupying lesions seem to fare better after resection *(32)*.

Stiff-Man Syndrome/Stiff-Person Syndrome

Stiff-man syndrome (SMS) or stiff-person syndrome, is a rare disorder of motor function characterized by involuntary stiffness of axial muscles and superimposed painful muscle spasms, which occur spontaneously or are provoked by startle or emotional stimuli *(33,34)*. An association has been reported between SMS and epilepsy, insulin-dependent diabetes, and a variety of organ-specific autoimmune disorders (pernicious anemia, thyroiditis, adrenalitis, ovarian failure, hypoparathyroidism) *(35)*. The prevalence of epilepsy is about 10%, mostly with generalized tonic-clonic seizures *(36,37)*. A functional impairment of γ-aminobutyric acid (GABA)-ergic neurons has been implicated in SMS and also may be of pathogenetic significance in some forms of epilepsy. Autoantibodies directed against glutamic acid decarboxylase (GAD) are detected only in about 60% of patients with SMS and suggest that the pathogenesis of this disorder may be heterogeneous. The pathogenetic role of antibodies directed against GAD, as well as a 128-kDa antigen, is unclear as both proteins are intracytoplasmic antigens concentrated at synapses. In one report epilepsy occurred only in SMS patients who had autoantibodies in serum and CSF against GABA-ergic neurons *(36)*. The etiology of SMS is obscure, and three patient groups can be identified: (1) patients with circulating GAD antibodies, islet-cell and other organ-specific autoantibodies, and the frequent association with an autoimmmune disease (autoimmune variant); (2) patients with associated neoplasm and circulating non-organ-specific autoantibodies but with neither GAD nor islet-cell autoantibodies (paraneoplastic variant); and (3) patients with no evidence of any known autoantibody or association with other clinically evident diseases (idiopathic variant) *(38,39)*. The routine EEG in a patient with SMS and seizures showed rare, sometimes sharp bilateral theta waves, and photic stimulation provoked a generalized tonic-clonic seizure *(37)*. The course of SMS seems to be one of slow progression or stabilization. Preliminary reports indicate a favorable response to plasma exchange and corticosteroid therapy. The cornerstone of symptomatic treatment is with diazepam combined with physical therapy and rehabilitation.

Other Systemic Immunologic Diseases

A diverse spectrum of neurologic symptoms and signs has been described in association with giant cell arteritis. For the most part, they are a consequence of focal ischemic or inflammatory lesions in various parts of the CNS. Seizures have no particular association with this disorder.

Sjøgren's syndrome is a chronic systemic inflammatory disorder of unknown cause, characterized by dryness of the eyes, mouth, and other mucous membranes and often associated with rheumatic disorders sharing certain autoimmune features in which lymphocytes infiltrate mucosal and other tissues. Involvement of the CNS occurs in 25% of patients and characteristically is a multifocal, recurrent, and progressive disorder that results in cumulative impairment over time *(40–42)*. More subtle abnormalities of personality and cognition may occur. Histologic studies show several types of CNS inflammatory lesions suggesting an immunologically mediated autoimmune disorder. CNS manifestations are protean, and seizures are not an outstanding feature. Seizures are usually the complex partial type of temporal lobe origin; secondary generalized tonic-clonic convulsions, focal motor seizures, status epilepticus (SE), and epilepsia partialis continua have been observed less commonly. Only about 40% of Sjøgren's syndrome patients with active CNS disease have serologic markers characteristic of autoimmune rheumatologic disorders. There are no differences in the CNS manifestations of seropositive and seronegative Sjøgren's disease patients.

Rheumatoid arthritis (RA) is a chronic syndrome characterized by nonspecific, usually symmetric inflammation of the peripheral joints, potentially resulting in progressive destruction of articular and periarticular structures, with or without generalized manifestations. RA complicated by vasculitis or rheumatoid nodules in the brain is rare. The prevalence of CNS involvement is unknown because no prospective studies are available and most descriptions are based on findings observed at autopsy. The most common symptom is non-specific altered mental status. Seizures, cranial nerve dysfunction, and hemiparesis or paraparesis occur less commonly but with approximately equal frequency. A literature review found that seizures have been reported in about 20% of patients with CNS involvement in RA *(43–45)*. Cerebral vasculitis usually occurs in the context of diffuse systemic vasculitis and may present with seizures. Rheumatoid nodules have been identified in the dura of the brain and choroid plexus and are associated with seizures. Temporal lobe epilepsy was described in a woman with diffuse leptomeningeal infiltration by lymphocytes and plasma cells, vasculitis, and multiple leptomeningeal nodules that affected the temporal lobes predominantly *(46)*.

Systemic sclerosis (SS) is a chronic disease of unknown cause, characterized by diffuse fibrosis, degenerative changes, and vascular abnormalities in the skin (scleroderma), articular structures, and internal organs. In a report of 32 patients with SS, 3 suffered neuropsychiatric symptoms such as encephalopathy, psychosis, and anxiety disorder. Secondary generalized tonic-clonic and focal motor seizures also occurred. Primary CNS involvement was not confirmed, as patients suffered concurrent or systemic complications of SS or had features that overlapped with other connective tissue diseases. EEGs were normal or showed only mild, nonspecific changes *(47)*. Seizures can occur as a complication of systemic necrotizing vasculitis with involved cerebral vessels *(48)*. Epilepsy has been described as a complication of the facial form of linear scleroderma. In a previous report, band-like sclerosis of the leptomeninges and associated vessels was found, with calcified and anomalous vessels in the adjacent brain parenchyma *(49)*.

Mitochondrial Disorders

Defects in mitochondrial DNA (mtDNA), a circular molecule of 16,569 base pairs that is exclusively maternally inherited, are associated with neurological disorders in man. The most striking feature of these disorders is their marked heterogeneity, which extends to their clinical, biochemical, and genetic characteristics. All of these disorders involve, at some level, a mitochondrial respiratory chain dysfunction. The relationship among mtDNA mutations, impairment of oxidative phosphorylation, and clinical phenotype remains poorly understood. Advances in the molecular analysis of mitochondrial diseases promise a rational genetic classification for this heterogeneous group of diseases.

MELAS

Mitochondrial encephalopathy, lactic acidosis, and stroke-like episodes (MELAS) is characterized by (1) stroke-like episodes (with computerized tomography [CT] or MRI evidence of focal brain abnormalities), (2) lactic acidosis, "ragged red fibers" on Gomori trichrome stain of muscle biopsy, or both, and, according to some studies, *(3)* focal or generalized seizures, dementia, recurrent headache and vomiting *(50–52)*. Biochemical studies of muscle have detected decreased activity of complex I and III, complex II and III, and complex IV. Most patients with typical MELAS have an A-to-G transition at nucleotide (nt) 3243 in the tRNA *(leu)* gene, and some patients have a T-to-C transition at nt 3271 in the same gene. Both mutations exhibit a heterogeneous phenotypic expression. A rare mutation also occurs at nt 3291 of the same gene. Maternal inheritance pattern is an important clinical clue. The pathogenic basis of the brain lesions and their unique distribution pattern is explained by a mitochondrial angiopathy of pial arterioles and small arteries up to 250 μm in diameter; this can occur less frequently but more severely in larger pial arteries, intracerebral arterioles, and small arteries. Stroke-like episodes are characterized by recurrent, mostly transient (recovery over days to weeks) focal deficits such as hemiparesis (may alternate), aphasia, hemianopsia, or cortical blindness. Episodic vomiting is a noticeable feature. Imaging studies show reversible focal abnormalities that may not correspond to vascular distribution. Seizures are focal or secondary generalized and include myoclonic seizures. Seizures may be followed by residual neurologic deficits that resolve partially or completely over weeks (53). Nonepileptic myoclonus does not occur. Occipital lobe seizures may occur in MELAS patients, as in myoclonic epilepsy with ragged red fibers (MERRF) patients (54). Occipital lobe seizures and elementary visual phenomena may be a presenting feature. Patients with MELAS have a history of photosensitivity and often have occipital lobe EEG abnormalities. At times, seizures become intractable, leading to epilepsia partialis continua or partial SE.

Myoclonic Epilepsy with Ragged Red Fibers

MERRF is characterized by myoclonus, seizures, cerebellar ataxia, and mitochondrial myopathy. Additional, less common signs include dementia, hearing loss, optic atrophy, peripheral neuropathy, and spasticity. Evidence for a maternal inheritance pattern is an important feature. Onset can be in childhood or in adult life, and the course can be slowly progressive or rapidly downhill (50,51). Biochemical studies of muscle have given inconsistent results, with defects reported of complex III (cytochrome b), complexes II and IV, complexes I and IV, complexes I, III, and IV, or complex IV (cytochrome c oxidase) alone. The mitochondrial mutation associated most commonly with MERRF is an A-to-G transition at nt 8344 in the tRNA (lys) gene of mtDNA. A second mutation at nt 8356 in the same gene has been described in two families (55). Tonic-clonic seizures are the most common variety and may be preceded by visual or somatosensory auras (54,56). Patients with MERRF may also present with occipital lobe seizures and elementary visual phenomena. Patients have a history of photosensitivity and often have occipital lobe EEG abnormalities, including slowing of background rhythm. Interictal epileptiform abnormalities include single or brief bursts of generalized, bilaterally synchronous epileptiform activity, irregular, atypical spike-and-wave bursts, multiple spike-and-wave or sharp-and-slow-wave discharges, or independent focal epileptiform abnormalities. Ictal recordings in patients with generalized seizures show a generalized ictal electrographic onset, either spontaneous or provoked by photic stimulation. The relationship between clinical myoclonus and EEG discharges is inconsistent. Spontaneous bilateral massive myoclonus is associated with generalized spike-and-wave discharges. Generalized atypical spike-and-wave discharges are markedly attenuated during NREM sleep. Arm myoclonus has been described associated with photically induced, synchronous, occipitally dominant spikes. Action and intention myoclonus, the more prominent and disabling form of myoclonus, has no clear correlation with observed EEG discharges. Seizures are usually easy to control. However, at times the epilepsy becomes intractable, leading to epilepsia partialis continua or partial SE.

Leigh Syndrome

The subacute necrotizing encephalomyelopathy, Leigh syndrome, is a progressive neurodegenerative disorder with onset usually in infancy or early childhood. Frequently encountered clinical signs include motor and/or intellectual retardation and regression, and signs of brainstem dysfunction such as respiratory abnormalities, nystagmus, and ophthalmoparesis. Other features include ataxia, dystonia, and optic atrophy. Typically, symptoms begin in the first months and progress to death within 2 years. The characteristic neuropathology consists of spongiform lesions, with vacuolation of the neuropil and relative preservation of neurons, associated with demyelination, gliosis, and capillary proliferation, distributed bilaterally and symmetrically especially in the brainstem. Leigh syndrome is genetically heterogeneous *(57,58)*. A universally accepted classification of Leigh syndrome, based on genetic and biochemical defects, does not exist. Biochemical studies have determined defects in all of the pyruvate dehydrogenase complex (PDHC) subunits, or of its activating enzyme pyruvate dehydrogenase phosphate. Respiratory chain enzyme defects include cytochrome *c* oxidase (complex IV), complex I, complex I and IV, complex II, and complex V (mtDNA adenosine triphosphatase [ATPase] 6). Point mutations of mtDNA descibed in this syndrome include T8993G, A8344G, T9176C, and mtDNA deletions. No consistent relationship has been detected between clinical phenotype and underlying biochemical or genetic defect. However, onset may be earlier and seizures more frequent in patients with PDHC deficiency and in those with the T8993G point mutation in the ATP synthase 6 gene. In a large study of 67 patients with Leigh syndrome, 32 suffered seizures *(59)*. The seizure types were not specified. Epilepsia partialis continua has also been reported. Epilepsy occurred when MRI of the head showed cortical lesions typically associated with congenital lactic acidosis.

Neuropathy, Ataxia, and Retinitis Pigmentosa

Neuropathy, Ataxia, and Retinitis pigmentosa (NARP) is a maternally inherited syndrome characterized by developmental delay, retinitis pigmentosa, dementia, seizures, ataxia, proximal neurogenic muscle weakness, and sensory neuropathy *(60)*. It is associated with a point mutation in the ATPase

6 gene at nt 8993. The mutation is heteroplasmic, and the clinical severity of the disease is dependent on the proportion of mutant mtDNA (61). Adults with this syndrome suffer generalized seizures. Infants suffer infantile spasms associated with hypsarrhythmia on the EEG. Tonic seizures with apneic spells also have been described. EEG abnormalities documented include spike-and-wave bursts on progressively abnormal, low-voltage background activity.

Kearns–Sayre Syndrome

This mitochondrial disease is characterized by progressive external oph-thalmoplegia, pigmentary degeneration of the retina with age of onset before 20 years, in addition to at least one of the following: heart block, cerebellar dysfunction, or CSF protein concentration >100 mg% (52). Deafness, myopathy, diabetes mellitus, and dementia can occur. The disease is almost invariably sporadic and is associated with large heteroplasmic mtDNA dele-tions. In a review of published cases, no patient had focal neurologic signs, episodic vomiting, cortical blindness, or myoclonus (62). Seizures occurred only in a few patients with concomitant hypoparathyroidism, and, therefore, are not a manifestation of uncomplicated CNS involvement by the mitochon-drial illness.

Reye's Syndrome

This syndrome of acute encephalopathy and fatty infiltration of the liver is associated with viral infections (e.g., influenza A or B, varicella virus), exoge-nous toxins (e.g., Aspergillus flavus aflatoxin), salicylates, and intrinsic meta-bolic defects. Patients with Reye's syndrome have defects of multiple mitochondrial enzymes, and an acute defect of protein translocation has been postulated but remains to be documented. Although the disease occurs pri-marily among children, histologically confirmed cases are described in adults. The reported incidence of seizures varies from 33% to 100% in different series (63,64). Seizures are uncommon in stage I disease (lethargy). In stage II (stupor), generalized seizures may develop and are usually brief and limited in number. SE is rare. In stage III (coma), convulsions occur in 33–50% of patients and can be generalized, focal, multifocal, or myoclonic in type. In infants <1 yr old, the prodromal illness may be followed suddenly by repeti-tive seizures progressing to coma. Seizures should not be confused with the intermittent extensor posturing of stage IV disease. The incidence of neuro-logic sequelae, including epilepsy, is as high as 30% in patients who devel-oped convulsions and extensor posturing during the acute phase of the illness. Residual epileptic syndromes include infantile spasms and the Lennox–Gastaut syndrome. However, even patients who suffered SE during the acute illness may recover well, and seizures per se do not appear to affect outcome.

A few case histories associate the use of the anticonvulsant valproic acid with Reye's syndrome in young children. This drug should not be used in children <2 yr of age because of a significant risk of severe hepatotoxicity. The dominant pathology is moderate to severe cerebral cytotoxic edema, with less vasogenic edema. Severe cases show cortical neuronal degeneration. Inflammation is absent. Viral particles or inclusion bodies are not seen, and the mitochondria appear normal.

Inherited Metabolic Disease

Acute Porphyria

Porphyrias are inherited metabolic disorders characterized by an impairment of heme synthesis. Acute attacks of hepatic porphyria often present with abdominal or psychiatric complaints, and neurologic manifestations include peripheral neuropathy and seizures. The nature of these attacks is identical, regardless of the specific type of porphyria. Furthermore, despite the different sites in the defects of heme biosynthesis in these disorders, during acute attacks all patients have marked overproduction and overexcretion of δ-aminolevulinic acid (ALA) *(65)*. Acute attacks of porphyria are precipitated by many medications (most commonly barbiturates, griseofulvin, hydantoins, meprobamate, oral contraceptives, sulfonamides), ethanol excess, low-calorie or low-carbohydrate diets, and stress (due to infections, other illnesses, surgical treatments, and psychological problems). Seizures affect up to 15% of patients. A recent population-based study of acute intermittent porphyria (AIP) in Sweden determined a lifetime prevalence of any seizures at 3.7%: 2.2% if only AIP-associated seizures were included, and 5.1% if only AIP-associated seizures in cases with manifest AIP were included *(66)*. These rates are lower than hospital-based studies in which there is a selection bias for more severe cases. Seizures generalized from onset are mainly tonic-clonic, but myoclonic and atypical absence seizures have also been observed. Partial seizures are less frequent. Convulsions usually occur during the acute attack but may be delayed for up to 28 days after crisis. Seizures during acute attacks may be caused by hyponatremia or hypomagnesemia. Seizures may also occur in otherwise asymptomatic porphyric patients in whom it may be impossible to determine whether they are the result of some other cause or are a manifestation of porphyria per se. Symptoms of porphyria rarely begin before puberty, but some children with idiopathic epilepsy have typical attacks of porphyria after receiving anticonvulsant therapy. Management is difficult because the usual drugs of choice for seizures (phenytoin, carbamazepine, valproic acid, most benzodiazepines, barbiturates) are contraindicated in acute porphyria *(67)*. During acute porphyric attacks complicated by seizures, therapy should be directed at the porphyria, avoiding anticonvulsants if possible and concentrating on conventional therapy, such as high carbohydrate intake and supportive measures. Hematin infusions may offer dramatic remissions. There is renewed interest in using bromide anticonvulsant treatment in porphyrics, and careful monitoring of serum levels may avert toxic effects. SE can be controlled with IV diazepam or paraldehyde per rectum. Maintenance antiepileptic drugs including barbiturates, phenytoin, carbamazepine, and ethosuximide should be avoided, given their likelihood of precipitating a crisis. Valproate and clonazepam have demonstrated in vitro porphyrogenicity that may predict attacks in humans *(68)*. Diazepam or magnesium sulfate appear safe but are not useful in the chronic treatment of epilepsy. Reports indicate seizure control with gabapentin or vigabatrin, which do not induce a porphyric crisis, as these drugs are not cytochrome P450 inducers *(69)*. The pathogenesis of the neurologic manifestations of acute porphyria remains unsettled, and the most likely hypotheses include direct CNS effects of ALA or porphobilinogen (PBG) or dysfunction due to a deficiency of heme in neural tissues.

Hematologic Diseases

Fat Embolism Syndrome

Subclinical systemic fat embolism probably occurs after almost all long-bone fractures, but the incidence of the clinically apparent syndrome has been reported in 1–5% of fracture patients *(70)*. The full syndrome develops 12–72 h after the injury and is manifested by respiratory distress, encephalopathy, cutaneous petechiae, and, less often, anemia, coagulopathy, fever, or urinary fat globules. Infrequently, encephalopathy (even coma) may occur in the absence of respiratory failure *(71)*. Generalized tonic-clonic seizures have been reported in as many as 25% of patients with systemic fat embolism; focal seizures are rare *(72,73)*. Seizures usually precede the onset of coma. Tests to identify this clinical entity include chest radiograph, arterial blood gas analysis, complete blood count, coagulation profile, and search for petechiae. Examination of urine, sputum, or CSF is neither sensitive nor specific enough to be of diagnostic help. The pathogenesis of the syndrome is controversial *(74)*. The mechanical theory proposes that intramedullary veins are damaged by trauma, allowing marrow fat to intravasate and embolize to the lungs and from there to the brain via the pulmonary capillary bed and arteriovenous shunts. The biochemical hypothesis suggests that fat emboli are composed of aggregated chylomicrons and very-low-density lipoproteins that coalesce within the vasculature after trauma, with the formation of fat globules. High intramedullary pressure is the main causative factor for fatty marrow release into the circulation during intramedullary nailing and hip and knee replacements. Prophylactic steroids have been shown to reduce the incidence of fat embolism in patients with long-bone fractures. The mainstay of treatment is respiratory support. Coma is the single most important factor that predicts a poor prognosis.

Dysbarism

Seizures are not a feature of decompression sickness when defined as a symptom complex that implicates a particular spinal cord region, if symptoms are characteristically progressive in nature, if symptoms begin after the diver surfaces, or if the diver's time at depth exceeds the maximum advised in diving tables *(75)*. Generalized tonic-clonic seizures occur in <10% of divers with a diagnosis of cerebral air embolism, defined as manifesting primarily cerebral symptoms. This occurs if there is breath-holding or panic on ascent, or if symptoms are already present on completion of the dive. The neurologic manifestations of altitude decompression occur through lack of attention to, or failure of, pressure suits or cabins beyond an altitude of 9300 m *(76,77)*. The incidence and severity of symptoms depend on the altitude attained, rate of ascent, duration at altitude, and frequency of repeated ascents within 24 h. A diffuse encephalopathy, with various degrees of altered levels of arousal, may be complicated by partial or generalized convulsions. Hyperbaric oxygen toxicity occurs during hyperbaric oxygen therapy (for anaerobic infections, X-ray therapy, hypoxic and ischemic conditions, and in the treatment of air embolism) and while breathing pure oxygen below a 7.5- to 9-m depth. Symptoms include syncope and generalized tonic-clonic convulsions. Oxygen syncope or convulsions may start beyond 2 atmospheric pressure (atm) of pure oxygen, but a considerable range of individual tolerance exists and a precise susceptibility curve cannot be drawn. An increased susceptibility to convulsions appears with elevated external temperature (>25°C), activity and exertion, poor health, acidosis, increased inhaled pCO_2, hyperthyroidism, water immersion, or continuous exposure. A decreased incidence of convulsions occurs with use of CNS depressants or sodium succinate, hypothermia, or intermittent exposure. The exact pathogenesis of hyperbaric oxygen toxicity is not known.

Thrombotic Thrombocytopenic Purpura

Thrombotic thrombocytopenic purpura (TTP) is characterized by microangiopathic hemolytic anemia, thrombocytopenia, neurological symptoms, renal failure, and fever. Pathologically, TTP shows widespread arteriolar and capillary thrombosis, which spares venules. Inflammation is absent. Nervous system involvement is the presenting feature in up to 60% of patients and eventually occurs in up to 90%. Fluctuating neurologic dysfunction is one of the most frequent presentations. EEGs can be normal in TTP, even with overt neurologic dysfunction. Seizures are the presenting manifestation in 12.5% and eventually occur in about 30% of patients with neurologic involvement *(78–81)*. Generalized seizures are most frequent. Seizures are usually attributed to vascular disease and metabolic derangement, including uremia, hyponatremia, and fever; some may follow cerebral hemorrhage. Seizures can also be a late sign and herald the onset of terminal coma. Fluctuating stupor in TTP is often ascribed to microvascular occlusive disease, but nonconvulsive SE (NCSE) is a treatable condition that can cause a similar picture *(82,83)*. TTP patients are at an increased risk for NCSE, as NCSE may follow generalized convulsions; severe medical illness with encephalopathy may increase the likelihood of NCSE. Probably about 10% of patients with TTP may have NCSE as a cause of, or associated with, their altered mental status. If patients have altered mental status it is prudent to perform an EEG to rule out NCSE before subjecting them to the laborious process of plasmapheresis. Early recognition and treatment may result in neurologic improvement.

Sickle Cell Disease

Neurological manifestations of sickle cell disease occur in up to 26% of patients *(84–86)*. Stroke develops in 5–17% of patients, and seizures occur in 12–16%. Seizures are mostly of the generalized type and less commonly are of the partial or complex partial type *(87)*. Patients with unprovoked seizures may have had cortical strokes and exhibit epileptiform foci on EEG. Such patients should be treated with anticonvulsant medication. Patients with stroke, particularly embolic and cortical thrombotic ones, are predisposed to seizures. The majority of epileptic sickle cell patients have non-focal CT or MRI studies but demonstrate focal EEG abnormalities. It is likely that sickle cell patients with renal failure are more predisposed to developing seizures. Meperidine, a narcotic analgesic preferred for crisis pain, may be associated with seizures in up to 7% of patients. Myoclonus is also a common side effect of meperidine but does not appear to be a seizure-related phenomenon. Meperidine-induced seizures are not associated with underlying structural brain lesions, such as stroke, and the EEG usually does not show interictal epilepliform activity. Therefore, a narcotic other than meperidine is preferred for crisis pain in patients with stroke or renal failure. A minority of patients may have idiopathic epilepsy, with a positive family history of seizures.

Infectious Disease

Whipple's Disease

Whipple's disease is a relapsing systemic illness characterized by migratory polyarthralgias, chronic diarrhea, and fever *(88)*. The pathogen, *Tropheryma whippelii,* is an intracytoplasmic Gram-negative bacillus. Although

5% of patients present with neurological manifestations, symptomatic CNS involvement eventually occurs in 6–43% *(89)*. Prompt diagnosis is imperative. If untreated, CNS disease may have a fulminant course and death occurs in 1 month. In a literature review of 84 patients with CNS Whipple's disease, 23% of patients had seizures and 25% developed myoclonus during the illness *(90)*. Other neurologic signs (with frequency) included cognitive change (71%), vertical supranuclear gaze palsy without or with a horizontal gaze palsy in 37.5% and 50%, respectively, altered level of consciousness (50%), psychiatric signs (44%), long tract signs (37%), hypothalamic manifestations (31%), cranial nerve abnormalities (25%), ataxia (20%), and oculomasticatory and facial myorhythmia (20%).

Diagnosis of CNS Whipple's disease is based on finding typical periodic acid–Schiff stain (PAS)-positive macrophages in the lamina propria, or typical PAS-positive macrophages with electron microscopic evidence of typical bacilli in extraintestinal sites; however, intestinal biopsy results are negative in 30% of patients, and the false-negative rate for any tissue is 11%. A polymerase chain reaction (PCR)-based approach may improve ability to diagnose CNS Whipple's disease antemortem *(91);* PCR of intestinal tissue, or brain tissue from an enhancing lesion seen on neuroimaging, is of value. PCR evaluation of CSF and other tissue fluid may turn out a less invasive option *(92)*. The brain histopathological hallmark is the presence of PAS-positive staining macrophages *(93)*. Extensive granulomatous inflammation is often seen in the hypothalamus, hippocampus, periaquaductal gray matter, thalamus, and putamen; less common sites are mesencephalon, rhinencephalon, and diencephalon. A large number of antibiotics have been used with variable efficacy *(90)*. Initial treatment of CNS Whipple's disease has been successful using parenteral procain penicillin (1.2 million U/d) plus streptomycin (1g/d) for 14 days. The third-generation cephalosporin, ceftriaxone (2g IV twice daily for 2 wk), is a preferred alternative to penicillin *(94,95)*. An effective alternative is 960 mg IV trimethoprim–sulfamethoxazole (TMP-SMX) twice daily for 2 wk. Follow-up treatment for 1 yr should consist of 960 mg oral TMP-SMX, twice daily, or 400 mg oral cefixime once daily. Treatment of the underlying disease may not prevent seizures, which may require anticonvulsant therapy in a suspension or elixir because malabsorption is a significant problem.

References

1. McCune WJ, Golbus J. Neuropsychiatric lupus. *Rheum Dis Clin North Am* 1988;14:149–167.
2. Janssen BA, Bruyn GAW. Nervous system involvement in systemic lupus erythematosis, including the antiphospholipid antibody syndrome. In: Aminoff MJ, Goetz CG (eds.), *Handbook of Clinical Neurology.* Amsterdam: Elsevier Science, 1998, vol 71, pp 35–58.

3. Kovacs JAJ, Urowitz MB, Gladman DD. Dilemmas in neuropsychiatric lupus. *Rheum Dis Clin North Am* 1993;19:795–814.
4. Herranz MT, Rivier G, Khamashta MA, Blaser KU, Hughes GRV. Association between antiphospholipid antibodies and epilepsy in patients with systemic lupus erythematosis. *Arthritis Rheum* 1994;37:568–571.
5. Bonfa E, Golombek SJ, Kaufman LD, Skelly S, Weissbach H, Brot N, Elkon KB. Association between lupus psychosis and anti-ribosomal-P antibodies. *New Engl J Med* 1987;317:265–271.
6. Golombek SJ, Graus F, Elkon KB. Autoantibodies in the cerebrospinal fluid of patients with systemic lupus erythematosus. *Arthritis Rheum* 1986;29:1090–1097.
7. Mevorach D, Elkon KB. Neuropsychiatric lupus: getting beyond the barrier of the brain. (editorial) *Lupus* 1996;5:173–174.
8. Toubi E, Khamashta MA, Panarra A, Hughes GRV. Association of antiphospholipid antibodies with central nervous system disease in systemic lupus erythmatosus. *Am J Med* 1995;99:397–401.
9. Hughes GRV. Anticardiolipin antibodies: risk factor for venous and arterial thrombosis. *Lancet* 1985;1:912.
10. Verrot D, San-Marco M, Dravet C, et al. Prevalence and signification of antinuclear and anticardiolipin antibodies in patients with epilepsy. *Am J Med* 1997;103:33–37.
11. Liou HH, Wang CR, Chen CJ, et al. Elevated levels of anticardiolipin antibodies and epilepsy in lupus patients. *Lupus* 1996;5:307–312.
12. Ford RG, Siekert RG. Central nervous system manifestations of periarteritis nodosa. *Neurology* 1965;15:114–122.
13. Moore PM, Fauci AS. Neurologic manifestations of systemic vasculitis. *Am J Med* 1981;71:517–524.
14. Tervaert JWC, Kallenberg C. Neurologic manifestations of systemic vasculitis. *Rheum Dis Clin North Am* 1993;19:913–940.
15. Drachman DD. Neurological complications of Wegener's granulomatosis. *Arch Neurol* 1963;8:145–155.
16. Fauci AS, Haynes BF, Katz P, Wolff SM. Wegener's granulomatosis: prospective clinical and therapeutic experience with 85 patients for 21 years. *Ann Intern Med* 1983;98:76–85.
17. Nishino H, Rubino FA, DeRemee RA, Swanson JW, Parisi JE. Neurological involvement in Wegener's granulomatosis: an analysis of 324 consecutive patients at the Mayo Clinic. *Ann Neurol* 1993;33:4–9.
18. Nishino H, Rubino FA, Parisi JE. The spectrum of neurologic involvement in Wegener's granulomatosis. *Neurology* 1993;43:1334–1337.
19. Kaklamani VG, Vaiopoulos G, Kaklamanis PG. Behcet's disease. *Semin Arthritis Rheum* 1998;27:197–217.
20. Goodin DS. Behcet's disease. In: Aminoff MJ, Goetz CG (eds.), *Handbook of Clinical Neurology.* Amsterdam: Elsevier Science, 1998, vol 71, pp 209–231.
21. Al-Dalaan AN, Al Balaa SR, El Ramahi K, et al. Behcet's disease in Saudi Arabia. *J Rheumatol* 1994;21:658–661.
22. Aron AM, Freemen JM, Carter S. The natural history of Sydenham's chorea: a review of the literature and long-term evaluation with emphasis on cardiac sequelae. *Am J Med* 1965;38:83–95.
23. Ch'ien LT, Economides AN, Lemmi H. Sydenham's chorea and seizures. *Arch Neurol* 1978;35:382–385.

24. Nausieda PA, Grossman BJ, Koller WC, Weiner WJ, Klawans HL. Sydenham's chorea: an update. *Neurology* 1980;30:331–334.
25. Krumholz A, Stern BJ. Neurological manifestations of sarcoidosis. In: Aminoff MJ, Goetz CG (eds.), *Handbook of Clinical Neurology.* Amsterdam: Elsevier Science, 1998, vol 71, pp 463–499.
26. Scott TF. Neurosarcoidosis: progress and clinical aspects. *Neurology* 1993;43:8–12.
27. Stern BJ, Krumholz A, Johns C, Scott P, Nissim J. Sarcoidosis and its neurological manifestations. *Arch Neurol* 1985;42:909–917.
28. Krumholz A, Stern B, Stern EG. Clinical implications of seizures in neurosarcoidosis. *Arch Neurol* 1991;48:842–844.
29. Pentland B, Mitchell JD, Cull RE, Ford MJ. Central nervous system sarcoidosis. *Q J Med New Series* 1985;220:457–465.
30. Delaney P. Seizures in sarcoidosis: a poor prognosis. *Ann Neurol* 1980;7:494.
31. Luke RA, Stern B, Krumholz A, Johns CJ. Neurosarcoidosis: the long-term clinical course. *Neurology* 1987;37:461–463.
32. Nishizaki T, Iwamoto F, Uesugi, Akimura T, Yamashita K, Ito H. Idiopathic cranial pachymeningoencephalitis focally affecting the parietal dura mater and adjacent brain parenchyma: case report. *Neurosurgery* 1997;40:840–843.
33. Lorish TR, Thorsteinsson G, Howard FM. Stiff-man syndrome updated. *Mayo Clin Proc* 1989;64:629–636.
34. McEvoy KM. Stiff-man syndrome. *Mayo Clin Proc* 1991;66:300–304.
35. Solimena M, Folli F, Denis-Donini S, et al. Autoantibodies to glutamic acid decarboxylase in a patient with stiff-man syndrome, epilepsy, and type I diabetes mellitus. *N Engl J Med* 1988;318:1012–1020.
36. Solimena M, Folli F, Aparisi R, Pozza G, DeCamilli P. Autoantibodies to GABA-ergic neurons and pancreatic beta cells in stiff-man syndrome. *N Engl J Med* 1990;322:1555–1560.
37. Martinelli P, Pazzaglia P, Montagna P, et al. Stiff-man syndrome associated with nocturnal myoclonus and epilepsy. *J Neurol Neurosurg Psychiatry* 1978;41:458–462.
38. Grimaldi LME, Martino G, Braghi S, et al. Heterogeneity of autoantibodies in stiff-man syndrome. *Ann Neurol* 1993;34:57–64.
39. Folli F, Solimena M, Cofiell R, et al. Autoantibodies to a 128-kd synaptic protein in three women with the stiff-man syndrome and breast cancer. *N Engl J Med* 1993;328:546–551.
40. Alexander EL, Provost TT, Stevens MB, Alexander GE. Neurologic complications of primary Sjøgren's syndrome. *Medicine* 1982;61:247–257.
41. Alexander E. Central nervous system disease in Sjøgren's syndrome: new insights into immunopathogenesis. *Rheum Dis Clin North Am* 1992;18:637–672.
42. Alexander EL. Neurologic disease in Sjøgren's syndrome: mononuclear inflammatory vasculopathy affecting central/peripheral nervous system and muscle. *Rheum Dis Clin North Am* 1993;19:869–908.
43. Bathon JM, Moreland LW, DiBartolomeo AG. Inflammatory central nervous system involvement in rheumatoid arthritis. *Semin Arthritis Rheum* 1989;18:258–266.
44. Gupta VP, Ehrlich GE. Organic brain syndrome in rheumatoid arthritis following corticosteroid withdrawal. *Arthritis Rheum* 1976;19:1333–1338.
45. Beck DO, Corbett JJ. Seizures due to central nervous system rheumatoid meningovasculitis. *Neurology* 1983;33:1058–1061.
46. Ouyang R, Mitchell DM, Rozdilsky B. Central nervous system involvement in rheumatoid disease. *Neurology* 1967;17:1099–1105.

47. Hietaharju A, Jååskelåinen S, Hietarinta M, Frey H. Central nervous system involvement and psychiatric manifestations in systemic sclerosis (sleroderma): clinical and neurophysiological evaluation. *Acta Neurol Scand* 1993;87:382–387.
48. Pathak R, Gabor AJ. Scleroderma and central nervous system vasculitis. *Stroke* 1991;22:410–413.
49. Chung MH, Sum J, Morrell MJ, Horoupian DS. Intracerebral involvement in scleroderma en coup de sabre : report of a case with neuropathologic findings. *Ann Neurol* 1995;37:679–681.
50. Pavlakis SG, Phillips PC, DiMauro S, DeVivo DC, Rowland LP. Mitochondrial myopathy, encephalopathy, lactic acidosis, and strokelike episodes: a distinctive clinical syndrome. *Ann Neurol* 1984;16:481–488.
51. DiMauro S, Moraes CT. Mitochondrial encephalomyopathies. *Arch Neurol* 1993; 50:1197–1208.
52. DiMauro S. Mitochondrial encephalomyopathies. In: Rosenberg RN, Prusiner SB, DiMauro S, Barchi RL, Kunkel LM (eds.), *The Molecular and Genetic Basis of Neurological Disease.* Boston, MA: Butterworth-Heineman, 1993, pp 665–694.
53. Ciafaloni E, Ricci E, Shanske S, et al. MELAS: Clinical features, biochemistry, and molecular genetics. *Ann Neurol* 1992;31:391–398.
54. Kuzniecky R. Symptomatic occipital lobe epilepsy. *Epilepsia* 1998;39(Suppl 4): 24–31.
55. Graeber MB, Müller U. Recent developments in the molecular genetics of mitochondrial disorders. *J Neurol Sci* 1998;153:251–263.
56. So N, Berkovic S, Andermann F, Kuzniecky R, Gendron D, Quesney LF. Myoclonic epilepsy and ragged red fibres (MERRF). Electrophysiological studies and comparison with other progressive myoclonic epilepsies. *Brain* 1989;112:1261–1276.
57. DiMauro S. Genetic heterogeneity in Leigh syndrome. *Ann Neurol* 1996;40:5–6.
58. Morris AAM, Leonard JV, Brown GK, et al. Deficiency of respiratory chain complex I is a common cause of Leigh disease. *Ann Neurol* 1996;40:25–30.
59. Rahman S, Blok RB, Dahl H-HM, et al. Leigh syndrome: clinical features and biochemical and DNA abnormalities. *Ann Neurol* 1996;39:343–351.
60. Holt IJ, Harding AE, Petty RKH, Morgan-Hughes JA. A new mitochondrial disease associated with mitochondrial DNA heteroplasmy. *Am J Hum Genet* 1990; 46:428–433.
61. Måkelå-Bengs P, Suomalainen A, Majander A, et al. Correlation between the clinical symptoms and the proportion of mitochondrial DNA carrying the 8993 point mutation in the NARP syndrome. *Ped Res* 1995;37:634–639.
62. Rowland LP, Hays AP, DiMauro S. Diverse clinical disorders associated with morphological abnormalities of mitochondria. In: Cerri C, Scarlato G (eds.), Mitochondrial pathology in muscle diseases. Padua: Piccin Editore, 1983, pp 141–158.
63. Huttenlocher PR, Trauner DA. Reye's syndrome. In: Vinken PJ, Bruyn GW (eds.), *Handbook of Clinical Neurology.* Amsterdam: North-Holland, 1977, vol 29, pp 331–344.
64. Davis LE, Woodfin BM. Reye's syndrome. In: Goetz CG, Aminoff MJ (eds.), *Handbook of Clinical Neurology.* Amsterdam: Elsevier Science, 1998, vol 70, pp 267–298.
65. Bonkowsky HL, Schady W. Neurologic manifestations of acute porphyria. *Semin Liver Dis* 1982;2:108–124.
66. Bylesjø I, Forsgren L, Lithner F, Boman K. Epidemiology and clinical characteristics of seizures in patients with acute intermittent porphyria. *Epilepsia* 1996; 37:230–235.

67. Reynolds NC, Miska RM. Safety of anticonvulsants in hepatic porphyrias. *Neurology* 1981;31:480–484.
68. Bonkowsky HL, Sinclair PR, Emery S, Sinclair JF. Seizure management in acute hepatic porphyria: risks of valproate and clonazepam. *Neurology* 1980;30:588–592.
69. Tatum WO, Zachariah SB. Gabapentin treatment of seizures in acute intermittent porphyria. *Neurology* 1995;45:1216–1217.
70. Thomas JE, Ayyar DR. Systemic fat embolism: a diagnostic profile in 24 patients. *Arch Neurol* 1972;26:517–523.
71. Jacobson DM, Terrence CF, Reinmuth OM. The neurologic manifestations of fat embolism. *Neurology* 1986;36:847–851.
72. Pell ACH, Hughes D, Keating J, Christie J, Busuttil A, Sutherland G. Brief report: fulminating fat embolism syndrome caused by paradoxical embolism through a patent foramen ovale. *N Engl J Med* 1993;329:926–929.
73. Scopa M, Magatti M, Rossitto P. Neurologic symptoms in fat embolism syndrome: case report. *Trauma* 1994;36:906–908.
74. Hofmann S, Huemer G, Salzer M. Pathophysiology and management of the fat embolism syndrome. *Anaesthesia* 1998;53(Suppl 2):35–37.
75. Dick APK, Massey EW. Neurologic presentation of decompression sickness and air embolism in sport divers. *Neurology* 1985;35:667–671.
76. Aita JA. Neurologic manifestations of dysbarism. In: Vincken PJ, Bruyn GW (eds.), *Handbook of Clinical Neurology.* Amsterdam: North-Holland, 1972, vol 12, pp 665–676.
77. Gillen HW. Air embolism. In: Vinken PJ, Bruyn GW (eds.), *Handbook of Clinical Neurology.* Amsterdam: North-Holland, 1975, vol 23, pp 609–629.
78. O'Brien JL, Sibley WA. Neurologic manifestations of thrombotic thrombocytopenic purpura. *Neurology* 1958;8:55–64.
79. Amorosi EL, Ultmann JE. Thrombotic thrombocytopenic purpura: report of 16 cases and review of the literature. *Medicine* 1966;45:139–159.
80. Silverstein A. Thrombotic thrombocytopenic purpura. The initial neurologic manifestations. *Arch Neurol* 1968;18:358–362.
81. Ridolfi RL, Bell WR. Thrombotic thrombocytopenic purpura. Report of 25 cases and review of the literature. *Medicine* 1981;60:413–428.
82. Garrett WT, Chang CWJ, Bleck TP. Altered mental status in thrombotic thrombocytopenic purpura is secondary to nonconvulsive status epilepticus. *Arch Neurol* 1996;40:245–246.
83. Blum AS, Drislane FW. Nonconvulsive status epilepticus in thrombotic thrombocytopenic purpura. *Neurology* 1996;47:1079–1081.
84. Greer M, Schotland D. Abnormal hemoglobin as a cause of neurologic disease. *Neurology* 1962;12:114–123.
85. Portnoy BA, Herion JC. Neurologic manifestations in sickle cell disease. *Ann Internal Med* 1972;76:643–652.
86. Fabian RH, Peters BH. Neurologic complications of hemoglobin SC disease. *Ann Neurol* 1984;41:289–292.
87. Liu JE, Gzech DJ, Ballas SK. The spectrum of epilepsy in sickle cell anemia. *J Neurol Sci* 1994;123:6–10.
88. Ramaiah C, Boynton RF. Whipple's disease. *Gastroenterol Clin North Am* 1998;27:683–695.
89. Riggs JE, Schochet SS. Neurological dysfunction in Whipple disease. In: Goetz CG, Aminoff MJ (eds.), *Handbook of Clinical Neurology.* Amsterdam: Elsevier Science, 1998, vol 70, pp 239–248.

90. Louis ED, Lynch T, Kaufmann P, Fahn S, Odel J. Diagnostic guidelines in central nervous system Whipple's disease. *Ann Neurol* 1996;40:561–568.
91. Lynch T, Odel J, Fredericks DN, et al. Polymerase chain reaction-based detection of *Tropheryma whippelii* in central nervous system Whipple's disease. *Ann Neurol* 1997;42:120–124.
92. Delanty N, Georgescu L, Lynch T, Paget S, Stübgen J-P. Synovial fluid polymerase chain reaction as an aid to the diagnosis of central nervous system Whipple's disease. *Ann Neurol* 1999;45:137–138.
93. Knox DL, Green WR, Troncoso JC, Yardley JH, Hsu J, Zee DS. Cerebral ocular Whipple's disease: a 62-year odyssey from death to diagnosis. *Neurology* 1995; 45:617–625.
94. Schnider PJ, Reisiger EC, Gerschlager W. Long-term follow-up in cerebral Whipple's disease. *Eur J Gastroenterol Hepatol* 1996;8:899–903.
95. Schnider PJ, Reisinger EC, Berger T, Krejs GJ, Auff E. Treatment guidelines in central nervous system Whipple's disease. *Ann Neurol* 1997;41:561–562.

5

Seizures and Organ Failure

Jane Boggs, MD

Introduction

Seizures and epilepsy commonly occur in patients with organ system failure, either as a consequence of trophic effects on cerebral function or of therapies used in such conditions. Acute organ failure results in an abrupt, but often reversible, lowering of seizure threshold, whereas chronic organ failure results in more pervasive and indolent cerebral compromise, often permanently altering both the seizure threshold and the physiologic responses to antiepileptic drugs (AEDs). Failure of an organ system is not typically a sudden, all-or-none phenomenon but occurs in stages with variable susceptibility to seizures as the condition worsens or remits. Although the principles of diagnosis and management of seizures in adult and pediatric patients with a specific organ dysfunction are similar, the underlying etiologies and influences of comorbid conditions differ between adults and children. Adult organ failure often involves multiple systems to different extents and is superimposed on other chronic diseases of adulthood. Pediatric organ failure is usually the result of inherited metabolic disorders, infections, and unique pediatric susceptibilities to metabolic effects of medications (**Table 1**).

This chapter will address seizures occurring in patients with acute and chronic failure of the liver, kidneys, gastrointestinal tract, hematologic, endocrine, and immunologic systems. Seizures in the settings of cardiac, respiratory, and primary neurologic failures are discussed in Chapters 3, 4, 14, 19, 20, and 21.

Hepatic Failure and Seizures

Massive hepatic necrosis occurring within 8 weeks of onset of illness, or acute hepatic failure, is most commonly caused by acute infection or inflammation of the liver or pancreas, acute hypotension, toxin exposure, or

From: *Seizures: Medical Causes and Management*
Edited by: N. Delanty © Humana Press, Inc., Totowa, NJ

Table 1
**Typical Organ Failure Syndromes Associated with Seizures
in Adults and Children**

Organ System	Adult Diseases	Pediatric Diseases
Cardiovascular (CV)	Atherosclerotic CV disease, postcardiac arrest, arrhythmias, congestive heart failure, cardiomyopathy, myxoma, subacute bacterial endocarditis, transplantation	Congenital defects, cardiomyopathy, transplantation
Respiratory	Anoxic–hypoxic insults, chronic obstructive pulmonary disease, asthma, carcinoma	Anoxic–hypoxic insults, asthma, cystic fibrosis
Hepatic	Hepatitis, cirrhosis, acute hypotension, Wilson's, porphyria, toxins, transplantation, carcinoma	Hepatitis, Reye's, toxins, transplantation
Renal	Acute interstitial nephritis, nephrotic syndrome, acute tubular necrosis, chronic renal insufficiency, dialysis, carcinoma	Congenital defects, toxins, dialysis
Gastrointestinal	Esophageal stricture, gastro-esophageal reflux, dumping syndrome, ileus, inflammatory bowel disease, Whipple's, celiac disease, gastric surgery	Pyloric stenosis, congenital defects, inflammatory bowel disease, celiac disease
Hematologic	Sickle cell anemia, HbSC, polycythemia, paraproteinemias, hyperleukocytosis, factor VIII deficiency, factor IX deficiency, drugs and toxins, DIC, anticardiolipin antibodies, TTP, essential thrombocythemia	Hemorrhagic disease of the newborn, sickle cell anemia, HbSC, polycythemia, paraproteinemias, hyperleukocytosis, factor VIII deficiency, factor IX deficiency, drugs and toxins, DIC, anticardiolipin antibodies
Endocrine	Hypothyroidism, diabetes mellitus, hypopituitarism, hypoparathyroidism, adrenal failure	Congenital hypothyroidism, hypothalamic hamartomas, hypopituitarism, adrenal failure
Immunologic	Radiation, chemotherapy, aplastic anemia, neutropenia, HIV	Radiation, chemotherapy, aplastic anemia, neutropenia, HIV

fulminant primary liver disease. These conditions are associated with changes in glucose metabolism, ammonia production, and the ability of the liver to remove metabolites and toxins from the circulation. Progressive encephalopathy results, which is typically associated with cerebral edema, jaundice, coagulopathy, and other organ system failure. The combination of these effects can produce seizures by directly or indirectly precipitating neurologic complications. Chronic hepatic failure is characterized by progressive inflammatory reaction of the liver for at least 6 mo.

The biochemical mechanisms of hepatic encephalopathy are controversial, and have been hypothesized to result from enhanced GABA effects *(1)*, hyperammonemia *(2)*, abnormal glutamine metabolism *(3)*, and the contribution of false neurotransmitters *(4)*, although there is inconclusive evidence in humans of a dominant pathogenic process. The incidence of seizures in hepatic encephalopathies varies from 2–33% in the literature *(5)*.

The degree of alteration of consciousness varies with the severity of hepatic encephalopathy. Bickford and Butt *(6)* have described three classical phases of EEG change with worsening hepatic coma, often correlating with increasing arterial ammonia. The first stage is a diffuse theta pattern, followed by a second stage with surface-positive, often sharp or spike morphology triphasic waveforms. Although it is during this stage that most seizures occur, clinically obvious seizures are not common in hepatic encephalopathy and occur much less frequently than in renal disease. Differentiation of ictal patterns from rhythmic epochs of triphasic waves, however, can be quite difficult. Disappearance of triphasic waves with the onset of sleep patterns may be helpful in determining that the EEG is nonictal. Administration of short-acting benzodiazepines intravenously can eliminate the triphasic waves and show improvement of the background to faster theta, indicating that the medication has treated an ictal pattern. Caution must be exercised with such an interpretation, as benzodiazepines lower the amplitude of paroxysmal nonictal patterns as well as elicit beta patterns obscuring the background. The final stage of hepatic encephalopathy shows arrhythmic delta with poor bilateral synchrony. Convulsive seizures are unusual in this stage, but potentially ictal patterns may be found in up to 25% of comatose patients' EEGs *(7)*. Asterixis can produce a rhythmic artifact on the EEG, requiring careful documentation by the technologist or application of accelerometers to avoid misinterpretation of these clinical movements as seizures.

Wilson's disease, or hepatolenticular degeneration, is a rare, autosomal recessive disease of copper metabolism. Associated liver disease varies from cirrhosis to fulminant hepatic necrosis. Neurologic manifestations can predominate, usually in cases presenting late in the second decade. Seizures occur infrequently, although unusual movement disorders occur that may require investigation by EEG.

Reye's syndrome is almost exclusively a disorder of children associated with aspirin exposure in the context of a flu-like illness. The condition is associated with rapid neurologic deterioration culminating in convulsions and coma, typically correlating with marked progressive elevations of liver transaminases and hyperammonemia.

The hepatic porphyrias pose unique clinical problems to the neurologist. Acute intermittent porphyria, variegate porphyria, and hereditary coproporphyria result from differing enzymatic deficiencies in heme synthesis, but all have similar neurologic manifestations. Acute exacerbations, which can be triggered by use of phenytoin, barbiturates, and meprobamate, among other drugs, result in seizures or bizarre behavioral abnormalities, autonomic dysfunction, aphasia, and hemiparesis, which can mimic seizures. Management of seizures in pophyrics requires supportive treatment of the underlying disease, avoidance of precipitants, and use of AEDs that are unlikely to provoke exacerbations (e.g., gabapentin, topiramate).

Many factors can contribute to altered AED metabolism in liver failure. Cirrhosis results in overall, progressive loss of total hepatic blood flow, hepatocellular mass, and hepatocyte function. Acute viral and alcoholic hepatitis can result in increased total hepatic blood flow in some patients or result in overall impairment of hepatocyte function. When infectious disorders become chronic, hepatocellular mass may increase, or in alcoholic hepatitis, increase or decrease. Hypoalbuminemia and altered binding of drugs to plasma proteins contribute to the increased appearance of AED toxicity at lower than expected drug levels *(8)*.

Renal Failure and Seizures

Acute renal failure is characterized by a rapid decline in the glomerular filtration rate, often a consequence of acute medication toxicities precipitating acute interstitial nephritis and acute tubular necrosis. Oliguria and extracellular fluid accumulation produce edema, hypertension, and congestive heart failure. Associated electrolyte abnormalities include hyperkalemia, hyponatremia, acidosis, and secondary hyperparathyroidism. All of these primary and secondary effects of acute renal failure can contribute to the development of uremic encephalopathy and seizures.

The clinical neurologic features of uremic encephalopathy typically relate more to the rate of development of renal failure rather than to the degree of laboratory abnormality. Chronic renal failure may be associated with greater degrees of azotemia than acute renal failure, but it has more insidious neurologic manifestations. Such progressive, permanent loss of renal function does not typically cause uremic symptoms until the glomerular filtration rate has declined to 25% of normal. In one study, seizures were reported in 5 of 13 patients with acute renal failure, typically occurring between the eighth and eleventh day of illness and were frequently multiple *(9)*. Seizures in chronic renal failure usually are a late manifestation and occur in approx. 10% of patients *(10)*.

Uremic encephalopathy, as in other metabolic encephalopathies, is accompanied by declining cerebral utilization of oxygen with concomitant reduction of glycolysis and energy utilization *(11)*. Organic acids share a common transport mechanism between the proximal renal tubule and the choroid plexus. These neurotoxins, which are usually excluded from the brain due to poor lipid solubility and plasma protein binding, gain entry to the brain in uremia and have been found to elicit convulsions and myoclonus in animal models *(12)*.

The EEG in uremic encephalopathy often shows nonspecific patterns seen in other metabolic encephalopathies, typified by large amounts of theta and delta frequencies indicative of overall impaired cerebral metabolism. Such patterns, as in hepatic disease, can become rhythmic and must be distinguished from ictal abnormalities. Bilateral spike-and-wave patterns have been reported in 8–9% of patients on chronic hemodialysis, with no known occurrence of seizure *(13)*.

Seizures also occur in hemodialysis as part of the dysequilibrium syndrome, typically toward the end of a dialysis session and up to 24 h later. The name of this syndrome originated with the incorrect idea that blood urea falls more rapidly than brain urea, resulting in an osmotic dysequilibrium. It is more plausible that production of idiogenic osmoles, or unidentified osmotically active solids, causes abrupt shift of water into brain tissue *(14)*. Chronic ambulatory peritoneal dialysis (CAPD) is rarely associated with seizures.

AED pharmacokinetics can be altered significantly in uremia, resulting in difficulties in treating such patients who develop seizures. The volume of distribution of drugs is increased, resulting in lower total plasma levels. Higher unbound AED levels, however, owing to decreased protein binding in renal failure, result in a greater AED effect in the CNS. Newer AEDs with a significant proportion of renal elimination (gabapentin, topiramate, oxcarbazepine) require lower doses in renal failure because of slower clearance. Such medications may be highly dialyzable, however, increasing the risk of acute withdrawal seizures if dosing is inappropriately timed relative to dialysis. Anticonvulsants that have been associated with minimally increased risk for renal stone formation (topiramate, zonisamide, acetozolamide) should be used with caution when the etiology of acute renal failure is undiagnosed.

Gastrointestinal Tract Failure and Seizures

The gastrointestinal (GI) tract extends from the oropharynx to the anus, and acute failure of this system can be the result of obstruction, dysmotility, or malabsorption. Although such disorders do not primarily cause seizures, the complications of dehydration, electrolyte disruptions, and nutritional deficiencies can lower the seizure threshold. In addition, treatment of patients with pre-existing or new-onset seizures can be difficult by limiting AEDs to those available in parenteral or mucosally absorbed formulations.

Acute upper GI failure typically is the result of esophageal obstruction or dysmotility. Large AED pills (e.g., divalproex sodium, felbamate) may worsen obstructions and should be avoided; liquid, chewable, opened capsules or sprinkle preparations are preferable if appropriate pharmacokinetic adjustments are made in dosing. Slowed gastric motility may be drug induced or may occur subsequent to a surgical procedure and requires avoidance of any enteral preparations. Only AEDs appropriate for parenteral administration (e.g., phenytoin/fosphenytoin, phenobarbital, valproic acid, benzodiazepines), or those with efficient absorption on mucosal surfaces (rectal or sublingual), should be used until normal GI function resumes.

Patients who have had gastric resection, diversion, or plication rarely develop seizures. Those patients requiring treatment for pre-existing epilepsy, of course, will be unable to utilize AEDs, which are highly absorbed in the stomach. Most delayed-release, enteric, coated, or sprinkle formulations have at least some absorption in more distal regions of the GI tract and are easier to use, if parenteral agents are impractical. AEDs primarily absorbed in the stomach can still be used successfully, however, if interdose intervals are significantly shortened.

Inflammatory diseases of the GI tract may be associated with diffuse inflammatory processes that can result in encephalopathy and seizures. Whipple's disease is a multisystem disorder with diagnostic inflammatory changes found on jejunal biopsy. Similar pathology can be found in the 10% of patients with neurologic manifestations, including seizures *(15)*. The relationship of celiac disease to increased incidence of seizures is controversial *(16,17)*, but some case reports have identified associated cerebral vasculitis, with seizures *(18)*. Inflammatory bowel disease (Crohn's disease and ulcerative colitis) may be associated with an increased risk for seizures due to vascular events, dehydration, or infection *(19)*.

Hematologic Failure and Seizures

Abnormalities of cellular, platelet, or clotting function, as well as altered rheological blood properties, can result in CNS hemorrhage or hypoperfusion. Any focal or generalized disturbance of brain perfusion can result in seizures. Seizures accompany up to 12.5–20% of acute strokes and are associated most commonly with etiologies causing acute subarachnoid or cerebral hemorrhage, or cortical emboli.

EEGs in patients with localization-related seizures caused by acute hematologic events may show focal slowing, especially persistent interictal delta waves. Periodic lateralized epileptiform discharges (PLEDs) are commonly encountered in patients with these events and are frequently associated with seizures. Controversy exists regarding whether PLEDs themselves consistently represent an ictal pattern and whether they should be treated in all cases with AEDs.

Seizures are the second most common neurologic complication of patients with sickle cell anemia, usually caused by vaso-occlusive events from the sickling of cells in acute crises *(20)*. Sickle cell trait is rarely associated with seizures, although HbSC (sickle-C) disease may have an increased incidence of seizures and other CNS complications relative to controls *(21)*.

Hyperviscosity syndromes, including polycythemia vera, Gaisbock's syndrome (pseudopolycythemia), paraproteinemias (e.g. Waldenstrom's macroglobulinemia, multiple myeloma), and hyperleukocytosis can increase the risk for cerebral thrombosis and resultant seizures. Abnormal thrombosis in these disorders can also increase risk for hemorrhagic transformation of lesions or disseminated intravascular coagulopathy (DIC), which also lowers the threshold for focal seizures.

Intracranial bleeding is the leading cause of death in factor VIII and factor IX deficiency, and seizures occur in 25% of survivors of those with intracranial hemorrhage (ICH) *(22)*. The risk for ICH in von Willebrand's disease, in contrast, is relatively low, occurring most commonly in the setting of head trauma. Iatrogenic thrombolysis or anticoagulation is also a well-known cause of ICH. Lupus anticoagulants and anticardiolipin antibodies prolong the partial thromboplastin time (PTT) and have been associated with a variety of neurologic conditions, including seizures *(23)*.

Hemorrhagic disease of the newborn is most commonly associated with prematurity and breech delivery, especially in the setting of maternal AED use, which iatrogenically interfere with vitamin K-dependent clotting factors. Uncontrolled hemolysis may result, with tearing of the bridging veins likely caused by molding of the head as it passes through the birth canal. Prenatal vitamin K supplementation of the mother and sometimes perinatal supplementation of the neonate are recommended.

Thrombotic thrombocytopenic purpura (TTP) may present with neurologic manifestations in up to 60% of cases but more commonly manifest as headache and confusion rather than seizures or focal abnormalities *(24)*. DIC, which may be precipitated by cerebral injury, is characterized by fibrin thrombi in small vessels and hemorrhagic lesions. Both of these diseases can result in ICH as a cause of seizures.

Essential thrombocythemia is a myeloproliferative disorder causing massive increases in platelet production. This disorder has a high incidence of embolic transient ischemic attacks and cerebral infarcts. The former can mimic seizures, and the latter can cause them.

Endocrine Failure and Seizures

Thyroid Failure

Chronic hypothyroidism, which may be the result of thyroid failure (primary hypothyroidism) or pituitary or hypothalamic disease (secondary hypothyroidism) may lead to acute thyroid failure and myxedema coma. The latter may be precipitated by cold exposure, trauma, infection, and certain drugs (e.g., narcotics, lithium). Decreased serum T_4 is common to all hypothyroidism, but serum thyroid-stimulating hormone (TSH) is increased in primary, while either normal or decreased in secondary, hypothyroidism.

Hypothyroid encephalopathy may include symptoms caused by dementia, depression, and other psychiatric diseases, and severe untreated myxedema can manifest as florid psychiatric symptoms or coma. Asher described myxedema madness as irritability, paranoia, hallucinations, delirium, and psychosis *(25),* which has been found to be exquisitely sensitive to treatment with triiodothyronine *(26).*

Both seizures and syncope may occur at a high incidence in untreated hypothyroid patients *(27).* As these reactive seizures typically respond to hormonal treatments, chronic anticonvulsants are infrequently required, and may be unwise, as the recurrence of seizure may be a useful harbinger of impending hypothyroid crisis. A prolonged postictal state, however, is not unusual and must be distinguished from ongoing nonconvulsive seizure activity by EEG.

The EEG typically is slow with impaired photic driving *(28).* Severe hypothyroidism can result in overall attenuation or lessened modulation of alpha rhythm *(29),* although generalized periodic complexes have been reported *(30).* Infants with severe myxedema may have slow, low-voltage patterns, as well as delayed maturation, especially of sleep spindles *(31).* Low-voltage patterns may evolve through more obviously interictal or ictal patterns with thyroid repletion and typically normalize even before the encephalopathy and thyroid profiles. Thus, serial EEGs can provide useful prognostic information during treatment of hypothyroidism.

Although phenytoin and carbamazepine have been found to alter thyroid levels, healthy patients usually remain clinically euthyroid *(32).* As increased peripheral metabolism of thyroid hormones occurs in patients treated with carbamazepine, increased doses of thyroxine may be needed in hypothyroid patients who have no other option for their AED therapy *(33).*

Diabetes Mellitus

CNS complications of diabetes mellitus increase with the severity and chronicity of disease. Most seizures result from severe metabolic abnormalities associated with nonketotic hyperosmolar hyperglycemia (NHH), diabetic ketoacidosis (DKA), hypoglycemia, or from an increase in cerebrovascular disease affecting diabetics.

Six percent of NHH patients present with focal motor seizures, and 25% of NHH patients eventually develop seizures *(34).* Seizures in NHH occur early in hyperglycemia, and osmolality is increased only modestly, with minimally decreased sodium levels, and usually when consciousness is preserved *(35).*

Neuroimaging of these patients reveals that some are not due to structural abnormalities but were caused solely by metabolic dysfunction. In contrast, seizures are rare in DKA, although altered mental status is seen frequently. Such a clinically ambiguous neurologic state, of course, can mimic or mask seizures and mandates performance of an EEG during the symptomatic interval. Hypoglycemia induces generalized seizures in up to 20% of adults and more frequently in children *(36)*. These occur commonly at night, as nocturnal hypoglycemia is common in diabetics.

The EEG is more responsive to acute hypoglycemia than hyperglycemia. Generalized seizures with high-voltage spike activity, as well as focal discharges, can be seen in metabolic disorders causing acute hypoglycemia such as insulinomas *(37)*. In severe hyperglycemia, pronounced slowing is typical, although focal abnormalities can be seen. Exaggerated responses to hyperventilation and accentuation of underlying interictal patterns can be seen during hypoglycemia.

As diabetes affects multiple organs systems, the use of AEDs in this disease must take the effects of altered renal, hepatic, GI, and vascular function into consideration. Insulin secretion may be decreased in some diabetics treated with phenytoin, although the majority of patients receiving long-term phenytoin therapy maintain normal carbohydrate metabolism *(38)*.

Pituitary Failure

Failure of the posterior pituitary occasionally can result in seizures through disorders affecting water balance, such as diabetes insipidus or as part of panhypopituitarism caused by tumors, primary hypoplasia, and pituitary apoplexy. Hypothalamic hamartomas result in pituitary dysfunction and characteristically present with seizures in infancy. Gelastic (pathologic laughter) seizures, in particular, are associated with these tumors. Extension of pituitary adenomas laterally can deform the uncinate gyrus, resulting in temporal lobe seizures *(39)*.

Parathyroid Failure

Hypoparathyroidism is characterized by hypocalcemia, which results in excitability of neuronal membranes and seizures. Seizures may occur at any age, usually precede the clinical appearance of tetany, and are usually generalized tonic-clonic, although partial seizures have been reported *(40)*. Children may manifest congenital hypoparathyroidism, which occurs in DiGeorge syndrome, Hallermann–Strieff syndrome, 10p deletion syndrome, familial nephrosis with nerve deafness, and a syndrome of growth failure and mental retardation *(41)*. EEGs may show irregular high-voltage delta rhythm increased by hyperventilation, as well as paroxysmal abnormalities *(42)*.

Adrenal Failure

Adrenal failure may be primary or result secondarily from pituitary failure or withdrawal from exogenous corticosteroids. Chronic adrenal failure is often associated with psychiatric symptoms, and although the EEG commonly appears encephalopathic, seizures are uncommon. If concomitant electrolyte disturbances are uncorrected, however, seizures may be intractable to steroid replacement. Although ACTH and steroids have been used to treat infantile spasms and other childhood epileptic syndromes, it is likely that these agents exert their antiseizure effects centrally, rather than by modulation of adrenal cortical function. AEDs that induce hepatic enzymes can increase clearance of corticosteroids and may lessen the response to exogenous steroids in patients with adrenal failure.

Immunologic Failure and Seizures

Acute immunologic failure may be seen in the setting of therapeutic or toxic ionizing radiation and chemotherapy for various diseases. There may be difficulty distinguishing whether subsequent seizures result from the underlying disease process or one of these treatments. Acute and chronic immuno-compromise can also result in seizures from opportunistic infections and medications used in HIV and post-transplant patients. These latter two situations will be addressed in Chapters 5 and 8.

Acute encephalopathy from radiation usually follows initial cranial irradiation and is less likely to occur with ensuing doses. Typical symptoms are of increased intracranial pressure, which can diminish with concomitant steroids. Early delayed encephalopathy typically occurs 2–3 mo after irradiation and is believed to be related to demyelination, with clinical manifestations suggested by the descriptor radiation somnolence syndrome *(43)*. The EEG is slow, and focal neurologic signs, including seizures, are uncommon in the absence of other clinical factors. Late delayed radiation necrosis may begin as long as 2 yr after completing radiation. Imaging reveals abnormalities affecting large focal areas near the original tumor, especially of the white matter. Symptoms mimic those of tumor recurrence, including seizures. In severe cases, the EEG reveals prominent slowing, high-voltage spikes, and electroclinical seizures.

Leukopenia is defined as a total leukocyte count of $<4300/\mu L$, with neutropenia as an absolute neutrophil count of $<2500/\mu L$ (although there is usually no significant increased risk in bacterial infection unless $<1000/\mu L$). These disorders may predispose patients to seizures by allowing opportunistic infections of the nervous system to occur. In patients with a history of aplastic anemia or clinically significant leukopenia, avoidance of any medications, including AEDs, with a high reported incidence of these idiosyncratic reactions is prudent. The AED associated most commonly with aplastic anemia is felbamate (27/100,000). Transient leukopenia occurs in 10–20% of carbamazepine-treated patients, is persistent in only 2% *(44),* and is unrelated to more serious reactions. Carbamazepine has been observed to result in aplastic anemia in only 2/575,000, or 0.34/100,00 patients *(45).* Occurrence of aplastic anemia has been described with all older generation AEDs and has no yet known association with the AEDs marketed since felbamate.

Summary

Seizures or epilepsy coexist with failure of every organ system discussed, as well as in cardiac and respiratory failure **(Table 1).** With progressive clinical involvement of each organ system, the likelihood that other systems will also fail increases. Thus, initial organ failure must be treated aggressively to avert the more difficult situation of managing seizures in multisystem failure. Neurologists must not only work closely with internal medicine specialists but must also be acutely aware of the interaction of seizures and non-neurologic disease. Because of the complexity of managing such patients, it is inappropriate for neurologists to be unknowledgeable about these medical conditions, and they must also fully involve themselves with the critical care team.

References

1. Lockwood AH. Hepatic encephalopathy: experimental approaches to human metabolic encephalopathy. *CRC Crit Rev Neurobiol* 1987;3:105–133.
2. Gabuzda GJ. Ammonium metabolism and hepatic coma. *Gastroenterology* 1967;53:806–810.
3. Duffy TE, Vergara F, and Plum R. Alpha-ketoglutarate in hepatic encephalopathy. In: Plum F (ed.), *Brain Dysfunction in Metabolic Disorders,* New York: Raven, 1974, pp 339–352.
4. Fischer JE. False neurotransmitters and hepatic coma. In: Plum F (ed.), *Brain Dysfunction in Metabolic Disorders,* New York: Raven, 1974, pp 353–373.
5. Plum F, Posner JB. (eds.) *Diagnosis of Stupor and Coma.* Philadelphia, PA: TA Davis, 1984, pp 222–225.
6. Bickford RG, Butt HR. Hepatic coma: the electroencephalographic pattern. *J Clin Invest* 1955;34:790–799.
7. Boggs JG, Towne A, Smith J, DeLorenzo RJ. Frequency of potentially ictal patterns in comatose ICU patients. *Epilepsia* 1994;35 (Suppl 8):135. (abstract).
8. Boggs JG, Waterhouse EJ, DeLorenzo RJ. The use of antiepileptic medications in renal and liver disease, In: E. Wyllie (ed.), *The Treatment of Epilepsy: Principles and Practice,* 3rd ed. Lea and Febiger, 2000, in press.
9. Locke S, Merrill JP, Tyler HR. Neurologic complications of uremia. *Arch Intern Med* 1961;108:519–522.
10. Tyler HR, Tyler KL. Neurologic complications. In: Eknoyan G, Knochel JP (eds.), *The Systemic Consequences of Renal Failure,* New York: Grune and Stratton, 1994, p 311.

11. Van den Noort S, Ekel RE, Brine KL, Hrdlicka J. Brain metabolism in experimental uremia. *Arch Intern Med.* 1970;126:831–834.
12. Fishman RA, Raskin NH. Experimental uremic encephalopathy:permeability ion exchange, and brain spaces. *Trans Am Neurol Assoc* 1965;90:71–75.
13. Hughes, JR. EEG in uremia. *Am J EEG Technol.* 1984;24:1–10.
14. Arieff AL, Massry SG, Barrientos, Kleeman CR. Brain water and electrolyte metabolism in uremia:effects of slow and rapid hemodialysis. *Kidney Int* 1973;4:177–187.
15. Halperin JJ, Landis DMD, Kleinman GM. Whipple disease of the nervous system. *Neurology* 1982;32:612–617.
16. Gobbi G, Bouquet F, Greco L, Lambertini A, Tassinari CA, Ventura A, Zaniboni MG. Coeliac disease, epilepsy and cerebral calcifications. Report from the Italian Working Group on Coeliac Disease and Epilepsy. *Lancet* 1992;340:439–443.
17. Hanly JG, Stassen W, Whelton M, Callaghan N. Epilepsy and celiac disease. *J Neurol Neurosurg Psychiatry* 1982;45:729–730.
18. Rush PJ, Inman R, Berstein M, Carlen P, Resch L. Isolated vasculitis of the central nervous system in a patient with celiac disease. *Am J Med* 1986;81:1092–1094.
19. Lossos A, River Y, Steiner I. Neurologic aspects of inflammatory bowel disease. *Neurology* 1995;45:416–421.
20. Portnoy BA, Herion JC. Neurologic manifestations in sickle cell disease. *Ann Int Med* 1972;76:643–652.
21. Fabian RH, Peters BH. Neurologic complications of hemoglobin SC disease. *Arch Neurol* 1984;41:289.
22. Gilchrist GS, Piepgras DG. Neurologic complications in hemophilia. *Prog Pediatr Hematol Oncol* 1977;1:79.
23. Levine J, Welch KMA. The spectrum of neurologic disease associated with antiphospholipid antibodies. *Arch Neurol* 1987;44:876–883.
24. Ridolfi RL, Bell WR. Thrombotic thrombcytopenic purpura:report of 25 cases and review of the literature. *Medicine* 1981;60:413–428.
25. Asher R. Myxoedematous madness. *Br Med J* 1949;2:555–560.
26. Cook DM, Boyle PJ. Rapid reversal of myxedema madness with triiodothyronine. *Ann Int Med* 1986;104:893, 894.
27. Evans EC. Neurologic complications of myxedema:convulsions. *Ann Inten Med* 1960;52:434–436.
28. Lansing RW, Trunnel JB. Electroencephalographic changes accompanying thyroid deficiency in man. *J Clin Endocrinol Metab* 1983;23:470.
29. Ross DA, Schwab RJ. The cortical alpha rhythm in thyroid disorders. *Endocrinology* 1939;25:75–79.
30. Wynn D, Lagerlund T, Mokri B, Westmoreland B. Periodic complexes in hypothyroidism masquerading as Jakob-Creutzfeldt disease:a case report. *Electroencephalogr Clin Neurophysiol* 1989;72:31 (abstract).
31. Schultz MA, Schulte FJ, Akiyama Y, Parmelee AH. Development of EEG sleep phenomena in hypothyroid infants. *Electroencephalogr Clin Neurophysiol* 1968; 25:351–358.
32. Rootwelt K, Ganes T, Johannessen SI. Effect of carbamazepine, phenytoin and phenobaritone on serum levels of thyroid hormones and thyrotropin in humans. *Scand J Lab Invest.* 1978;38:731–736.
33. De Luca F, Arrigo T, Pandullo E, Siracusano MF, Benvenga S, Trimarchi F. Changes in thyroid function tests induced by 2 month carbamazepine treatment in L-thyroxine-substituted hypothyroid children. *Eur J Pediatr* 1986;145:77–79.

34. Grant C, Warlow C. Focal epilepsy in diabetic nonketotic hyperglycemia. *Br Med J* 1985;290:1204, 1205.
35. Singh BM, Strobos RJ. Nonketotic hyperglycemia associated with epilepsia partialis continua. *Arch Neurol* 1973;29:187–190.
36. Malouf R, Brust JC. Hypoglycemia:causes, neurologic manifestations and outcome. *Ann Neurol* 1985;17:421–430.
37. Scarpino O, Mauro AM, Del Pesce M. Partial seizures and insulinoma: a case report. *Electroencephalogr Clin Neurophysiol* 1985;61:90 (abstract).
38. Levin SR, Booker J, Smith DF, Grodsky GM. Inhibition of insulin secretion by diphenylhydantoin in the isolated perfused pancreas. *J Clin Endocrinol.* 1970; 30:400–401.
39. Bairamian D, Di Chiro G, Blume H, Ehrenberg B. Pituitary adenoma with seizures:PET demonstration of reduced glucose utilization in the medial temporal lobe. *J Comput Assist Tomogr* 1986;10:529–532.
40. Graham K, Williams BO, Rowe MJ. Idiopathic hypoparathyroidism:a cause of fits in the elderly. *Br Med J* 1979;6176:1460–1461.
41. Kalam MA, Hafeez W. Congenital hypoparathyroidism, seizure, extreme growth with developmental delay and dysmorphic features. *Clin Genet* 1992;42:110–113.
42. Kurtz D. The EEG in parathyroid dysfunction. In: A. Redmond (ed.), *Handbook of Electroencephalography and Clinical Neurophysiology,* Amsterdam: Elsevier, vol 15C, pp 77–87.
43. Freeman JE, Johnston PGB, Voke JM. Somnolence after prophylactic cranial irradiation in children with acute lymphoblastic leukemia. *Br Med J* 1973;4:523–525.
44. Hart RB, Easton JD. Carbamazepine and hematological monitoring. *Ann Neurol* 1982;11:309–312.
45. Seetharam MN, Pellock JM. Risk-benefit assessment of carbamazepine in children. *Drug Safety* 1991;6:148–158.

6

Seizures and Electrolyte Imbalance

Alvaro R. Gutierrez, MD and Jack E. Riggs, MD

Introduction

Although electrolyte imbalance is commonly encountered in clinical practice, associated seizures occur infrequently. Indeed, the finding of an electrolyte imbalance in the setting of new-onset seizure activity should not preclude a search for other potential causes of seizures. An important clinical caveat is that seizures secondary to electrolyte abnormalities can be either partial or generalized. In this chapter, disturbances of serum sodium, magnesium, potassium, and calcium will be reviewed with regard to their propensity to provoke seizures. The causes of electrolyte imbalance and the pathogenesis and treatment of associated seizures will be discussed.

Sodium Imbalance

Abnormalities of serum sodium typically produce central, rather than peripheral, neurological manifestations *(1)*. Because the brain has considerable ability to adapt to changes in serum osmolality, the propensity of hyponatremia or hypernatremia to produce neurologic symptoms typically depends on the rapidity with which the serum sodium abnormality develops *(1)*.

Hyponatremia

The clinical manifestations of hyponatremia are highly variable and not stereotyped *(1)*. In the setting of hyponatremia, neurological symptoms, including seizures, usually manifest when serum sodium has fallen quickly to below 120 mmol/L *(2)*. Conversely, in chronic hyponatremia, similarly low serum sodium levels may be observed in patients who are neurologically asymptomatic *(2)*. In a series of 73 hyponatremic patients, 33% had no

From: *Seizures: Medical Causes and Management*
Edited by: N. Delanty © Humana Press, Inc., Totowa, NJ

symptoms referable to the central nervous system (CNS), 33% had confusion only, and 14% patients had associated seizures *(2)*. Thirteen patients had focal neurological signs, including hemiparesis, monoparesis, tremors, and ataxia, which reversed with correction of the hyponatremia *(2)*. In another series of 84 hyponatremic patients, 76% had confusion (including 11% with coma), 6% had long tract signs, 1% had intellectual impairment or psychosis, and 3.3% had associated seizures *(3)*. As a general rule, seizures are only seen in association with severe hyponatremia. However, neurologic symptoms and morbidity are only grossly correlated with either the magnitude or duration of the hyponatremia *(4)*.

Etiology of Hyponatremic Seizures

Hyponatremic seizures potentially may be seen in a variety of clinical situations.

HYPONATREMIC SEIZURES IN ICU PATIENTS

Although infrequent, new-onset seizures do occur in intensive care unit (ICU) patients *(5)*. Shivering, myoclonic jerks, and periodic decorticate posturing can be misinterpreted as seizure activity in ICU patients. Withdrawal from benzodiazepines and narcotics is apparently a relatively common cause of new-onset seizures in ICU patients *(5)*. Drug-induced seizures have accounted for about 15% of new-onset seizures in ICU patients *(5)*. However, metabolic alterations, most frequently acute hyponatremia, may account for as many as one-third of all new-onset seizures in surgical and medical ICUs *(5)*. Inadequate monitoring of fluid management may contribute to many cases of severe hyponatremia in the ICU. With the exception of neurosurgical patients, neuroimaging studies seldom demonstrate the cause of seizures in the ICU setting. Guillain-Barré syndrome, massive fluid shifts in severe burn patients *(6)*, and liver transplant patients account for only a small proportion of hyponatremic patients in the ICU. An important observation to keep in mind is that hospitalized patients with hyponatremia have a severalfold increased risk of mortality compared to those without hyponatremia *(7)*.

HYPONATREMIC SEIZURES IN HEALTHY POPULATIONS

Seizures are not unusual in the healthy general population. The cumulative incidence of all unprovoked seizures through age 74 was 4.1% in one longitudinal study *(8)*. Young children and the elderly have the highest risk of a new-onset seizure *(8)*. Of 56 pediatric cases of new-onset seizures seen in an emergency room, only two children had hyponatremia *(9)*. In the first 2 yr of life, however, hyponatremia may account for about one-half of all afebrile seizures *(10)*. Moreover, even in febrile seizures, hyponatremia increases the risk of seizure recurrence *(11)*. In infants younger than 6 mo who present with a new-onset seizure without another readily identifiable cause, hyponatremia has been present in the majority *(12)*. Water intoxication is the most common underlying cause of hyponatremia in infants and young children and is most often caused by substituting water for infant formula *(13)*. Incorrectly mixed infant formula *(14)* and commercial bottled drinking water given to infants *(15)* have also been implicated in causing water intoxication. Accidental water intoxication resulting from the treatment of diarrhea and gastroenteritis are also occasional causes of hyponatremia in infants. In older children, hyponatremic seizures have been described in a child made to ingest large amounts of water as punishment *(16)*, following the use of intranasal desmopressin for nocturnal enuresis *(17)* and even following the ingestion of large amounts of water during swimming lessons *(18)*.

In young adults, the causes of hyponatremic seizures are substantially different. The hyponatremia associated with exercise develops when poorly trained athletes retain large volumes of excess fluid *(19)*. The syndrome of inappropriate antidiuretic hormone (SIADH), "third spacing," and abnormal regulation of extracellular fluid are suggested mechanisms of hyponatremia associated with exercise *(19)*. The "squash drinking syndrome" is caused by excessive intake of high energy fluids during or following exercise *(20)*.

HYPONATREMIC SEIZURES IN PSYCHIATRIC PATIENTS

Epilepsy often coexists with psychotic conditions *(21)*. When seizures and hyponatremia are encountered in psychiatric patients, several possible conditions should be considered. The psychosis, intermittent polydipsia, and hyponatremia syndrome is well-recognized and often leads to seizures. Arguing against an iatrogenic etiology for this hyponatremia, studies from the pre-neuroleptic era suggested that up to 25% of patients with untreated schizophrenia had polydipsia *(22)*. In a recent series of long-term hospitalized psychiatric patients, the prevalence of polydipsia was 42%, and 5% of these patients had a history of water intoxication *(23)*. Compulsory water drinking leading to water intoxication, as the mechanism of hyponatremia in psychiatric patients, has fallen out of favor *(24)*. A central mechanism, such as enhanced vasopressin secretion, may be important in psychogenic polydipsia with hyponatremia and seizures in psychiatric patients *(25)*. Medications and medical comorbidities may also have a role in producing polydipsia with hyponatremia and seizures in psychiatric patients *(26–28)*. Treatment strategies to prevent seizures in the polydipsia–hyponatremia syndrome associated with psychiatric disease include behavioral modification and the use of medications that oppose the central release or renal action of antidiuretic hormone (ADH) *(29)*.

HYPONATREMIC SEIZURES ASSOCIATED WITH DRUGS

Numerous reports of hyponatremic seizures caused by drugs exist (**Table 1**). The most notorious agents reported to induce hyponatremic seizures are the thiazide diuretics *(30)*. Other diuretics have also been implicated in causing hyponatremic seizures.

The SIADH syndrome has been linked to many drugs and may result in hyponatremic seizures (**Table 1**). These drugs may induce pituitary release of ADH in a nonphysiological manner and include oral hypoglycemic agents (such as chlorpropamide and tolbutamide), antineoplastic agents (such as vincristine, cyclophosphamide, and cisplatin *[31]*), psychoactive drugs (such as the neuroleptics, tricyclic antidepressants, and serotonin reuptake inhibitors *[32,33]*), and miscellaneous drugs (such as lisinopril and clofibrate *[34]*).

Some drugs either mimic ADH activity or increase renal sensitivity to ADH. Intranasal desmopressin for nocturnal enuresis *(35)* and intravenous desmopressin for surgical hemostasis *(36)* has been associated with hyponatremic seizures. Oxytocin-augmented labors have been complicated by maternal hyponatremic seizures *(37)*. Carbamazepine and oxcarbazepine are anticonvulsants that can also cause hyponatremic seizures *(38)*. Serum sodium levels should be measured in epileptics on these anticonvulsants if "breakthrough" seizures occur.

The transurethral resection of prostate syndrome is the clinical manifestation of the resorption of a large amount of glycine and irrigating fluid during that surgical procedure *(39)*. Confusion and seizures have been reported *(40)*. The pathophysiology of this syndrome may involve the development of acute hyponatremia (sometimes dissociated from hypo-osmolality), toxicity of glycine and its metabolites glyoxylic and glycolic acids, and hyperammonemia *(39,41)*. These different pathogenic mechanisms may be synergistic. Cerebral edema may not be the predominant pathophysiological aspect, as this syndrome can occur under isotonic conditions *(42)*.

HYPONATREMIC SEIZURES IN NEUROSURGICAL PATIENTS

Hyponatremia and seizures have been observed following trans-sphenoidal surgery for pituitary tumors *(43)* and suprasellar lesions, such as craniopharyngioma and Rathke's cyst *(44)*. Hyponatremia is also a common complication of subarachnoid hemorrhage, head injury, intracranial tumors, intracranial infections, and stroke *(45,46)*. Hyponatremia in acute brain disease has been attributed to two distinct entities: the cerebral salt-wasting syndrome (CSWS) and SIADH *(47)*. CSWS is characterized by hyponatremia, excessive renal loss of sodium without an increase in total body fluid (actually, a decrease in extracellular fluid volume may occur) *(48)*. In unselected neurosurgical patients who fulfilled the laboratory criteria for SIADH, most

Table 1
Drugs Causing Hyponatremia

Drugs that sensitize kidney to ADH
  Hypoglycemic agents
    chlorpropamide
    tolbutamide
  Antiepileptic drugs
    carbamazepine[a]
    oxcarbazepine[a]
  Indomethacin
Drugs that stimulate release of ADH
  Diuretics
    thiazides and thiazide-like diuretics*
    furosemide
    ethacrynic acid
  Antineoplastic agents
    cyclophosphamide[a]
    vincristine[a]
    cisplatin[a]
  Sedatives
    barbiturates
    morphine
  Miscellaneous
    clofibrate
    lisinopril[a]
Drugs with a direct ADH effect
  desmopressin[a]
  oxytocin[a]
Other drugs
  Psychotropic agents
    thioridazine and neuroleptics[a]
    amitriptyline and tricyclic antidepressants[a]
    serotonin reuptake inhibitors[a]
    monoamine oxidase inhibitors

[a]Reported association with hyponatremic seizures.

had decreases in plasma volume, red blood cell mass, and total blood volume *(49)*. These observations raise the issue that in intracranial disease, CSWS may be a better explanation for hyponatremia than is SIADH (which is either a euvolemic or hypervolemic state). Increasing evidence suggests that the hyponatremia of CSWS may be the result of sustained elevations of atrial natriuretic peptide *(50)*. Accurate diagnosis and management of CSWS are critical, as its treatment (salt and water supplementation) is the opposite of the usual treatment of the dilutional hyponatremia associated with SIADH *(51)*.

POSTOPERATIVE HYPONATREMIC
ENCEPHALOPATHY OF MENSTRUATING WOMEN

A dramatic clinical syndrome consisting of postoperative hyponatremia, encephalopathy with permanent brain damage, seizures, and respiratory arrest has been described in menstruating women *(52)*. This syndrome, however, was not observed in a recent retrospective study of over 290,000 surgical procedures from 1976 to 1992 at the Mayo Clinic *(53)*.

Pathophysiology of Hyponatremic Seizures

The pathophysiological basis for seizure induction in hyponatremia is likely multifactorial. Indeed, no conclusive evidence exists that hyponatremia, in and of itself, leads to epileptogenesis *(54)*. The decrease in serum osmolality in hyponatremia is essential in initiating the chain of events leading to neurological symptoms and seizures. When the decrease in serum osmolality is acute, passive water influx occurs in CNS cellular compartments (neurons and glial cells) with an associated contraction of the extracellular space. The rat hippocampal slice experimental model has shed some light on these processes *(55)*. In this model, osmotically induced extracellular volume contraction enhances epileptiform bursts from CA1 pyramidal cells even when chemical synaptic transmission is blocked *(55)*. Rapid lowering of the osmolality also increases field potential amplitude of CA3 region cells, which is probably caused by the increased proximity of these cell bodies leading to larger field effects and associated neuronal synchronization *(55)*.

Intracellular recordings document no change in resting membrane potentials, cell resistance, and action potential thresholds of the CA3 cell body with lowered osmolality *(56)*. However, a gradual increase in the amplitude of excitatory postsynaptic potentials does take place in most of the cell recordings. These observations occur independent of the field effect changes. Spontaneous endogenous bursting is also more frequent under conditions of hypo-osmolality. All of these changes are reversible by rapidly raising the extracellular osmolality with mannitol, suggesting a causal relationship *(56)*.

Synaptic mechanisms may also have a role in hyponatremic seizures. When exposed to a hypo-osmolar bathing solution, an increase in the amplitude of a delayed rectifier potassium current in inhibitory interneurons of hippocampal slices is observed *(57)*. Antagonists of the chloride cotransporter, such as furosemide, can block epileptiform activity *(57)*. Manipulation of the ionic environment with drugs has not been exploited as an antiepileptic strategy *(57)*.

Treatment of Hyponatremic Seizures

Seizures in a patient with hyponatremia should be managed in the same manner as with any other patient with a new-onset seizure. Treatment of the hyponatremia is usually dependent on removing the factors producing the hyponatremia. One word of caution, central pontine myelinolysis (osmotic demyelination syndrome) may occur if hyponatremia is corrected too rapidly, particularly if the hyponatremia has been chronic *(1)*.

Hypernatremia

Hypernatremia (serum sodium level >145 mmol/L) can cause several CNS manifestations. Abnormalities of sensorium are common; seizures are unusual. Dehydration leading to hypernatremia can also be responsible for serious intracranial structural lesions (such as cortical vein thrombosis and subdural hematomas) that can potentially cause seizures. Potential alternative etiologies for seizures in the setting of hypernatremia should always be considered. Rehydration in the treatment of hypernatremia can also lead to seizures if not properly controlled. Thus, not only is hypernatremia often iatrogenic, its correction can also induce seizures iatrogenically.

Etiology of Hypernatremic Seizures

Hypernatremic seizures may potentially be seen in many different clinical situations.

HYPERNATREMIC SEIZURES WITH VOLUME DEPLETION

Hypernatremia in nonhospitalized patients is predominantly a disease of the elderly and is commonly a manifestation of infection or inadequate nursing care *(58)*. Hospital-acquired hypernatremia, on the other hand, occurs in a population that reflects the general hospitalized population *(58)*. Approximately 1% of all inpatients who are at least 60 yr old have been found to be hypernatremic; and of those, one-half developed the hypernatremia while in the hospital *(59)*.

In a recent series of 103 hypernatremic hospitalized patients, "18 patients were hypernatremic on hospital admission, and 85 developed hypernatremia during hospitalization. Eighty-nine percent of patients who developed hypernatremia during hospitalization had urine-concentrating defects, primarily as the result of the use of diuretics or of solute diuresis, whereas only 50% of patients who were hypernatremic on admission could be shown to have concentrating defects. Fifty-five percent of all hypernatremic patients had increased insensible water losses, and 35% had increased enteral water losses. Eighty-six percent of patients with hospital-acquired hypernatremia lacked free access to water, 74% had enteral water intake of less than 1 L/day, and 94% received less than 1 L of intravenous electrolyte-free water per day during the development of hypernatremia. No supplemental electrolyte-free water was prescribed during the first 24 h of hypernatremia in 49% of patients" *(60)*. Hospital mortality rates range from approx. 40% to more than 60% in hospitalized patients with hypernatremia *(58)*. These observations emphasize the iatrogenic nature and seriousness of this condition. Often water deficits are associated with sodium deficits such as in uncompensated profuse sweating or diabetic hyperosmolar states. Many drugs, such as lithium, methicillin, cisplatin, and amphotericin B, inhibit the effect of ADH on the kidney (nephrogenic diabetes insipidus) and can also produce dehydration and hypernatremia.

HYPERNATREMIC SEIZURES FROM SODIUM EXCESS

Exogenous intake of salt is seldom the cause of hypernatremia. Oral overloads or mistaken intravenous infusion of hypertonic sodium chloride or bicarbonate solutions have been reported to cause hypernatremia *(61)*. Peritoneal dialysis is another potential cause of sodium overload and hypernatremia.

HYPERNATREMIC SEIZURES IN PEDIATRIC PATIENTS

In infants, enteral water losses owing to infectious diarrhea constitute the majority of the cases of hypernatremia. Inappropriate preparation of formula (e.g., substitution of sugar by salt) has also been implicated *(62)*. Hypernatremic dehydration can also occur as a result of insufficient breast milk volume *(63)*. The pathophysiology of this entity is complex, and alterations in the ratio of lactose to sodium in breast milk may have some role in addition to the low volume of breast milk *(63)*.

HYPERNATREMIC SEIZURES IN NEUROSURGICAL PATIENTS

Postoperative neurosurgical patients or severe stroke victims can develop hypernatremia as a result of being on high-protein tube feedings. These patients develop hypernatremia because of urea diuresis, which is compounded by their inability to ingest water. Diabetes insipidus can occur in patients with brain trauma, subarachnoid hemorrhage, intracranial masses, intracranial inflammatory disease, and cerebrovacular disease. Surprisingly, many patients with diabetes insipidus can maintain their serum osmolality despite massive diuresis, as long as they have access to fluids. Consequently, obtundation puts patients with diabetes insipidus at great risk of hypernatremic dehydration.

Pathophysiology of Hypernatremic Seizures

Normally, increases in serum tonicity stimulate thirst and ADH secretion. Thirst and the stimulation of water intake represent the primary defense mechanisms against hypernatremia. Hypernatremia occurs when individuals cannot respond to thirst by drinking or when they do not experience thirst. Defects in thirst may result from focal lesions involving the hypothalamic osmoreceptors. Neurologic lesions that impair higher cortical processes may also interfere in thirst perception and water ingestion. Mineralocorticoid excess and drug side effects may also lead to thirst deficiency *(64)*. The obtunded patient, either because of anesthesia or intercurrent illness, is often unable to request or drink water. Hospital-acquired hypernatremia is largely a result of inadequate fluid management *(65)*. Essential hypernatremia is a rare and poorly characterized condition. "In response to hypernatremia, the brain undergoes adaptive responses to minimize osmotic shrinkage. Initially there is a rapid uptake of electrolytes, while a slower adaptive phase involves the accumulation of organic osmolytes" *(58)*. If hypernatremia progresses, severe neuronal cell volume loss and functional impairment can occur.

Treatment of Hypernatremia and Rehydration Seizures

The management of hypernatremia depends on the mechanism that produced the hypernatremia. The degree and the rate of volume loss also have therapeutic implications. Because the brain tends to accumulate organic osmolytes over time to maintain cell volume, the sudden availability of water can initiate a pathological shift of water into the intracellular compartment. This process can occur even when serum osmolality would not appear to warrant such water movement. The organic osmolytes accumulated will either be degraded or eliminated at a rate that is likely to follow, but lag significantly behind, extracellular osmolality changes *(58)*. The rate of rehydration in hypernatremia is, therefore, very important. If the rate of rehydration is too fast, a rapid movement of free water into the brain parenchyma will occur. Brain edema, produced in such a manner, can result in increased intracranial pressure, decreased sensorium, and rehydration seizures *(62)*. Under experimental conditions, rehydration seizures appear to be correlated with the brain water content when rehydration occurs over several hours *(66)*. A direct correlation exists between the incidence of seizures and the rate of administration of intravenous (IV) solutions. In an animal model, rehydration seizures were less frequent when using fructose, rather than glucose, solutions for acute volume replacement *(66)*. Accordingly, a controlled drop in serum sodium avoided rehydration seizures in 40 infants with severe hypernatremic dehydration *(67)*. A desired rate of fall in serum sodium has been suggested to be less than 0.5 mmol/L per hour *(67)*. Although apparently much less common, the osmotic demyelination syndrome has also been described with rapid lowering of serum osmolality in the treatment of hypernatremia *(68)*. The recommendation to control the rate of serum osmotic shift applies to the correction of both hyponatremia and hypernatremia.

Magnesium Imbalance

Magnesium is an important intracellular ion that is required for the activation of a wide range of intracellular enzymes and exerts significant effects on synaptic transmission *(1)*. Abnormalities of magnesium are being recognized increasingly, although this electrolyte remains relatively neglected *(69)*. Part of the reason for this neglect is that magnesium is often not included in the standard electrolyte panel, thus precluding widespread experience in the range of clinical manifestations associated with alterations in serum magnesium *(70)*.

Hypomagnesemia

Hypomagnesemia is conventionally defined as serum levels of magnesium less than 1.2 meq/L. However, because less than 2% of total body magnesium is extracellular, serum magnesium levels do not accurately reflect tissue magnesium stores. Moreover, tissue magnesium depletion may be organ selective. Magnesium, potassium, and phosphorus cellular stores tend to deplete simultaneously, even if only one of the electrolytes is deficient. For example, unrecognized hypomagnesemia is occasionally the abnormality underlying refractory hypokalemia.

Hypomagnesemia has been associated with several clinical abnormalities including cardiac arrhythmias, sudden death, tetany, and seizures *(71)*. Dietary deprivation of normal volunteers leads to symptoms within weeks. Gastrointestinal symptoms and weakness are followed by higher cortical function deficits and sensorium abnormalities. Symptoms brought on by associated hypocalcemia can become prominent. Hypocalcemia is the result of the effect of severe hypomagnesemia on calcium metabolism. The hypokalemia that accompanies hypomagnesemia can also become symptomatic. The rate of fall of tissue magnesium levels is also likely to influence the clinical presentation.

In a prospective study of hypomagnesemia, tremor and fasciculations were seen only in patients with coexisting hypocalcemia. Tetany was not observed. Many signs and symptoms of hypomagnesemia are not specific and may be attributable to other concomitant electrolyte abnormalities *(72)*. Nevertheless, seizures may be directly related to hypomagnesemia. Auditory and tactile stimuli can precipitate neurologic symptoms and seizures in humans with hypomagnesemia as has been documented in experimental animals *(73,74)*.

Hypomagnesemia is an uncommon but treatable cause of acute intractable seizures in humans *(75)*. Hypomagnesemic seizures might be responsible for some sudden deaths in humans, as has been observed in laboratory animals *(74)*. Ataxia, dysphagia, and psychiatric disturbances (including delirium and coma) have also been reported in hypomagnesemia *(76)*. Among hospitalized patients, the incidence of hypomagnesemia is as high as 10%. If other electrolyte abnormalities are present, the incidence of hypomagnesemia is much higher *(77)*. Among patients entering an ICU, the incidence of hypomagnesemia is around 20% *(78)*.

Etiology of Hypomagnesemic Seizures

Hypomagnesemic seizures can occur in many clinical situations. Stress from any cause can decrease serum magnesium levels without affecting tissue stores. This observation adds a confounding variable, as most other causes of hypomagnesemia are also associated with stress. The mechanism of stress-induced hypomagnesemia involves the release of catecholamines. IV epinephrine given to normal volunteers will lower levels of serum magnesium *(79)*. Seizures also cause the release catecholamines. Consequently, postictal serum magnesium levels can be transiently depressed and be mistaken for a cause of the seizure. These theoretical considerations, however, should not deter the clinician from correcting hypomagnesemia when encountered in patients with a new-onset seizure.

During the first few weeks of life, infants with primary familial hypomagnesemia (an extremely rare disease) develop their initial seizures associated with hypocalcemia and hypomagnesemia. Early identification and treatment with oral magnesium appears to improve neurological outcome *(80)*. In the neonatal period, as many as one-half of the infants with seizures brought on by hypocalcemia and hypomagnesemia have associated severe congenital heart disease *(81)*. Congenital causes of renal magnesium loss include Bartter's and Gitelman's syndrome. Renal magnesium loss also accompanies hypercalcemia and diuretic usage. Aminoglycosides, pentamidine, foscarnet, and cyclosporin also cause renal magnesium loss *(82)*. Cisplatin chemotherapy causes magnesium diuresis and hypomagnesemia in more than one-half of patients receiving this drug when studied prospectively *(83)*. A plethora of unrelated diseases have in common the depletion of magnesium tissue stores. These conditions include diabetes, parenteral nutrition, chronic and acute alcoholism *(84)*, diarrheal diseases, and intestinal malabsorption *(85)*. A variety of rare endocrine disorders can also manifest as hypomagnesemic seizures **(Table 2)**.

Pathophysiology of Hypomagnesemic Seizures

The incidence of sudden death in rats treated with magnesium-deficient diets is much higher than those on control diets when subjected to in vivo electrophysiologic studies *(86)*. During these studies, sudden, unexpected asystolic deaths were observed in hypomagnesemic rats. Interestingly, the deaths were preceded by seizures following exposure to auditory stimuli. These observations suggest that some sudden unexplained deaths in humans might also be related to seizure activity in hypomagnesemia.

An apparent threshold for low magnesium levels in the CNS must be exceeded for the development of seizures to take place. Magnesium concentrations readily equilibrate between the cerebrospinal fluid, extracellular fluid, and other magnesium repositories *(73)*. Cerebrospinal fluid magnesium levels

Table 2
Causes of Hypomagnesemia

Stress hypomagnesemia
Diabetic ketoacidosis
Chronic alcoholism
Dietary insufficiency
Total parenteral nutrition
Gastrointestinal disorders
Drugs that enhance magnesium renal excretion
Severe congenital heart disease
Parathyroid dysfunction
Renal failure
Magnesium-losing nephropathy
Bartter's syndrome
Gitelman's syndrome
Primary hypomagnesemia
Primary hypomagnesemia with secondary hypocalcemia

are higher than serum levels due to active transport of magnesium across the blood–brain barrier. Under physiological conditions, magnesium blocks *N*-methyl-D-aspartamate (NMDA) receptors in neurons by exerting voltage-dependent regulation of the ion channel *(87)*. Glutamate or NMDA binding at the NMDA receptor results in a conformational change that opens the channel. Glycine has a separate binding site on the NMDA receptor that interacts allosterically with the glutamate binding site. Binding of glutamate or glycine on the NMDA receptor enhances binding of the other ligand. Thus, glutamate and glycine appear to function as excitatory coagonists on the NMDA receptor *(88)*. Glycine does exert an inhibitory influence on the strychnine-sensitive chloride channel. Abnormal and excessive stimulation of the NMDA receptors can precipitate seizures. However, experimental evidence does not show that the impairment of this inhibitory effect of magnesium is responsible for the seizures associated with hypomagnesemia. Nevertheless, epileptiform activity due to magnesium deficiency can be blocked by NMDA receptor antagonists, suggesting that hypomagnesemic seizures may be dependent on NMDA receptor activation *(86)*. Other biochemical pathways that might have a role in epileptogenesis in magnesium deficiency include alterations in Na/K ATPase, cAMP/cGMP activity, and pre- and postsynaptic calcium currents *(89)*.

Many rat strains become susceptible to noise-induced seizures after being deprived of dietary magnesium for 15–30 days *(90)*. These seizures have essentially the same features as genetic audiogenic seizures. The susceptibility to hypomagnesemic seizures can be quantified by changing the intensity of the noise stimulus *(91)*. The nutritional model of magnesium deficiency-dependent audiogenic seizures has been used to test the therapeutic effect of standard antiepileptic drugs. Phenytoin, carbamazepine, phenobarbital, valproic acid, ethosuximide, and diazepam are effective in preventing these seizures *(92)*. However, late epileptiform activity in this model may become insensitive to valproic acid *(93)*. Ethanol inhibits NMDA receptor activity. The role of magnesium in this interaction has not been fully characterized *(94)*.

Treatment of Hypomagnesemic Seizures

When patients present with seizures and hypomagesemia, alternative etiologies for the seizures should be pursued. Nevertheless, the clinician should correct serum magnesium levels and check the levels of other frequently associated electrolyte abnormalities (such as potassium, calcium, and phosphorus). For rapid replacement, IV magnesium sulfate is the agent of choice and is ideally delivered using an infusion pump. In the adult, an initial dose of 4 g magnesium sulfate is given at a rate not exceeding 1 g/min. If convulsions persist, another 2 g of magnesium sulfate can be given after 15 min. During the first day, 4 g of magnesium sulfate every 6 h is a standard approach. During magnesium administration, urine output should be carefully monitored. Loss of the patellar reflex is an early sign of magnesium intoxication. IV calcium gluconate should be given to treat symptomatic magnesium intoxication. However, studies have not demonstrated the efficacy of acute magnesium replacement in the treatment of acute seizures associated with hypomagnesemia. Therefore, patients who are seizing should also be treated with conventional antiepileptic therapy. Phenytoin and benzodiazepines are effective in the nutritional model of magnesium deficiency-dependent audiogenic seizures *(92)*. The efficacy of valproic acid in the treatment of protracted hypomagnesemic seizures in the laboratory is limited *(93)*.

Magnesium sulfate is standard treatment of eclamptic seizures. Indeed, magnesium appears to be superior to either phenytoin or diazepam in the treatment of eclamptic seizures. However, because there are no significant differences in serum or cerebrospinal fluid magnesium levels between normal pregnant and pre-eclamptic women *(95)*, magnesium deficiency may not have a role in eclampsia.

Hypermagnesemia

Hypermagnesemia is usually encountered in the setting of acute or chronic renal failure and excessive intake of magnesium. Refractory hypotension, sensorium abnormalities, and respiratory arrest can occur in hypermagnesemia. The neurological manifestations of hypermagnesemia are secondary to central and peripheral nervous system depression. Lethargy and confusion occur at serum magnesium levels of 8–10 meq/L *(96)*. However, in experimental human subjects, CNS signs and symptoms did not manifest even at serum magnesium levels of 15 meq/L *(97)*. Seizures have not been reported in association with hypermagnesemia in clinical observations or animal experimental conditions. The predominant peripheral nervous system manifestation of hypermagnesemia is muscular paralysis. The most effective treatment of severe hypermagnesemia is renal dialysis.

Another relatively frequent occurrence of hypermagnesemia is the transient neonatal hypermagnesemia caused by magnesium sulfate administration to women with eclampsia in labor. Newborns with hypermagnesemia are more likely to be hypotonic and to have lower Apgar scores *(98)*. Seizures attributable to hypermagnesemia in newborns have not been reported.

Potassium Imbalance

Hypokalemia and hyperkalemia rarely affect the CNS. Although hypokalemia may occasionally be associated with seizures, this usually reflects coexisting undetected hypomagnesemia *(1)*. Hypokalemia refractory to potassium repletion is often the consequence of decreased magnesium tissue stores and is not correctable until the magnesium deficit is addressed *(99)*. Hyperkalemia will produce fatal cardiac rhythm disturbances before CNS manifestations can occur *(1)*. Moreover, CNS manifestations are not present in hyperkalemic periodic paralysis *(1)*.

Changes in extracellular potassium concentration will alter various parameters that are considered conducive to seizure activity in rat hippocampal slice preparations *(100)*. When extracellular potassium is increased, spontaneous bursting is observed more readily. The combination of increased extracellular potassium and decreased extracelluar calcium increases seizure susceptibility in a synergistic manner in this rat model *(101)*. Finally, benign familial neonatal convulsions is a type of epilepsy that results from mutations in voltage-sensitive potassium channels *(101)*.

Calcium Imbalance

Because calcium stabilizes excitable membranes, neurological symptoms are not unexpectedly associated with disorders of calcium *(1)*.

Hypocalcemia

Symptomatic hypocalcemia is correlated with serum-ionized calcium concentrations (true hypocalcemia). Ionized serum calcium is related to serum protein concentration and pH. Hypocalcemia occurs in many conditions **(Table 3).** The neurological manifestations of hypocalcemia are usually peripheral (such as perioral and limb paresthesias, carpopedal spasms, laryngeal stridor, and tetany) *(1)*. Occasionally, papilledema, mental status

Table 3
Causes of Hypocalcemia

Repeated transfusions
Plasmapheresis
Heparin
Critical illness
Sepsis
Acute pancreatitis
Post-thyroidectomy
Fat embolism
Crush injury
Rhabdomyolysis
Hypomagnesemia
Chronic renal failure
Acute renal failure
Hypoparathyroidism
Pseudohypoparathyroidism
Primary hypomagnesemia with secondary hypocalcemia
Vitamin D deficiency
Drugs (such as pentamidine, foscarnet, and chemotherapy)

changes, and seizures occur with very low serum-ionized calcium levels. Hypocalcemic seizures often follow a generalized tetanic response and consist of generalized convulsions and status epilepticus. Prolonged spike and wave stupor has been reported *(102)*.

Pathophysiology of Hypocalcemic Seizures

In rat hippocampal slices, reduction of extracellular calcium induces spontaneous epileptic activity characterized by rhythmic burst firing of CA1 neurons *(103)*. Because this epileptogenic activity can propagate in the face of synaptic blockade, a nonsynaptic mechanism of spread is suggested *(104)*.

Treatment of Hypocalcemic Seizures

In severe hypocalcemia associated with seizures, the treatment should include IV calcium chloride or calcium gluconate in addition to IV anticonvulsants. For example, management of symptomatic hypocalcemia can be treated with a slow IV bolus of 15 ml of 10% calcium gluconate solution followed by a slow IV infusion (10 ml/h) of 10% calcium gluconate solution. Because concentrated calcium solutions are very irritating, the calcium gluconate solution is often diluted. When giving IV calcium, cardiac monitoring should be done, particularly if the patient is on digitalis. Coexisting electrolyte abnormalities, like hypomagnesemia or hyperphosphatemia, should be addressed.

Hypercalcemia

The most prominent neurological manifestation of hypercalcemia is decreased sensorium leading to stupor and coma. Psychiatric symptomatology may precede the onset of obtundation. Easy fatigability and muscle weakness often accompany CNS symptoms. Convulsions, either generalized or focal, can also occur in hypercalcemia. The most common cause of hypercalcemia in the general population is primary hyperparathyroidism. Hyperparathyroidism is usually chronic and relatively benign. However, acute seizures and coma, as part of a "parathyroid storm," have been described *(105,106)*. Hypercalcemia is a complication of many types of malignancy and can produce an oncological emergency *(107,108)*. In children with solid tumors and hypercalcemia, focal seizures may occur *(109)*. In uremic patients, the presence of dysarthria, seizures, myoclonic jerks, and behavioral and sensorium abnormalities suggests dialysis dementia. However, in a few patients, this constellation of signs and symptoms has been attributed to hypercalcemia associated with renal disease *(110)*. Lithium occasionally causes hypercalcemia that may be related to increased humoral concentrations of parathyroid hormone *(111)*. Immobilization hypercalcemia is a rare cause of hypercalcemic seizures *(112)*.

Pathophysiology of Hypercalcemic Seizures

Electroencephalographic abnormalities can occur before clinical manifestations in hypercalcemia. These abnormalities consist of nonspecific slowing of the background and the presence of intermittent rhythmic delta activity. At the cellular level, increases in extracellular calcium reduce the tendency toward multiple spiking in hippocampal slices *(113)*. Because of this finding, the development of seizures in the face of increased rather than decreased extracellular calcium remains a paradox.

Treatment of Hypercalcemic Seizures

The seizures associated with hypercalcemia are usually controlled with its reversal. Severe hypercalcemia is a medical emergency when neurological manifestations are present. IV fluids are crucial in the treatment of hypercalcemia. Dialysis may also be necessary to lower serum calcium in some situations. Seizures should also be treated with standard anticonvulsants.

Concluding Remarks

Electrolyte abnormalities are generally rare causes of seizures. The presence of a severe electrolyte abnormality in the setting of a new-onset seizure does not invariably imply a causal relationship. Consequently, vigilance for other potential causes of seizures is always recommended.

References

1. Riggs JE. Neurologic manifestations of fluid and electrolyte disturbances. *Neurol Clin* 1989;7:509–523.
2. Daggett P, Deanfield J, Moss F. Neurological aspects of hyponatremia. *Postgrad Med J* 1982;58:737–740.
3. Ellis SJ. Severe hyponatremia: complications and treatment. *Q J Med* 1995;8:905–909.
4. Arieff AI, Llach F, Massry SG. Neurological manifestations and morbidity of hyponatremia: correlation with brain water and electrolytes. *Medicine* 1976;55:121–129.
5. Wijdicks EFM, Sharbrough FW. New-onset seizures in critically ill patients. *Neurology* 1993;43:1042–1044.
6. Cohen BJ, Jordan MH, Chapin SD, Cape B, Laureno R. Pontine myelinolysis after correction of hyponatremia during burn resuscitation. *J Burn Care Rehabil* 1991;12:153–156.
7. Tierney WM, Martin DK, Greenlee MC, Zerbe RL, McDonald CJ. The prognosis of hyponatremia at hospital admission. *J Gen Intern Med* 1986;1:380–385.
8. Hauser WA, Annegers JF, Kurland, LT. Incidence of epilepsy and unprovoked seizures in Rochester, Minnesota: 1935–1984. *Epilepsia* 1993;34:453–468.
9. Landfish N, Gieron-Korthals M, Weibley RE, Panzarino V. New onset childhood seizures. Emergency department experience. *J Fla Med Assoc* 1992;79:697–700.
10. Corneli HM, Gormley CJ, Baker RC. Hyponatremia and seizures presenting in the first two years of life. *Pediatr Emerg Care* 1985;1:190–193.
11. Hugen CA, Oudesluys-Murphy AM, Hop WC. Serum sodium levels and probability of recurrent febrile convulsions. *Eur J Pediatr* 1995;154:403–405.
12. Farrar HC, Chande VT, Fitzpatrick DF, Sherma SJ. Hyponatremia as the cause of seizures in infants: a retrospective analysis of incidence, severity, and clinical predictors. *Ann Emerg Med* 1995;26:42–48.
13. Keating JP, Schears GJ, Dodge PR. Oral water intoxication in infants. An American epidemic. *Am J Dis Child* 1991;145:985–990.
14. Grant CC, Rive SJ, Duncan KM. Water intoxication secondary to incorrectly mixed infant formula. *NZ Med J* 1994;107:359–360.
15. Bruce RC, Kliegman RM. Hyponatremic seizures secondary to oral water intoxication in infancy: association with commercial drinking water. *Pediatrics* 1997;100:1024–1025.
16. Tilelli JA, Ophoven JP. Hyponatremic seizures as a presenting symptom of chid abuse. *Forensic Sci Int* 1986;30:213–217.
17. Donoghue MB, Latimer ME, Pillsbury HL, Hertzog JH. Hyponatremic seizures in a child using desmopressin for nocturnal enuresis. *Arch Pediatr Adolesc Med* 1998;152:930–931.
18. Bennett HJ, Wagner T, Fields A. Acute hyponatremia and seizures in an infant after a swimming lesson. *Pediatrics* 1983;72:125–127.
19. Noakes TD. The hyponatremia of exercise. *Int J Sport Nutr* 1992;2:205–228.
20. Hope SA, Foote KD. Morbidity from excessive intake of high energy fluids; the 'squash drinking syndrome.' *Arch Dis Child* 1995;73:277.
21. McKenna PJ, Kane JM, Parrish K. Psychotic syndromes in epilepsy. *Am J Psychiatry* 1985;142:895–904.

22. Vieweg WV, David JJ, Rowe WT, Peach MJ, Veldhuis JD, Kaiser DL, Spradlin WW. Psychogenic polydipsia and water intoxication—concepts that have failed. *Biol Psychiatry* 1985;20:1308–1320.
23. de Leon J, Dadvand M, Canuso C, Odom-White A, Stanilla J, Simpson GM. Polydipsia and water intoxication in a long-term psychiatric hospital. *Biol Psychiatry* 1996;40:28–34.
24. Verghese C, de Leon J, Josiassen RC. Problems and progress in the diagnosis and treatment of polydipsia and hyponatremia. *Schizophr Bull.* 1996;22:455–464.
25. Goldman MB, Robertson GL, Luchins DJ, Hedeker D, Pandey GN. Psychotic exacerbations and enhanced vasopressin secretion in schizophrenic patients with hyponatremia and polydipsia. *Arch Gen Psychiatry* 1997;54:443–449.
26. Siegler EL, Tamres D, Berlin JA, Allen-Taylor L, Strom BL. Risk factors for the development of hyponatremia in psychiatric inpatients. *Arch Intern Med* 1995;155:953–957.
27. Santonastaso P, Sala A, Favaro A. Water intoxication in anorexia nervosa: a case report. *Int J Eat Disord* 1998;24:439–442.
28. Yassa R, Iskandar H, Nastase C, Camille Y. Carbamazepine and hyponatremia in patients with affective disorder. *Am J Psychiatry* 1998;145:339–342.
29. Vieweg WV. Treatment strategies in the polydipsia-hyponatremia syndrome. *J Clin Psychiatry* 1994;55:154–160.
30. Johnson C, Webb L, Daley J, Spathis GS. Hyponatremia and Moduretic-grand mal seizures. *J Roy Soc Med* 1990;83:479–483.
31. Mead GM, Arnold AM, Green JA, Macbeth FR, Williams CJ, Whitehouse JM. Epileptic seizures associated with cisplatin administration. *Cancer Treat Rep* 1982;66:1719–1722.
32. Spigset O, Hedenmalm K. Hyponatremia and the syndrome of inappropriate antidiuretic hormone secretion (SIADH) induced by psychotropic drugs. *Drug Safety* 1995;12:209–225.
33. Goldstein L, Barker M, Segalll F, Asihene R, Balser S, Lautenbach D, McCoy M. Seizure and transient SIADH associated with sertraline. *Am J Psychiatry* 1996;153:732.
34. Subramanian D, Ayus JC. Case report: severe symptomatic hyponatremia associated with lisinopril therapy. *Am J Med Sci* 1992;303:177–179.
35. Williford SL, Bernstein SA. Intranasal desmopressin-induced hyponatremia. *Pharmacotherapy* 1996;16:66–74.
36. Shepherd LL, Hutchinson RJ, Worden EK, Koopmann CF, Coran A. Hyponatremia and seizures after intravenous administration of desmopressin acetate for surgical hemostasis. *J Pediatr* 1989;114:470–472.
37. McKenna P, Shaw RW. Hyponatremic fits in oxytocin-augmented labors. *Int J Gynaecol Obstet* 1979;17:250–252.
38. Kloster R, Borresen HC, Hoff-Olsen P. Sudden death in two patients with epilepsy and the syndrome of inappropriate antidiuretic hormone secretion (SIADH). *Seizure* 1998;7:419–420.
39. Tauzin-Fin P, Sanz, L. Prostate transurethral resection syndrome. *Ann Fr Anesth Reanim* 1992;11:168–177.
40. Clement P, Paulet C. Resorption of the lavage fluid during transurethral resection of the prostate. Apropos of 13 cases. *Ann Urol (Paris)* 1990;24:565–568.
41. Mahul P, Molliex S, Auboyer C, et al. Neurotoxic role of glycocolle and derivatives in transurethral resection of the prostate. *Ann Fr Anesth Reanim* 1993;12:512–514.

42. Rothenberg DM, Berns AS, Ivankovich AD. Isotonic hyponatremia following transurethral prostate resection. *J. Clin. Anesthesiol.* 1990;2:48–53.
43. Yamaki T, Tano-oka A, Takahashi A, Imaizumi T, Suetake K, Hashi K. Cerebral salt wasting syndrome distinct from the syndrome of inappropriate secretion of antidiuretic hormone (SIADH). *Acta Neurochir. (Wien)* 1992;115:156–162.
44. Atkin SL, Coady AM, White MC, Mathew B. Hyponatremia secondary to cerebral salt wasting syndrome following routine pituitary surgery. *Eur. J. Endocrinol.* 1996;135:245–247.
45. Hasan D, Schonck RS, Avezaat CJ, Tanghe HL, van Gijn J, van der Lugt PJ. Epileptic seizures after subarachnoid hemorrhage. *Ann Neurol* 1993;33:286–291.
46. Fox JL, Falik JL, Shalhoub RJ. Neurosurgical hyponatremia: the role of inappropriate antidiuresis. *J Neurosurg* 1971;34:506–514.
47. Kroll M, Juhler M, Lindholm J. Hyponatremia in acute brain injury. *J Intern Med* 1992;232:291–297.
48. Harrigan MR. Cerebral salt wasting syndrome: a review. *Neurosurgery* 1996;38:152–160.
49. Nelson PB, Seif SM, Maroon JC, Robinson AG. Hyponatremia in intracranial disease: perhaps not the syndrome of inappropriate secretion of antidiuretic hormone (SIADH). *J Neurosurg* 1981;55:938–941.
50. Isotani E, Susuki R, Tomita K, et al. Alterations in plasma concentrations of natriuretic peptides and antidiuretic hormone after subarachnoid hemorrhage. *Stroke* 1994;25:2198–2203.
51. Uygun MA, Ozkal E, Acar O, Erongun U. Cerebral salt wasting syndrome. *Neurosurg Rev* 1996;19:193–196.
52. Ayus JC, Wheeler JM, Arieff AI. Postoperative hyponatremic encephalopathy in menstruant women. *Ann Intern Med* 1992;117:891–897.
53. Wijdicks EF, Larson TS. Absence of postoperative hyponatremia syndrome in young women. *Ann Neurol* 1994;38:696–697.
54. Andrew RD. Seizure and acute osmotic change: clinical and neurophysiological aspects. *J Neurol Sci* 1991;101:7–18.
55. Dudek FE, Obenaus A, Tasker JG. Osmalality-induced changes in extracellular volume alter epileptiform bursts independent of chemical synapses in the rat: importance of non-synaptic mechanisms in hippocampal epileptogenesis. *Neurosci Lett* 1990;120:267–270.
56. Saly V, Andrew RD. CA3 neuron excitation and epileptiform discharge are sensitive to osmolality. *J Neurophysiol* 1993;69:2200–2208.
57. Schwarzkroin PA, Baraban SC, Hochman DW. Osmolarity, ionic flux and changes in brain excitability. *Epilepsy Res.* 1998;32:275–285.
58. Palevsky PM. Hypernatremia. *Semin Nephrol* 1998;18:20–30.
59. Snyder NA, Feigal DW, Arieff AI. Hypernatremia in elderly patients. A heterogeneous, morbid, and iatrogenic entity. *Ann Intern Med* 1987;107:309–319.
60. Palevsky PM, Bhagrath R, Greenberg A. Hypernatremia in hospitalized patients. *Ann Intern Med* 1996;124:197–203.
61. Moder KG, Hurley DL. Fatal hypernatremia from exogenous salt intake: report of a case and review of the literature. *Mayo Clin Proc* 1990;65:1587–1594.
62. Hogan GR. Hypernatremia—problems in management. *Pediatr Clin North Am* 1976;23:569–574.
63. Mercier JC, Outin S, Paradis K, et al. Breast feeding and hypernatremic dehydration. 3 case studies. *Arch Fr Pediatr* 1986;43:465–470.

64. Farley PC, Lau KY, Suba S. Severe hypernatremia in a patient with psychiatric illness. *Arch Intern Med* 1986;146:1214–1215.

65. Sadat A, Paulman PM, Mathews M. Hypernatremia in the elderly. *Am Fam Physician* 1989;40:125–128.

66. Hogan GR, Pickering LK, Dodge PR, Shepard JB, Master S. Incidence of seizures that follow rehydration of hypernatremic rabbits with intravenous glucose or fructose solutions. *Exp Neurol* 1985;87:249–259.

67. Kahn A, Blum D, Casimir G, Brachet E. Controlled fall in natremia in hypertonic dehydration: possible avoidance of rehydration seizures. *Eur J Pediatr* 1981;135:293–296.

68. Go M, Amino A, Shindo K, Tsunoda S, Shiozawa Z. A case of central pontine myelinolysis and extrapontine myelinolysis during rapid correction of hypernatremia. *Rinsho Shinkeigaku* 1994;34:1130–1135.

69. Workman ML. Magnesium and phosphorus: the neglected electrolytes. *AACN Clin Issues Crit Care Nurs* 1992;3:655–663.

70. Whang R, Hampton EM, Whang DD. Magnesium homeostasis and clinical disorders of magnesium deficiency. *Ann Pharmacother* 1994;28:220–226.

71. Tso EL, Barish RA. Magnesium: clinical considerations. *J Emerg Med* 1992;10:735–745.

72. Kingston ME, Al-Siba'i MB, Skooge WC. Clinical manifestations of hypomagnesemia. *Crit Care Med* 1986;14:950–954.

73. Langley WF, Mann D. Central nervous system magnesium deficiency. *Arch Intern Med* 1991;151:593–596.

74. Nakamura M, Abe S, Goto Y, Chishaki A. Sudden sound-induced death in magnesium-deficient rats after repetitive episodes of seizures result from brain dysfunction. *Magnes Res* 1995;8:47–53.

75. Nuytten D, Van Hees J, Meulemans A, Carton H. Magnesium deficiency as a cause of acute intractable seizures. *J Neurol* 1991;238:262–264.

76. Flink EB. Magnesium deficiency. Etiology and clinical spectrum. *Acta Med Scand Suppl* 1981;647:125–137.

77. Whang R. Routine serum magnesium determination—a continuing unrecognized need. *Magnesium* 1987;6:1–4.

78. Reinhart RA, Desbiens NA. Hypomagnesemia in patients entering the ICU. *Crit Care Med* 1985;13:506–507.

79. Ryzen E, Servis KL, Rude RK. Effect of intravenous epinephrine on serum magnesium and free intracellular red blood cell magnesium concentrations measured by nuclear magnetic resonance. *J Am Coll Nutr* 1990;9:114–119.

80. Shalev H, Phillip M, Galil A, Carmi R, Landau D. Clinical presentation and outcome in primary familial hypomagnesemia. *Arch Dis Child* 1998;78:127–130.

81. Lynch BJ, Rust RS. Natural history and outcome of neonatal hypocalcemic and hypomagnesemic seizures. *Pediatr Neurol* 1994;11:23–27.

82. Sutton RA, Domrongkitchaiporn S. Abnormal renal magnesium handling. *Miner Electrolyte Metab* 1993;19:232–240.

83. Stewart AF, Keating T, Schwartz PE. Magnesium homeostasis following chemotherapy with cisplatin: a prospective study. *Am J Obstet Gynecol* 1985;153:660–665.

84. Schmickaly R, Nickel B, Jarisch M, Kursawe HK, Sachs E, Karson A. Electrolyte disorders, EEG changes and epileptic seizures in alcohol withdrawal delirium. *Psychiatr Neurol Med Psychol (Leipzig)* 1989;41:722–729.

85. al-Ghamdi SM, Cameron EC, Sutton R. Magnesium deficiency: pathophysiologic and clinical overview. *Am J Kidney Dis* 1994;24:737–752.

86. Nakamura M, Abe S, Goto Y, Chishaki A, Akazawa K, Kato M. In vivo assessment of prevention of white-noise-induced seizure in magnesium-deficient rats with N-methyl-D-aspartamate receptor blockers. *Epilepsy Res* 1994;17:249–256.

87. Nowak L, Bregestovski P, Ascher P, Herbet A, Prochiantz A. Magnesium gates glutamate-activated channels in mouse central neurones. *Nature* 1984;307:462–465.

88. Curras MC, Pallotta BS. Single-channel evidence for glycine and NMDA requirement in NMDA receptor activation. *Brain Res* 1996;740:27–40.

89. Morris ME. Brain and CSF magnesium concentrations during magnesium deficit in animals and humans: neurological symptoms. *Magnes Res* 1992;5:303–313.

90. Buck DR, Mahoney AW, Hendricks DG. Preliminary report on the magnesium deficient rat as a model of epilepsy. *Lab Anim Sci* 1978;28:680–685.

91. Bac P, Tran G, Paris M, Binet P. Characteristics of the audiogenic convulsive crisis in mice made sensitive by magnesium deficiency. *CR Acad Sci III* 1993; 316:676–681.

92. Bac P, Maurois P, Dupont C, et al. Magnesium deficiency-dependent audiogenic seizures (MDDASs) in adult mice: a nutritional model for discriminatory screening of anticonvulsant drugs and original assessment of neuroprotection properties. *J Neurosci* 1998;18:4363–4373.

93. Dreier JP, Heinemann U. Late low magnesium-induced epileptiform activity in rat entorhinal cortex slices becomes insensitive to the anticonvulsant valproic acid. *Neurosci Lett* 1990;119:68–70.

94. Michaelis ML, Michaelis EK. Effects of ethanol on NMDA receptors in brain: possibilities for MG(2+)-ethanol interactions. *Alcohol Clin Exp Res* 1994; 18:1069–1075.

95. Fong J, Gurewitsch ED, Volpe L, Wagner WE, Gomillion MC, August P. Baseline serum and cerebrospinal fluid magnesium levels in normal pregnancy and preeclampsia. *Obstet Gynecol* 1995;85:444–448.

96. Alfrey AC, Terman DS, Brettschneider L. Hypermagnesemia after renal homotransplantation. *Ann Intern Med* 73:367–371.

97. Somjen G, Hilmy M, Stephen CR. Failure to anesthetize human subjects by intravenous administration of magnesium sulfate. *J Pharmacol Exp Ther* 1996; 154:652–659.

98. Riaz M, Porat R, Brodsky NL, Hurt H. The effects of maternal magnesium sulfate treatment on newborns: a prospective controlled study. *J Perinatol* 1998; 18:449–454.

99. Whang R, Whang DD, Ryan MP. Refractory potassium repletion. A consequence of magnesium deficiency. *Arch Intern Med* 1992;152:40–45.

100. Stringer JL, Lothman EW. Epileptiform discharges induced by altering extracellular potassium and calcium in the rat hippocampal slice. *Exp Neurol* 1988;101:146–157.

101. Ryan SG. Ion channels and the genetic contribution to epilepsy. *J Child Neurol* 1999;14:58–66.

102. Nagashima C, Kubota S. Parathyroid epilepsy with continuous EEG abnormality. *Clin Electroencephalogr* 1981;12:133–138.

103. Haas HL, Jefferys JG. Low-calcium field burst discharges of CA1 pyramidal neurones in rat hippocampal slices. *J Physiol (London)* 1984;354:185–201.

104. Yaari Y, Konnerth A, Heinemann U. Spontaneous epileptiform activity of CA 1 hippocampal neurons in low extracellular calcium solutions. *Exp Brain Res* 1983;51:153–156.
105. Sallman A, Goldberg M, Wombolt D. Secondary hyperparathyroidism manifesting as acute pancreatitis and status epilepticus. *Arch Intern Med* 1981;141:1549–1550.
106. Bayat-Mokhtari F, Palmieri GM, Moinuddin M, Pourmand R. Parathyroid storm. *Arch Intern Med* 1980;140:1092–1095.
107. Markman J. Common complications and emergencies associated with cancer and its therapy. *Cleve Clin J Med* 1994;61:105–114.
108. Silverman P, Distelhorst CW. Metabolic emergencies in clinical oncology. *Semin Oncol* 1989;16:504–515.
109. Leblanc A, Hartmann O, Pons G, Caillaud JM, Couanet D, Lenoir G, Lemerle J. Hypercalcemia associated with tumors in children. 20 cases. *Arch Fr Pediatr* 1984;41:551–555.
110. Rivera-Vazquez AB, Noriega-Sanchez A, Ramirez-Gonzalez R, Martinez-Maldonado M. Acute hypercalcemia in hemodialysis patients: distinction from 'dialysis dementia.' *Nephron* 1980;25:243–246.
111. Komatsu M, Shimizu H, Tsuruta T, et al. Effect of lithium on serum calcium level and parathyroid function in manic-depressive patients. *Endocr J* 1995;42:691–695.
112. Hauser GJ, Gale AD, Fields AI. Immobilization hypercalcemia: unusual presentation with seizures. *Pediatr Emerg Care* 1989;5:105–107.
113. Stringer JL, Lothman EW. In vitro effects of extracellular calcium concentration on hippocampal pyramidal cell responses. *Exp Neurol* 1988;101:132–146.

7

Seizures and Endocrine Disorders

Cormac A. O'Donovan, MD and Ramel A. Carlos, MD

Introduction

Derangement in endocrine homeostasis can result in many different neurological signs and symptoms *(1)*. Seizures are a common neurological presentation of changes in endocrine function **(Table 1),** which may be difficult to control until the underlying etiology is uncovered and addressed. Hypoglycemia and hyperglycemia are important common defects of endocrine disorders encountered in clinical practice *(2,3)*. Glucose is the primary energy substrate of the brain, and any disturbance of normal glucose concentration may cause altered cerebral function and result in irreversible neuronal damage if the process is prolonged. Seizures may also occur as a result of electrolyte imbalance secondary to primary endocrine disorders, such as hypocalcemia *(4)* from hypoparathyroidism and hyponatremia from primary adrenal insufficiency *(5)*. Recognition and correction of the underlying metabolic disturbance are of utmost importance in the management of such cases **(Table 2).**

Seizures and Hypothalamic–Pituitary Adrenal Axis

The mechanism of the effects of seizures on the hypothalamic–pituitary axis is unknown. Changes in the levels of pituitary hormones are known to occur after different types of seizures. Prolactin (PRL) elevation occurs most frequently after generalized tonic-clonic seizures but also after complex partial seizures and, to a lesser extent, with simple partial seizures. This change in serum PRL does not appear to occur after multiple seizures. Seizures of extratemporal origin are less likely to produce elevated PRL, suggesting that the limbic pathway has an important role in PRL elevation. Leuteinizing

From: *Seizures: Medical Causes and Management*
Edited by: N. Delanty © Humana Press, Inc., Totowa, NJ

Table 1
Different Types of Seizure and Overall Incidence in Patients with Endocrine Disorders

	Gen. Tonic Clonic[a]	Complex Partial[a]	Absence[a]	Akinetic[a]	Atonic[a]	Gazed Evoked[a]	Overall Incidence
Nonketotic Hyperglycemia	+ (10)	+ (3,11)	–	–	–	+ (12,13)	20–25% (2,15)
Hypoglycemia							
diabetes mellitus	+ (15)	+ (9)	–	–	–	–	7% (15)
hyperinsulinism	+ (28)	+ (23–25)	–	–	–	–	12% (28)
adrenal insufficiency	+ (38)	–	–	–	–	–	20% (38)
Hyperthyroidism	+ (47–49)	+ (47–49)	–	–	–	–	10% (47–49)
Hypothyroidism	+ (2,15)	+ (15)	–	–	–	–	20–25% (15)
Pheochromocytoma	+ (41)	+ (42)	–	–	–	–	5% (41,42)
Hypoparathyroidism	+ (63)	+ (15)	+ (15)	+ (15)	–	–	30–70% (63)
Hypothalamic Hamartoma	+ (71)	+ (77)	–	–	+ (75)	–	ND[b]

[a]Presence (+) or absence (–) of seizures. Reference citations are in parentheses.
[b](ND) no data.

Table 2
Response of Seizures to AEDs, Surgery, and Correction
of Metabolic Derangements in Endocrine Disorders

	Response to AEDs[a,b]	Response to Surgery[b]	Response to Endocrine Treatment[b]
Ketotic and nonketotic hyperglycemia	−	ND	+ Insulin and rehydration with 0.45% hypotonic solution *(1)*
Hypoglycemia diabetes mellitus	−	ND	+ IV glucose *(10)*
hyperinsulism	−	± *(29)* (pancreatectomy)	± IV glucose *(28)*
adrenal insufficiency	−	ND	+ Hydrocortisone *(1)*
Hyperthyroidism	−	ND	+ Antithyroid drugs (propylthiouracil [PTU], methimazole) *(1)*
Hypothyroidism	−	ND	+ Thyroid hormone (L-thyroxine) *(1)*
Pheochromocytoma	−	+ *(41)*	ND
Hypoparathyroidism	± *(15)*	ND	+ IV calcium *(15)*
Hypothalamic hamartoma	−	± *(77–80)*	ND

[a]AEDs = Antiepileptic drugs.
[b](+) Effective; (±) Variable; (−) Ineffective or refractory; (ND) no data.

hormone, adrenocorticotropic hormone, and growth hormone also show significant increases after a seizure *(6)*.

Seizures and Altered Glucose Levels

The difference in the effect of rapid changes in serum glucose level compared to the absolute serum glucose level in the causation of seizures is not known. Marked alteration of serum glucose level produces profound neurologic manifestations through many different mechanisms. Reversal of the deficit by correction of altered glycemia appears to be the primary determinant of clinical improvement. Anticonvulsants used at doses that control seizures in other clinical situations appear to be ineffective in treating seizures resulting from derangement of glucose levels. Impaired glucose transport across the blood–brain barrier during seizures may be a factor that causes seizures to persist. The reduction in transport of glucose across the blood–brain barrier during seizures suggests that cerebral glucose hypermetabolism during the ictus is independent of plasma glucose levels *(7)*. In animal models, seizures induced in the immature rat by hypoglycemia frequently cause focal brain lesions that are subsequently epileptogenic in the presence of normal serum glucose levels *(8)*.

Diabetes Mellitus

Diabetes mellitus is the most common cause of symptomatic hypoglycemia. Seizures occur in 7–20% of diabetic patients. Nonketotic hyperglycemia from diabetes mellitus may present with seizures that are unresponsive to anticonvulsants *(9)*. The presenting seizures are predominantly motor and include focal motor seizures and epilepsia partialis continua *(3)*, and status epilepticus *(10)*. The seizures may be induced by stimuli such as movement of a limb *(11)*. Gazed-evoked visual seizures have also been reported *(12,13)*. Neurological deficits, occurring in addition to the seizures, include speech arrest *(14)*, visual field defect, and hemiparesis but are usually transient *(15)*. Focal epileptiform and slow-wave disturbances are usually present on the electroencephalogram (EEG) and resolve with control of hypoglycemia *(13,14)*.

Seizures secondary to ketotic hyperglycemia are relatively rare compared to nonketotic hyperglycemia and occur mostly in severe cases *(11)*. Ketosis is thought to exert an anticonvulsant effect that is attributed to the production of γ-aminobutyric acid (GABA). The mechanism of increase in GABA production is related to the occurrence of intracellular acidosis, which enhances the activity of glutamic acid decarboxylase (GAD). This principle has been used in clinical practice through the use of ketogenic diet in intractable epilepsy *(2)*. Normalization of blood glucose level with insulin therapy and rehydration in ketotic hyperglycemia causes resolution of seizures *(11)*.

Hyperglycemia preceding ischemic insults to the brain results in exacerbation of ischemic brain damage *(16,17)* and postischemic generalized seizures *(16)*. Administration of insulin to hyperglycemic rats prior to induction of ischemia results in improved outcome. The induction of ischemia in hyperglycemic rats produces epileptiform activity on EEG that frequently progresses into status epilepticus *(17)*. The plasma glucose threshold at which hyperglycemic seizures are likely to occur is about 10–13 mmol/L (180–235 mg/100 ml). Glucose levels >16 mmol/L (290 mg/100 ml) are associated with seizures that result in high mortality *(18)*.

Hypoglycemia

Several endocrine disorders can lead to significant hypoglycemia, such as primary hypothalamic–pituitary insufficiency (growth hormone, adrenocorticotropic hormone, and thyroid stimulating hormone), primary adrenal insufficiency (Addison's disease), and primary hypothyroidism *(5)*. Seizures are the most common presenting neurological symptom of hypoglycemia at any age. Hypoglycemic seizures usually occur at serum glucose concentrations lower than 2.2 mmol/L (40 mg/100 ml) *(19)*.

Hypoglycemic episodes that occur with fasting and are associated with a blood glucose of less than 2.8 mmol/L (50 mg/100 ml), together with relief of symptoms following administration of intravenous glucose, constitute the Whipple's triad. These findings occur in cases of endogenous etiologies of hyperinsulinism, such as insulinomas. Insulinomas may present with hypoglycemic seizures *(20)* and are refractory to anticonvulsant medications *(21)*. These may present with nocturnal or early morning (fasting) complex partial seizures *(22–24)* and may be misdiagnosed as epilepsy *(25,26)*. In the early stages of hypoglycemic episodes secondary to insulinoma, the EEG shows slowing of background rhythms, progressing to generalized slowing in the delta range, if coma ensues. With the correction of hypoglycemia, the EEG returns to normal in minutes, but in severe cases, improvement may take hours to several days after symptoms are resolved *(27)*.

Islet cell dysfunction syndrome encompasses the diverse causes of persistent hyperinsulinemic hypoglycemia *(27,28)*. Histologically, the causes are described as islet cell hyperplasia, pancreatic adenomatosis, and nesidoblastoma *(27)*. Subtotal pancreatectomy is of limited value in control of glucose levels *(27)*, and near-total pancreatectomy has emerged as the procedure of choice *(28)*. Poorly controlled seizures occur in this condition and produce irreversible brain damage *(28,29)*. Hypoglycemia stimulates several neuroendocrine responses, such as secretion of glucagon, epinephrine, growth hormone, and cortisol *(30)*. The majority of signs and symptoms of hypoglycemia are attributed to excessive secretion of epinephrine. Neuroglycopenic episodes manifest as nervousness, hunger, flushed facies, headache, palpitation, anxiety, sweating, and trembling, in addition to seizure. Prolongation of the hypoglycemia produces confusion, focal neurological signs, and seizures. In diabetic subjects, the prodromal symptoms may not be manifest if severe neuropathy is present *(28)*.

Experimental and clinicopathological observations in postmortem studies of death resulting from hypoxia and hypoglycemia show comparable gross and microscopic findings in the brain suggestive of a common pathophysiology for these two conditions. The seizures occurring as a result of either insulin-induced hypoglycemia or hypoxia share a common pathway by disrupting cell membrane-bound Na^+K^+-activated ATPase and causing a net Na^+ influx into the brain. The resultant increase in sodium raises brain osmolality causing shifts from intracellular to extracellular space in the brain and producing cerebral edema. Other possible mechanisms of hypoglycemic coma are lack of specific energy-supplying substrate such as lactate and glutamate, which serve as the energy source for the brain under hypoglycemic conditions *(31)*.

Focal neurological deficits associated with hypoglycemia have been reported in children with and without diabetes mellitus. In those with diabetes mellitus, acute transient hemiplegia is believed to represent Todd's paralysis in the majority of cases due to unwitnessed seizures *(32)*. Patients with early onset diabetes and episodes of hypoglycemic convulsion are likely to show persistent electroencephalographic abnormalities *(32)*. The degree of metabolic control does not influence the occurrence of electroencephalographic findings during the early years of diabetes, but previous severe hypoglycemia and young age are important risk factors for permanent electroencephalographic abnormalities *(33)*. The effects of hypoglycemic and hyperglycemic seizures in the blood–brain barrier in rats show that blood–brain barrier dysfunction is worsened by electrographic seizures in moderately hypoglycemic animals *(34)*. Persistent memory deficits following seizures caused by hypoglycemia and other conditions may be secondary to disruption of cyclic AMP (cAMP) response element-binding protein (CREB)-dependent transcription. CREB is a critical factor for activation of protein synthesis required for long-term memory. In animal studies, hypoglycemia-induced seizures reduced CREB levels in the hippocampi of rats *(35)*. Acute starvation for 48–72 h increases seizure threshold. Increased ketone body formation is believed to be the pathway responsible for the elevation in seizure threshold *(36)*.

Hypoglycemia in diabetics taking prescribed insulin and oral hypoglycemic agents is common. This is the most significant adverse effect of sulfonylureas, such as chlorpropramide, which is frequently associated with severe and prolonged hypoglycemic episodes because of its long half-life *(37)*. Factitious hypoglycemia from either insulin or oral agents occurs as frequently as insulinoma. Newborns of mothers receiving these agents have been reported to have hypoglycemic episodes. Other drugs that can cause hypoglycemia are salicylates and propranolol. Salicylates can stimulate muscle glucose uptake, whereas propranolol presumably impairs glycogenolytic response and peripheral utilization. Propranolol may prevent recognition of impending hypoglycemia in diabetics by preventing epinephrine release and glucagon response to insulin-induced hypoglycemia *(10)*.

Adrenal Disorders

Hypoglycemia occurs in approximately one-fifth of children with primary adrenal insufficiency. Primary adrenocortical insufficiency or Addison's disease may present with hypoglycemic seizures *(38)* and cause fatalities in some cases *(39)*. Adrenal insufficiency may be clinically occult and present under certain situations such as surgery with the occurrence of symptomatic hyponatremia and seizures *(40)*. Seizures may occur in patients with pheochromo-cytoma. Generalized convulsions are the most common type and occur in synchrony with other symptoms of the disease. The degree of elevation of blood pressure seems to correlate with the occurrence of seizures in this condition *(41)*. Pheochromocytoma can present as complex partial seizures with prominent cardiovascular symptoms like "anginal pain" *(42)*. Hypoglycemia is rarely the initial manifestation of adrenocorticotropic hormone (ACTH) deficiency *(43)*. Hypoglycemic seizures and coma secondary to isolated ACTH deficiency have been reported in children but are uncommon in adults *(5)*.

Thyroid Disease

Thyroid disorders are usually associated with reversible neurologic signs and symptoms. Marked derangement of thyroid function may affect the nervous system and cause seizures *(44,45)*. Seizures occurring in patients with thyroid disease usually have underlying epilepsies and do not arise *de novo* in the hyperthyroid state *(46)*. Generalized and focal seizures can be seen in thyrotoxicosis and thyroid storm *(47–49)*. Coma, transient pyramidal tract signs, and mental status changes may also occur following these seizures. Approximately two-thirds of hyperthyroid patients exhibit abnormalities on EEGs. Generalized slow-wave activity, focal spike or slow waves, and triphasic waves may be seen. These abnormalities normalize after treatment of the hyperthyroidism *(46)*. The mechanism of the seizure activity in hyperthyroidism remains unclear. However, several theories have been proposed that include the direct effect of thyroxine on cerebral metabolism, changes in ion channels that regulate flow between intra- and extracellular compartments, and upregulation of catecholamine receptors *(50)*.

Seizures are an unusual manifestation of myxedema *(2)* and may be the presenting sign *(51)*. Other neurological manifestations such as encephalopathy and coma are reported more commonly *(49)*. In myxedema coma, as many as 20–25% of patients experienced generalized convulsions. Complex partial seizures have been reported. The EEG in most cases demonstrates minor abnormalities with decreased voltage and mild generalized slowing *(15)*. Treatment of the thyroid dysfunction can control seizures and revert the abnormal EEG and encephalopathy to normal *(46)*.

Hashimoto's encephalopathy is a steroid-responsive relapsing thyroid disorder accompanied by high titers of antithyroid antibodies *(52)*. Patients may be euthyroid or hypothyroid. This presents with seizures and diffuse EEG abnormalities *(53,54)*. Seizures may be generalized *(52,55)* or partial *(55,56)*. The most common EEG abnormalities include slowing, which is generalized, rhythmic bifrontal, or temporal *(57)*, triphasic waves, and periodic sharp waves *(58)*. Other clinical features are confusion, myoclonus, and tremors

(59). Myoclonus and tremors can be induced by thyrotropin-releasing hormone in a dose-dependent manner. These symptoms can be controlled effectively with thyroxine replacement therapy *(60).* Myoclonus can also be seen in hyperthyroidism and improve after treatment of the thyroid disorder *(61).* Thyroid antibodies are elevated in all patients. The occurrence of seizures is independent of the degree of thyroid dysfunction and may occur with only elevated antibodies. CSF analysis is abnormal in 60% of patients with CSF protein or leukocytes being mildly elevated and oligoclonal bands or increased immunoglobulin G (IgG) index present (59).

The pathophysiology of Hashimoto's encephalopathy remains speculative *(59,62).* Autoimmune cerebral vasculitis or an antineural antibody-mediated reaction has been suggested as the mechanism. Thyroid antibodies may represent an epiphenomenon of another autoimmune process. Several investigators have proposed a toxic effect of thyroid-releasing hormone on the central nervous system. The response to steroids further supports an autoimune mechanism *(59).*

Hypoparathyroidism

Seizures secondary to hypocalcemia in hypoparathyroidism are the most common neurological manifestation in children *(15)* and may be difficult to control *(63).* Such seizures occur in 30–70% of patients and may be generalized tonic-clonic *(64),* focal, and less frequently consist of atypical absence and akinetic attacks *(15).* EEG abnormalities may include generalized slowing or focal epileptiform discharges. With therapy, improvement in the EEG frequently lags behind seizure control *(15).* Late-onset seizures have been reported on patients who developed chronic hypoparathyroidism, many years after thyroidectomy *(65).* Some patients with familial hypoparathyroidism do not experience seizures, even those with severe hypocalcemia *(66).* In some cases, seizures may be intractable despite fair control of serum calcium level and are therefore thought to be secondary to calcinosis in the brain *(67).* Seizures secondary to hypoparathyroidism have been reported in Fahr syndrome *(68)* and children with 22q11 deletion *(69).* Neonatal convulsions caused by hypoparathyroidism can be secondary to maternal hyperparathyroidism *(70).*

Seizures and Hypothalamic Hamartoma

Hypothalamic hamartomas are benign malformations of the brain consisting of heterotropic nervous tissue *(71).* They contain neurosecretory cells that produce luteinizing hormone-releasing hormone (LHRH), which can cause precocious puberty *(72).* Gelastic seizures are the most common type of seizure occurring *(73–75)* but tonic-clonic seizures *(72)* and atonic seizures *(76)* have also been reported. The origin and the pathophysiology of the epileptic attacks are obscure *(77).* It has been suggested in the past that gelastic seizures are symptoms owing to temporal lobe involvement, but temporal resections have been ineffective in controlling seizures *(78)*. Recent electrophysiologic evidence suggests that the epileptogenic discharges may originate in the hamartoma itself *(76–79)*. Removal of the lesions alters the endocrinological status *(80)* and improves seizure control in some patients *(80,81)*. Anterior corpus callosotomy results in a significant reduction in drop attacks in few patients *(82)*.

Conclusions

Seizures are commonly encountered in individuals with endocrine disorders. Such seizures may be the presenting symptom of the disorder, and many different types of seizures occur. These seizures tend to be resistant to anticonvulsant treatment but are controlled with treatment of the underlying abnormality. Delay in the diagnosis and treatment of the underlying disease may cause increased morbidity and mortality from seizures.

References

1. Singer MM. Endocrine Emergencies. Med Clin North Am, 1971;55:1315–1329.
2. Gilmore RL. Seizures associated with nonneurologic medical conditions. *In The Treatment of Epilepsy: Principles and Practice,* Wyllie, E (ed), Williams and Wilkins, pp. 654–665.
3. Delanty N, Vaughan JA. Medical causes of seizures. *Lancet* 1998;352:383–390.
4. Panagariya A, Sharma A, Chhabria H. Hypoparathyroidism—presenting as uncontrolled seizures. *J Assoc Physicians India* 1990;38:442 (abstract).
5. Samaan NA. Hypoglycemia secondary to endocrine deficiencies. *Endocrinol Metab Clin N Am* 1989;18:145–153.
6. Schachter SC. Neuroendocrine aspects of epilepsy. *Neurol Clin* 1994;12:31–37.
7. Cornford EM, Olendorf WH. Epilepsy and the blood brain barrier. *Adv Neurol* 1986;44:787–812.
8. Wasterlain CG, Dwyer BE. Brain metabolism during prolonged seizures in neonates. *Adv Neurol* 1983;34:241–260.
9. Whiting S, Camfield P, Arab D, Salisbury S. Insulin-dependent diabetes mellitus presenting in children as frequent, medically unresponsive, partial seizures. *J Child Neurol* 1997;12:178–180.
10. Malouf R, Brust JC. Hypoglycemia: causes, neurological manifestations, and outcome. *Ann Neurol* 1985;1985:421–430.
11. Hennis A, Corbin D, Fraser H. Focal seizures and non-ketotic hyperglycemia. *J Neurol Neurosurg Psychiatry* 1992;55:195–197.
12. Harden CL, Rosenbaum DH, Daras M. Hyperglycemia presenting with occipital seizures. *Epilepsia* 1991;32:221–224.
13. Duncan MB, Jabbari B, Rosenberg ML. Gaze-evoked visual seizures in non-ketotic hyperglycemia. *Epilepsia* 1991;32:221–224.
14. Carril JM, Guijarro C, Portocarrero JS, et al. Speech arrest as manifestation of seizures in non-ketotic hyperglycemia. *Lancet* 1992;340:1227.

15. Messing RO, Simon RP. Seizures as a manifestation of systemic disease. *Neurol Clin* 1986;4:563–579.
16. Warner DS, Gionet TX, Todd MM, McAllister AM. Insulin-induced normoglycemia improves ischemic outcome in hyperglycemic rats. *Strokes* 1992;23:1775–1781.
17. Uchino H, Smith ML, Bengzon J, Lundgren J, Siesjo BK. Characteristics of post-ischemic seizures in hyperglycemic rats. *J Neurol Sci* 1996;139:21–27.
18. Li PA, Shamloo M, Smith ML, Katsura K, Sisjo BK. The influence of plasma glucose concentrations on ischemic brain damage is a threshold function. *Neurosci Lett* 1994;177:63–65.
19. Ehrlich RM. Hypoglycemia in infancy and childhood. *Arch Dis Child* 1971;46:716–719.
20. Doherty GM, Doppman JL, Shawker TH, et al. Results of a prospective strategy to diagnose, locate, and resect insulinomas. *Surg Gynecol Obstet* 1991;163:509–512.
21. Ginsberg-Fellner F, Rayfield EJ. Metabolic studies in a child with a pancreatic insulinomas. *Am J Diseases Child* 1980;134:64–67.
22. Katz LB, Aufses AH, Rayfield E, Mitty H. Preoperative localization and intraoperative glucose monitoring in the management of patients with pancreatic insulinoma. *Surg Gynecol Obstet* 1986;163:509–512.
23. Fowler DL, Wood WG, Kontz PG. Endogenous hyperinsulinism. *J Gastroenterol* 1980;74:321–327.
24. van Heerden JA, Edis AJ, Service FJ. The surgical aspects of insulinomas. *Ann Surg* 1979;189:677–682.
25. Bjerk HS, Kelly RE, Geffner ME, Fonkalsurd EW. Surgical management of islet cell dysmaturation syndrome in young children. *Surg Gynecol Obstet* 1990;171:321–325.
26. Desai MP, Khatri JV. Persistent hyperinsulinemic hypoglycemia of infancy. *Indian Pediatr* 1998;35:317–328.
27. Service FJ, Dale AJ, Jiang AS. Insulinoma. *Mayo Clin Proc* 1976;51:417–427.
28. Lovvorn HN, Nance ML, Ferry RJ, et al. Congenital hyperinsulinism and the surgeon: lessons learned over 35 years. *J Surg* 1999;34:786–792.
29. Telander RL, Wolf SA, Simmons PS, Zimmerman D, Haymond MW. Endocrine disorders of the pancreas and adrenal cortex in pediatric patients. *Mayo Clin Proc* 1986;61:459–466.
30. Chiarelli F, Verrotti A, Catino M, Sabatino G, Pinelli L. Hypoglycemia in children with type I diabetes mellitus. *Acta Paediatr* 1999;88:31–34.
31. Arieff AI, Doerner T, Zelig H, Massry S. Mechanisms of seizures and coma in hypoglycemia. *J Clin Invest* 1974;54:654–663.
32. Wayne EA, Booth F, Teenbein M. Focal neurologic deficits associated with hypoglycemia in children with diabetes. *J Pediatr* 1990;117:575–577.
33. Soltesz G, Ascadi G. Association between diabetes, severe hypoglycemia, and electroencephalogarphic abnormalities. *Arch Dis Child* 1989;64:992–996.
34. Oztas B, Camurcu S. Blood brain barrier permiability after electrically induced seizures in normoglycemic, hypoglycemic and hyperglycemic rats. *Psychiatry Res* 1989;29:151–159.
35. Panickar KS, Purushotham K, Rajakumar G, Simpkins W. Hypoglycemia-induced seizures reduce cyclic AMP response element binding protein levels in rat hippocampus. *Neuroscience* 1998;83:1155–1160.

36. De Vivo DC, Malas KL, Leckie MP. Starvation and seizures; observation of the electroconvulsive threshold and cerebral metabolism of the starved adult rat. *Arch Neurol* 1975;32:755–760.

37. Ferner, RE, Neil AJ, Jiang AS. Sulfonylureas and hypoglycemia, *Br Med J Clin Res Ed* 1988;296:949–950.

38. Ntyonga-Pono M.P. Addison's disease revealed by hypoglycemic convulsion. *Med Trop* 1997;57:311–312.

39. Samantray SK. Fatal hypoglycemia: the sole presentation of Addison's disease. *Med J Australia* 1977;2:304.

40. Agura ED. Seizure in a normal marrow donor: Addison's disease unmasked. *Bone Marrow Transplant* 1994;13:215–216.

41. Thomas ET, Rooke D, Kvale WE. The neurologist's experience with pheochromocytoma. *J Am Med Assoc* 1996;197:100–104.

42. Devinsky O, Price BH, Cohen SI. Cardiac manifestations of complex partial seizures. *Am J Med* 1986;80:195–202.

43. Ehrlich RM. Hypoglycemia in infancy and childhood. *Arch Dis Child* 1971; 46:716–719.

44. Tonner DR, Schlechte JA. Neurologic complications of thyroid and parathyroid disease. *Med Clin North Am* 1993;77:251–263.

45. Smith DL, Looney TJ. Seizures secondary to thyrotoxicosis and high dosage Propranolol therapy. *Arch Neurol* 1983;40:457–458.

46. Primavera A, Brusa G, Novello P. Thyrotoxic encephalopathy and recurrent seizures. *Eur Neurol* 1990;30:186–188.

47. Aiello DP, DuPlessis AJ, Pattishall AC, Kulin HE. Thyroid storm: presenting with coma and seizures in 13 year old girl. *Clin Pediatr* 1989;28:571–574.

48. Rangel-Guerra R, Martinez HR, Garcia-Hernandez P, et al. Epilepsy and thyrotoxicosis in a 4-year-old boy. *Revisita Invest Clin* 1992;44:109–113.

49. Radetti G, Dordi B, Mengarda G, Biscaldi I, Larizza D, Severi F. Thyrotoxicosis presenting with seizures and coma in two children. *Am J Dis Child* 1993;1147:925–927.

50. Tonner DR, Schlechte JA. Neurologic complications of thyroid and parathyroid disease. *Med Clin North Am* 1993;77:251–263.

51. Bryce GM, Poyner F. (1992) Myxoedema presenting with seizures. *Postgrad Med J* 1992;68:35–36.

52. Bostantjopoulou S, Zafiriou D, Katsarou Z, Kazis A. Hashimoto's encephalopathy: clinical and laboratory findings. *Functional Neurol* 1996;11:247–251.

53. Kothbauer-Margreiter I, Sturzenegger M, Komor J, Baugartner R, Hess CW. Encephalopathy associated with Hashimoto's thyroiditis: diagnosis and treatment. *J Neurol* 1996;243:585–593.

54. Henchey R, Cibula J, Helveston W, Malone J, Gilmore RL. Electroencephalographic findings in Hashimoto's encephalopathy. *Neurology* 1995;45:977–981.

55. Shaw PJ, Walls TJ, Newman PK, Cleland PG, Cartlidge NE. Hashimoto's encephalopathy: a steroid responsive disorder associated with high anti-thyroid antibody titers. *Neurology* 1991;41:228–233.

56. Ghika-Schmid F, Ghika J, Regli F, et al. Hashimoto's myoclonic encepahlopathy: an underdiagnosed treatable condition? *Movement Disorders* 1996;11:555–562.

57. Peschen-Rosib R, Schabet M, Dichgans J. Manifestation of Hashimoto's encephalopathy years before the onset of thyroid disease. *Eur Neurol* 1999;41:78–84.

58. Henchey R, Cibula J, Helveston W, Malone J, Gilmore RL. Electrographic findings in Hashimoto's encephalopathy. *Neurology* 1995;45:977–981.
59. Vanconcellos E, Pina-Garza JE, Fakhoury T, Fenichel GM. Pediatric Manifestations of Hashimoto's encephalopathy. *Pediatr Neurol* 1999;20:394–398.
60. Desai J, Wadai N. Hashimoto's encephalopathy. *J Neurol Sci* 1999;163:202–203.
61. Ishii K, Hayashi A, Tamaoka A, Usuki S, Mizusawa H, Shoji S. Case report: Thyrotropin releasing hormone induced myoclonus and tremor in a patient with Hashimoto's encepahlopathy. *Am J Med Sci* 1995;310:202–205.
62. Liao KK, Wang SJ, Lin KP, Tsai CP. Myoclonus associated with hyperthyroidism and thymoma; a case report. *Chinese Med J* 1993;51:138–140.
63. Panagariya A, Sharma A, Chhabria H. Hypoparathyroidism presenting as uncontrolled seizures. *J Assoc Physicians India* 1990;38:442.
64. Mithal A, Menon PS, Ammini AC, Karmarkar MG, Ahuja MM. Spontaneous hypoparathyroidism: clinical, biochemical and radiologic features. *Indian J Pediatr* 1989;56:267–272.
65. Reddy ST, Merrick RD. Hypoparathyroidism, intracranial calcification and seizures, 61 years after thyroid surgery. *Tenn Med* 1999;92:341–342.
66. Watanabe T, Bai M, Lane CR, et al. Familial hypoparathyroidism: identification of a novel gain of function mutation in transmembrane domain 5 of calcium-sensing receptor. *J Clin Endocrinol Metab* 1998;83:2497–2502.
67. Fulop M, Zeifer B. Case report: extensive brain calcification in hypoparathyroidism. *Am J Med Sci* 1991;302:292–295.
68. el Maghraoui A, Birouk N, Zaim A, Slassi I, Yahyaoui M, Chkili T. Fahr syndrome and dysparathyroidism. 3 cases. *Presse Med* 1995;24:1301–1304.
69. Scire G, Dallapiccola B, Iannetti P, et al. Hypoparathyroidism as the major manifestation in two patients with 22q11 deletions. *Am J Med Genet* 1994;52:478–482.
70. Brisse F, Breton D, Gagey V, Cheron G. Convulsions and neonatal hypoparathyroidism revealing maternal hyperparathyroidism. *Archiv Pediatr* 1994;1:255–259.
71. Commentz JC, Helmke K. Precocious puberty and decreased melatonin secretion due to a hypothalamic hamartoma. *Hormone Res* 1995;44:271–275.
72. Machachoklertwattana P, Kaplan SL, Grumbach MM. The luteinizing hormone-releasing hormone-secreting hypothalamic hamartoma is a congenital malformation: natural history. *J Clin Endocrinol Metab* 1993;77:118–124.
73. Valdueza JM, Cristante L, Dammann O, et al. Hypothalamic hamartomas: with special reference to gelastic epilepsy and surgery. *Neurosurgery* 1994;34:949–958.
74. Acilona Echevarria V, Casado Chocan JL, et al. Gelastic seizures, precocious puberty and hypothalamic hamartomas: a case report and the contributions of Single Photon Emission Computed Tomography (SPECT). *Neurologia* 1994;9:61–64 (abstract).
75. Minns RA, Stirling HF, Wu FC. Hypothalamic hamartoma with skeletal deformities, gelastic epilepsy, and precocious puberty. *Dev Med Child Neurol* 1994;26:173–176.
76. Munari C, Kahane P, Francione S, et al. Role of hypothalamic hamartoma in the genesis of gelastic fits (a video-stereo-EEG study). *Electroencephalogr Clin Neurophysiol* 1995;95:154–160.
77. Kuzniecky R, Gurthrie B, Mountz J, Faught E, Gilliam F, Liu HG. Intrinsic epileptogenesis of hypothalamic hamartomas in gelastic epilepsy. *Ann Neurol* 1998;43:273–275.
78. Tasch E, Cendes F, Li LM, et al. Hypothalmaic hamartomas and gelastic epilepsy: a spectroscopic study. *Neurology* 1998;51:1046–1050.

79. Arroyo S, Santamria J, Sanmari F, et al. Ictal laughter associated with paroxysmal hypothalamopituitary dysfunction. *Epilepsia* 1997;38:114–117.
80. Nishio S, Fujiwara S, Aiko Y, Takeshita I, Fukui M. Hypothalamic hamartoma. Report of two cases. *J Neurosurg* 1989;70:640–645.
81. Georgakoulias N, Vize C, Jenkins A, Singounas E. Hypothalamic hamartoma causing epilepsy: two cases and a review of the literature. *Seizure* 1998;7:167–171.
82. Cascino GD, Andermann F, Berkovic SF, et al. Gelastic seizures and hypothalamic hamartomas: evaluation of patients undergoing chronic intracranial EEG monitoring and outcome of surgical treatment. *Neurology* 1993;43:747–750.

8

Seizures, Fever, and Systemic Infection

Kevin Murphy, MRCPI and Henry Fraimow, MD

Introduction

The concurrence of fever and seizure in a patient raises many questions, the most immediate and important being whether or not the patient has an infection. If present, infection may either be intrinsic to the central nervous system (CNS), may have spread to the CNS from a systemic source, or may remain extracranial. About 5% of patients with CNS infections experience an acute symptomatic seizure *(1,2)*. Infections of the CNS account for about 15% of all acute symptomatic seizures *(1,3)*. Fever can occur for reasons other than infection, including inflammatory and connective tissue disorders, tumors, heat stroke, tissue ischemia, reactions to therapeutic drug use and vaccinations, drugs of abuse (such as ecstasy, amphetamines, and cocaine), factitious fever, and that of unknown origin. Rarely, primary lesions of the hypothalamic thermoregulatory center may lead to fever. Importantly, fever can also occur following prolonged convulsive activity in the absence of infection. In a retrospective study of the temperature curves of patients hospitalized after a seizure, Wachtel et al. found that 43% were febrile during their hospital course *(4)*. Although no underlying infection was identified in two-thirds of these patients, fever persisting beyond 48 h after the seizure was a sensitive (100%) and specific (89%) indicator of infection. Furthermore, infection can result from a seizure (e.g., aspiration pneumonia), or be nosocomially acquired.

Although fever and infection commonly occur together, they are not synonymous. In practice, it is difficult to separate the clinical and pathological effects of fever from infection, at least in the acute phase. Fever, as one of the most common acute phase responses to infection, trauma, and other injuries, is not only a state of altered temperature but involves a variety of cellular and humoral defense responses *(5)*. The mechanism by which fever is induced by

From: *Seizures: Medical Causes and Management*
Edited by: N. Delanty © Humana Press, Inc., Totowa, NJ

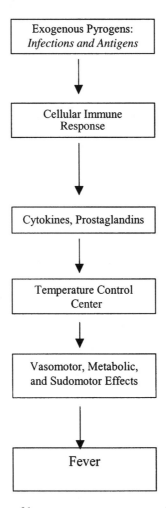

Fig. 1. Summary of how exogenous pyrogen induces fever *(5)*.

an exogenous pyrogen is complicated, not completely understood and involves a cascade of chemical responses **(Fig. 1).** This fever cascade is closely related to, and interwoven with, the pathogenetic sequence of events involved in the systemic inflammatory response to infection. This systemic inflammatory response syndrome (SIRS) involves activation of cytokine, complement, and coagulation cascades, resulting in structural and chemical changes that can lead to multiple organ system failure and death **(Fig. 2)** *(6)*. The release of mediators depends primarily on the severity of the infection and secondarily on the activation of the various cascades.

The possible clinical implications of, and relationships between, seizures, fever, and infection are diverse. In this chapter, we review the possible mechanisms whereby fever and systemic infection may cause neuronal injury and seizures. As the closest available in vivo paradigm of this subject, the clinical

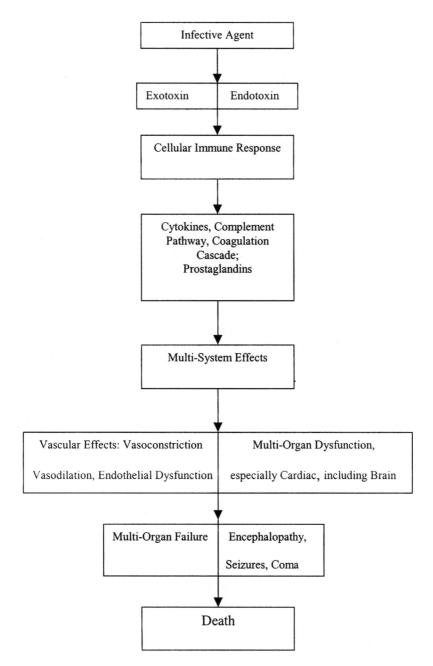

Fig. 2. How infection induces multi-organ failure, shock and death *(6)*.

phenomenon of febrile convulsions in children will be reviewed in some detail. In describing an approach to the patient who presents with seizures, fever, and possible infection, we discuss the clinical examples of human immunodeficiency virus (HIV) infection, cerebral abscess, and infective endocarditis to illustrate our subject matter.

Pathophysiology of Brain Injury in Fever and Infection

How Does Fever Damage the Brain and Cause Seizures? (see Definition of Terms)

The limited human studies available indicate that hyperthermia (and fever) can lead to initially reversible functional changes that may in turn produce anatomicopathological changes. Functionally, for example, somatosensory-evoked potentials disappear during sustained hyperthermia and reappear as the temperature drops *(15)*. Pathological studies of the human brain in fever are rare. Human neuropathological changes in fever are likely to be similar to those of patients who die from hyperthermia; however, such studies are also rare. Malamud et al. performed a clinicopathological study of heat stroke in 125 fatal cases in 1946, finding diffuse neuronal swelling and loss, glial proliferation, and microhemorrhages *(16)*. These changes were less marked in the white matter and basal ganglia.

Using a rat model to investigate the effects of whole body hyperthermia on brain function, Sharma et al. demonstrated that heat stress induced a selective increase in the permeability of the blood–brain barrier (BBB), a reduction in cerebral blood flow not correlated with the BBB changes, and regional brain edema, especially in the hippocampus *(8)*. Pathological and electron microscopic studies showed neuronal cell loss (especially in the hippocampal CA4 subfield), glial changes, myelin vesiculation, swollen synapses and axons, along with a selective increase in permeability in tight junctions and the microvasculature. Interestingly, young rats were more susceptible than adult rats to the changes induced by heat stress. The mechanisms underlying cellular injury in heat stress were similar to those following various types of CNS insults, such as ischemia, hypoxia, and trauma. In rats with neuronal migration disorders, hyperthermia resulted in hippocampal pyramidal cell loss independent of seizure activity, the extent of neuronal damage correlating positively with the duration of hyperthermia *(9)*.

Nevertheless, it is difficult to distinguish the effects on the brain of hyperthermia alone from the effects of hyperthermic seizures. In an immature rat model for febrile seizures, Toth et al. found that hyperthermic seizures, but not hyperthermia alone, resulted in numerous argyrophilic neurons in discrete regions of the limbic system within 24 h of seizures *(10)*. These physicochemical alterations, although transient, were profound and persisted for at least 2 wk. Pathological studies in rats who seized after exposure to a hot water jet on the head revealed ischemic changes in specific topographic areas like Sommer's sector in the hippocampus, layer 4 and 5 neurons of the cerebral cortex, and reticular neurons in the brain stem *(11)*. These pathological features were reminiscent of the human epileptic brain. Jiang et al. also found

Definition of Terms *(5,7)*

Fever is a state of raised core body temperature that is often part of a host's response to infection or other injury, causing activation of cold defense responses like skin vasoconstriction and shivering.

Hyperthermia is a state in which core temperature is above its set-range specified for the normal active state of the species, causing activation of heat defense responses like skin vasodilatation, sweating, and thermal panting.

Terminology: Fever and hyperthermia are two different conditions in which body temperature is raised above the normal range *(5,7)*. However, in the literature on fever, febrile convulsions (FCs) and hyperthermic brain injury, these terms are often used interchangeably, even synonymously *(8–14)*. For example, hyperthermia-induced seizures are the prototypical animal model for research in febrile seizures *(10–13)*. We also use the terms in a largely interchangeable way, distinguishing between them only in the interests of clarity.

a pattern of neurodegeneration similar to that observed in human temporal lobe epilepsy in rats who developed hyperthermia-induced status epilepticus *(12)*.

Although hyperthermia or fever may produce these pathological changes, the exact mechanisms producing neuronal injury and seizures are neither fully delineated nor understood. Many of the chemical mediators involved in the fever and SIRS cascades (**Figs. 1** and **2**) are known to affect neuronal function and excitability leading to neurological dysfunction and seizures. Disturbing the delicate balance between neuronal excitation and inhibition may lead to changes in ion channel function *(17)*. The activation of the *N*-methy-D-aspartate (NMDA) receptor has an important part in hyperthermia-induced seizures and kindling in rat models of febrile seizures *(13)*. Hypothermia may protect against glutamate and calcium toxicity *(18)*. Sharma et al. found increased plasma and brain serotonin level in heat-stressed rats *(14)*. Pretreating these rats with a serotonin synthesis inhibitor attenuated both the increased serotonin level and the increased BBB permeability induced by heat stress *(14)*. Kao and Lin also showed that brain serotonin depletion attenuated heat stroke-induced cerebral ischemia and cell death in rats *(19)*. Likewise, dopamine depletion protected striatal neurons from heat stroke-induced ischemia and cell death in rats *(20)*. Hyperthermia may disrupt mitochondrial function and facilitate the accumulation of oxygen species and free radicals *(21)*. Fever can disturb fluid and electrolyte balance in cerebrospinal fluid (CSF) and serum *(22)*. Although changes in CSF osmolality and electrolytes do not explain susceptibility to simple febrile seizures, hyponatremia may increase the risk for multiple convulsions during the same febrile illness *(23)*. Hypocarbia caused by fever-induced hyperpnea probably contributes to the generation of fever-induced seizures *(24)*. Although fever leads to an increase in CSF and blood glucose, even in the absence of seizures, this is probably not important in the genesis of febrile seizures *(25)*.

In summary, although the pathological data are limited and the exact pathogenesis is not fully understood, abnormal elevation of temperature can clearly disrupt brain function and, if prolonged, brain structure, leading to seizures.

How Do Infections Damage
the Brain and Cause Seizures?

Systemic infection can disrupt neuronal homeostasis in ways very similar to those just described for fever. However, infection without fever can damage the brain independently. The SIRS cascade (**Fig. 2**) is activated by many infections and involves many potent vascular and neurologic toxins. In severe adenoviral infection, for example, increases in interleukin 6 (IL6), IL8 and tumor necrosis α (TNF-α) factor are associated with hypoperfusion, febrile peaks, tonic-clonic seizures, and septic shock *(26)*. The neurotoxicity of bacterial products is illustrated in an animal model, whereby Shiga toxin and lipopolysaccharide (or endotoxin) together induced encephalopathy and seizures early in *Shigella* infections *(27)*. In some infections, the pathophysiology of CNS dysfunction and seizures remains unclear. In *Legionella pneumophilia* infection, for example, neurologic signs including seizures have been reported with usually unremarkable cranial computerized tomogram (CT) and CSF examinations, whereas neuropathological examination fails to demonstrate specific characteristics *(28,29)*.

The hemodynamic effects of infection, especially shock, can cause or exacerbate neuronal injury. Persistent hypotension, often combined with hypoxia, anemia, and multiple organ failure, worsens hypoxic-ischemic injury, especially to the hippocampus. Multiple organ failure of itself can lead to seizures. Clotting abnormalities, like disseminated intravascular coagulation (DIC), which are commonly seen in severe infections, can lead to cerebral hemorrhage or thrombosis, thereby precipitating seizures. Enteric verotoxin from *Escherichia coli* can cause the hemolytic uremic syndrome (HUS), which was associated with seizures in 17 out of 91 patients in one study *(30)*.

Numerous other metabolic abnormalities can exacerbate the neurological effects of infection. Pneumonia for example, can cause the syndrome of inappropriate antidiuretic hormone (SIADH) secretion, leading to hyponatremia and possibly seizures. Seizures have been reported secondary to hyponatremia in cholera *(31)*. Infection can also cause abnormalities of potassium, calcium, and magnesium, thereby predisposing to seizure occurrence *(17)*.

Systemic infection can also spread directly to the brain via the hematogenous route. Bacterial endocarditis can behave in this fashion. The CNS manifestations in such cases can be protean and include meningoencephalitis, septic embolic stroke, cerebritis, microabscesses, cerebral abscess, cerebral venous or sinus thrombosis, cerebral edema, mycotic aneurysms, and cerebral hemorrhage. Seizures occur either secondary to these manifestations or independently as a sign of systemic infection involving the brain.

In summary, there are potentially numerous direct and indirect mechanisms by which infection can disrupt brain function and structure, resulting in seizures.

Febrile Convulsions

The interesting and complex relationship between fever, infection, and seizures is well illustrated by the study of FCs in children. One of the difficulties surrounding the term FC has been its definition. Although at one time defined as "any seizure of cerebral origin which occurs in association with any feverish illness," *(32)* most investigators now do not regard FCs in children as being symptomatic of a known underlying neurological illness. The Commission on Epidemiology and Prognosis of the International League Against Epilepsy (ILAE) defined FC as "an epileptic seizure . . . occurring in childhood after age 1 mo, associated with a febrile illness not caused by an infection of the CNS, without previous neonatal seizures or a previous unprovoked seizure, and not meeting criteria for other acute symptomatic seizures" *(33)*. Simple FCs are those that last for less than 15 min and are generalized. Complex FCs are those that are partial, prolonged, or recurrent within 24 h. In the clinical setting, any child with a convulsion and fever cannot initially be assumed to have only a FC, as other more sinister causes of acute symptomatic seizures must be excluded. For this reason, the Royal College of Physicians in London distinguished between FCs and "convulsions with fever," the latter term including any convulsion in a child of any age with fever of any cause *(34)*. FCs are not like other acute symptomatic seizures because they are familial, have a unique age specificity, are common, universal, and have a largely benign outcome *(35)*. These unique features, however, have allowed the syndrome to be studied extensively.

Epidemiology of FCs

The refinement of the definition, along with the results of large, prospective, population-based studies, gives a more balanced view of the outcome of FCs compared to earlier studies, which were retrospective, hospital and tertiary referral center-based, and over-represented more extreme cases with the worst outcomes. Three studies in particular have provided very useful epidemiological information on FCs, namely the American National Collaborative Perinatal Project (NCPP) *(36)*, the Rochester Epidemiological Project in Minnesota (USA) *(37)* and the Child Health and Education Study (CHES) (UK) *(38)*. From these and other studies, it is clear that FCs are universal and common, occurring in 2–5% of all children under 5 yr of age in the USA,

South America, and Western Europe *(36–39)*. Rates as high as 9–14% have been reported in some populations, for example, in Japan *(40)*. Occurrence is slightly more common in boys. In about 20% of patients, the first febrile seizure is complex. The average age of onset is between 18 and 22 mo. Risk factors for the development of a first FC are family history of FCs, slow development, day care, higher temperature, and neonatal discharge at 28 d or later *(35,41,42)*. About one-third of children with a first FC experience a recurrence, usually within 1 yr. Risk factors for recurrences are young age at onset, family history of FCs, complex FCs, shorter duration of fever and a lower temperature before the first seizure, and probably a family history of afebrile seizures *(35,36,41)*.

Etiology of FCs

FCs have a genetic basis, believed to be either polygenetic or autosomal dominant with variable penetrance *(43)*. Recent linkage studies provide evidence that regions of chromosomes 8q and 19p contain FC susceptibility genes *(43–45)*. Infections with high fever in combination with genetics, age, and relatively low seizure threshold in the immature brain allow for the occurrence of FCs. Millichap has postulated a convulsive threshold beyond which the seizure is precipitated *(46)*. An otherwise benign and most commonly viral illness usually causes the fever associated with FCs. Tonsillitis, upper respiratory tract infections, otitis media, roseola infantum, and gastroenteritis, including that caused by echoviruses, rotaviruses, and *Shigella,* are infections commonly implicated in FCs. The specific etiological role of human herpesvirus 6 (HHV-6) in FCs is a matter of controversy and ongoing research. Whereas Barone et al. found that infection with HHV-6, the causative organism of roseola infantum, is more common in children with FCs than in controls *(47)*, Hukin et al. recently concluded that HHV-6 did not seem to be a major factor in the pathogenesis of first and second febrile seizures *(48)*.

Other findings give tantalizing but inconclusive insights into the etiology of FCs. Whether these are epiphenomena or have a more definitive role in the pathophysiology of FCs remains to be seen. In one study, serum and CSF zinc levels were reported to be decreased during infectious diseases, with the reduction being more significant in patients with FCs *(49)*. Hyponatremia has been correlated with the risk for, and associated with, the recurrence of FCs *(50)*. Arginine vasopressin, somatostatin, and γ-aminobutyric acid (GABA) may also be involved in the pathogenesis of FCs in different ways in rat pups *(51)*. The central histaminergic neuron system may be involved in inhibition of seizures associated with febrile illnesses in childhood *(52)*. Iron deficiency anemia may protect against the development of FCs *(53)*.

In summary, the etiology of FCs appears to be multifactorial, involving genetic and environmental factors in an age-susceptible population.

Pathology of FCs

Comprehensive pathological studies in otherwise healthy children with FCs are very limited. In children whose deaths were attributed to prolonged FCs, neuronal necrosis was described in the cerebral cortex, the hippocampi (especially in the pyramidal layer of CA1 or Sommer sector), the basal ganglia, and the Purkinje cells of the cerebellum *(54,55)*. However, these autopsy studies were of extreme cases that were not typical of FCs in general and most likely do not represent FCs as now defined by the ILAE *(33)*. More recent prospective, population-based studies do not report any deaths in association with FCs.

Prognosis of FCs

About 15% of children with epilepsy have a history of one or more FCs *(56)*. Although the relationship of FCs to the development of later temporal lobe epilepsy related to mesial temporal sclerosis (MTS) remains controversial (see below), there is agreement that epilepsy subsequently develops more frequently in children with FCs. Depending on the length of follow-up, a 2–7% incidence of later epilepsy occurs following FCs, which is 2–10 times greater than in the general population *(36,37,57–60)*. Risk factors for the later development of epilepsy are a complex first febrile seizure, abnormal development before first seizure, onset of FCs prior to 12 mo of age, multiple recurrences of FCs, and family history of epilepsy. If two or more risk factors were present in a child with FCs, the risk of subsequent epilepsy was estimated at 13% *(36)*. The British CHES group showed that the rate of epilepsy depends on the type of preceding complex FC, with a 4%, 6%, and 29% rate after multiple, prolonged, and focal FCs, respectively; overlap occurred as FCs that were focal tended to be prolonged as well *(38)*. The American NCPP study reported the risk for epilepsy as 3%, 4%, and 7% when the first FC was prolonged, multiple, and had focal features, respectively *(36)*. In the Rochester study, Annegers et al. found a 49% rate of epilepsy among those who had FCs with all three complex features *(37)*.

In trying to delineate the type of epilepsy that may follow FCs, the literature is somewhat confusing, as many investigators do not overtly distinguish between seizure types and epilepsy syndromes. In general, however, the type of afebrile seizure that later occurs after a FC can be of any kind. In a population study in Nova Scotia, Camfield et al. found that FCs more often preceded apparent generalized tonic-clonic afebrile seizures than seizures that were complex partial and partial with secondary generalization. While finding a strong relationship between prolonged FCs and intractable epilepsy of all kinds, they found that prolonged FCs rarely preceded intractable partial epilepsy *(56)*. Annegers et al., however, found a strong association between FCs with all three complex features and the subsequent occurrence of partial epilepsy *(37)*. In this latter study, subsequent generalized epilepsy was associated with the number of FCs and a family history of epilepsy, and the investigators proposed that this represented a predisposition to both simple FCs and generalized epilepsy.

The time at which subsequent afebrile seizures occur in those with a history of FCs is controversial. Lennox found that afebrile seizures, if they occur, tend to do so within 1 yr of the first FC *(61)*. Nelson and Ellenberg also suggested that the association of afebrile seizures with FCs diminishes with age *(58)*. However, Annegers et al. found no reduction with age in the relatively increased incidence of afebrile seizures in a long-term follow-up in the Rochester study *(37)*.

Intellectual and behavioral outcomes in children with FCs are good. No difference was found between children with and without a history of FCs in psychometric test results at the age of 7 yr in the NCPP *(62)*. Even children with a FC lasting longer than 30 min had a mean full-scale intelligence quotient (IQ) no different from their siblings. Recurrent FCs were also not associated with any deficit in IQ *(62)*. British population studies are similarly reassuring; Verity et al. concluded that children who had FCs showed no significant intellectual or behavioral deficit by 10 yr of age *(63)*. Therefore, other than a potential association with subsequent epilepsy, it has become clear from these large population studies that FCs have a largely benign outcome in most children.

Relationship of FCs to MTS

Controversy continues to surround the issue of the relationship among FCs, partial epilepsy, and MTS. Is partial epilepsy, especially mesial temporal lobe epilepsy, a consequence of FCs? If so, what is the role of FCs in causing MTS? Retrospective studies from tertiary epilepsy centers report that many adults with intractable mesial temporal lobe epilepsy gave a history of prolonged or atypical FCs in childhood *(64–66)*. Maher and McLachlan studied families with at least four members with FCs and found a strong association between the occurrence of FCs and temporal lobe epilepsy secondary to MTS, with a prolonged FC being the most important determinant *(67)*. In recent magnetic resonance imaging (MRI) and functional imaging studies, Vanlandingham et al. presented evidence that prolonged FCs can be associated with MTS in rare cases *(68)*. Definite abnormalities were seen in the postictal MRIs of 6 of 15 infants with focal complex FCs and in 0 of 12 infants with generalized complex FCs. Two of these six infants had chronic MRI abnormalities, consistent with preexisting hippocampal atrophy; interestingly, both of these infants had histories of perinatal insults. The remaining four infants showed MRI changes compatible with acute hippocampal edema, with their FCs lasting significantly longer than did those of infants with focal FCs without MRI changes. Follow-up MRIs 1 yr later showed MTS in three of these four infants *(69)*.

However, even if a causal relationship between FCs and MTS exists, its importance is unclear. In the study of Vanlandingham et al., for example, MRI changes occurred in only a minority of patients with FCs *(68)*. Conversely, in a study of patients with MRI evidence of hippocampal volume loss, 64% gave no history of FCs *(70)*. This implies that even if FCs can cause MTS, they are not the only or major cause. Shinnar speculates that preexisting pathology may in some way be responsible for the febrile illness, triggering a seizure that was both prolonged and focal, thereby causing the brain to be more susceptible to seizure-induced damage *(71)*. There is support for such concepts with the frequent pathological finding of heterotopias and subtle migration defects in the resected temporal lobes of patients with MTS and intractable complex partial seizures *(72–74)*. There is also experimental support for this hypothesis. Immature rats with induced neuronal migration defects have a lower seizure threshold to hyperthermia-induced seizures and are more susceptible to irreversible hippocampal neuronal damage than control immature rats without migration defects *(9)*.

Data from epidemiological and other clinical studies further cloud the association between FCs and MTS. Although population studies do show an increased incidence of epilepsy in those with a history of FCs, the subsequent afebrile seizure type is more likely to be generalized tonic-clonic than partial *(56)*. The UK CHES cohort data found no excess of subsequent complex partial seizures in those with a history of FCs *(38)*. Similar findings were reported in a Danish study which concluded that temporal lobe epilepsy was not a consequence of childhood FCs in Denmark *(60)*. Annegers et al. found that the occurrence of subsequent partial epilepsy was strongly associated with the concurrence of all three of the complex features of FCs; however, this association may reflect the presence of preexisting brain disease that is responsible for both the complex FCs and later partial seizures *(37)*.

Although the first afebrile seizure frequently occurs early after the first FC *(58,61)*, patients with both refractory mesial temporal epilepsy and a history of FCs who are being evaluated for epilepsy surgery typically give a history of FCs followed by a seizure-free interval of up to 15 yr with subsequent development of intractable complex partial seizures in adolescence *(64–66,72,73)*. The causal relationship between FCs and subsequent intractable partial epilepsy is weakened further by the finding that treatment can result in a reduction in the number of FCs without effect on the rate of subsequent epilepsy *(75)*.

In summary, although there is an association between FCs and MTS with intractable partial epilepsy, a direct causal relationship is far from certain. MTS is found in many patients with no history of FCs and has other known etiologies including prior CNS infection and head trauma. Epidemiological studies do not consistently support a causal relationship between FCs, even if prolonged, and subsequent MTS, indicating that hippocampal damage is rarely the consequence of FCs *(76)*.

Clinical Features of FCs

A FC usually occurs early in a febrile illness. It may be the first sign that a child is ill. It is the height of the elevated temperature rather than its rate of rise that is the important trigger *(42)*. The seizure can be generalized or partial, the most common being a tonic-clonic convulsion *(35)*. Other types of seizures include atonic seizures, staring with stiffness or limpness, focal stiffness, or jerking. There may be apnea. A prolonged seizure is more often focal, thereby fulfilling two of the criteria for complexity. Nelson and Ellenberg reported fewer than 8% of FCs lasting longer than 15 min, most last less than 6 min *(36)*. This results in most children not being brought to medical attention until after the FC is over.

Assessment, Management, and Treatment of FCs

Despite the generally benign outcome of FCs, a child with a suspected FC still requires a thorough assessment. FCs remain a diagnosis of exclusion, by definition and by clinical criteria. When first seen, a child is best considered as having convulsions with fever *(34)*, implying a convulsion in a child of any age with fever of any cause. This puts the onus on the physician to search for other causes of seizure and fever, rather than presuming a diagnosis of "benign" FC. A detailed history is mandatory, especially a description of the convulsion itself. Physical examination should include evaluation for signs of infection, especially intracranial infection. Routine laboratory tests are rarely helpful in an otherwise healthy child. In general, the neurologically normal child does not need neuroimaging. Whether the child who has just had a first FC should have a lumbar puncture to exclude CNS infection is a matter of some debate. However, if in doubt, it is better to err on the side of caution and perform a spinal tap. The role of the electroencephalogram (EEG) in assessment of the child with a FC is limited. Paroxysmal abnormalities in the EEG have varied in studies from 1.4% to 20%, their presence being of no value in predicting recurrence of FCs or their evolution to afebrile seizures *(77,78)*. EEG is most useful in the assessment of prolonged, focal, or recurrent FCs.

A child who has just had a FC should be kept under medical observation for at least 6–12 h. Parental anxiety is often understandably high, as many parents fear that their child is dying during the seizure. About 16% of children experience another FC within 24 h; *(35)* however, it is not possible to predict recurrence. The use of antipyretic agents and tepid sponging has not been proven to reduce recurrence of FCs *(79)*, although the use of acetaminophen may make the child more comfortable. Although multiple FCs are associated with subsequent epilepsy, there is no evidence that treatment to prevent recurrence of FCs reduces this small risk of subsequent epilepsy *(75)*. Intermittent or continuous use of phenobarbital is not effective in preventing recurrence of FCs and is poorly tolerated *(80,81)*. Similarly, the usefulness of continuous valproate or primidone to prevent recurrence is questionable, whereas use of carbamazepine and phenytoin is generally regarded as ineffective *(82)*. Intermittent use of either oral or rectal diazepam is effective in decreasing recurrences of FCs; however, it may cause ataxia and drowsiness and does not alter the generally benign long-term outcome in terms of subsequent epilepsy, neurological status, neuropsychological measures, or scholastic ability *(83)*. There is general agreement that prophylactic treatment rarely should be used in children with FCs *(35,84,85)*. Prophylactic treatment will also not prevent the majority of prolonged FCs, as most prolonged FCs occur as the first FC *(35)*. Most authorities would only consider the use of prophylaxis in young children with multiple FCs or recurrent prolonged FCs, or in children in isolated areas with poor access to medical care or where very high parental anxiety exists despite appropriate counseling and reassurance *(35,85)*. If intermittent treatment of an episode of FC is to be offered, the use of liquid rectal diazepam at the time of a FC is recommended. At all times, communication with and reassurance of parents is essential.

Approach to Patient with Seizure, Fever, and Possible Infection

In approaching the patient with seizure, fever, and possible infection, the emphasis should be on detailed clinical assessment, with further investigations being guided by the history and physical examination. In this section, we discuss three specific conditions that demonstrate the range of challenges faced when confronted by this clinical triad.

HIV-Related Seizures

CNS involvement in HIV infection can occur either directly from the HIV virus or from secondary complications including opportunistic infections, neoplasms, metabolic disturbances, and medications. Estimates of involvement of both the central and peripheral nervous system in the course of HIV infection range from 40% to 70% *(86)*. MRI abnormalities are found in about 70% of patients with the acquired immunodeficiency syndrome (AIDS), regardless of neurological symptoms, whereas neuropathological changes at autopsy are reported at 70–80% *(87)*. About 40% of neurological involvement in HIV infection is estimated to be the result of opportunistic infection (88).

Retrospective studies have estimated seizure occurrence in HIV infection to be 11–17% *(89,90)*. A prospective study from Spain reported new onset seizures in 3% (17 of 550) of an HIV-infected patient cohort, recruited and studied over a 1-yr period *(91)*. However, these patients were only followed up until death or study end. Van Paesschen et al. reported a 4% incidence of seizures in hospitalized HIV-infected patients *(92)*. Generalized seizures are encountered most commonly; focal seizures usually but not always indicate a structural brain lesion *(91)*. Both simple and complex partial seizures are seen in patients with diffuse brain disease, such as HIV encephalopathy and meningoencephalitis. The incidence of convulsive status epilepticus has been reported to be between 8% and 18% in different studies *(89,92,93)*. Seizures are not usually the presenting sign of HIV infection, being reported as the signal of such infection in only 0–18% of patients *(88,91)*. Most reports agree that seizures occur more frequently in patients with severe immunosuppression *(89,92–94)*. Fifty-five to 91% of patients have already been diagnosed with AIDS prior to their first seizure *(88,91)*. Pascual-Sedano et al. reported a mean latency of 60.7 ± 37.6 mo between diagnosis of HIV infection and the occurrence of first seizure with a mean CD4+ cell count of 115 ± 16/mm^3 in the same group *(91)*. Seizures usually portend a poor prognosis. During a 1-yr study period of 550 HIV-infected patients, 17 developed new onset seizures. Of these 17 patients, 8 died during the study period, with a mean survival of 3 mo from time of first seizure *(91)*. With the availability of highly active antiretroviral therapy (HAART), the prognosis of HIV infection has now improved.

Opportunistic infections are the single largest cause of neurological involvement in HIV-infected patients and should be the first consideration when seizures occur, even in the absence of fever. Many such opportunistic infections are highly treatable once an accurate diagnosis is made. The most common opportunistic infection in HIV-infected patients with new onset seizures is a mass lesion resulting from CNS toxoplasmosis, estimated as the cause in 12–28% of cases *(92,93,95)*. Conversely, seizures have been reported as an early sign in 15–40% of patients with a cerebral toxoplasma mass lesion *(90,96–98)*. Early treatment with sulfadiazine and pyrimethamine generally results in rapid clinical improvement. Other infectious mass lesions in AIDS likely to produce seizures include tuberculous, cryptococcal and nocardial abscesses, as well as syphilitic gummas. Seizures have been reported as the presenting neurological sign of progressive multifocal leukoencephalopathy (PML) in 1–20% of HIV-infected patients with PML *(93,99,100)*, with the latter study reporting seizure occurrence in one-third of HIV-infected PML patients. Meningitis and encephalitis account for 12–16% of causes of new onset seizures in HIV-infected patients *(88)*. Cryptococcal meningitis is the most frequent cause of meningoencephalitis producing seizures, with other less frequent causes including aseptic meningitis, neurosyphilis, herpes simplex, herpes zoster, *Toxoplasma gondii,* and cytomegalovirus *(88,95).* Subacute sclerosing panencephalitis can cause seizures and encephalopathy in HIV-infected children *(101).*

Conditions other than opportunistic infections also cause seizures in HIV-infected patients. Primary CNS lymphoma is the second most common cause of an AIDS-related mass lesion and is also the second most common mass lesion giving rise to seizures in HIV infection. Cerebral infarction with edema can also cause seizures in AIDS *(102).* Toxic and metabolic factors, such as hypoglycemia, hypomagnesemia, and drug toxicity, were causative in more than half of new onset seizures in one study *(91).* The drugs implicated were foscarnet, ceftazidime, sulfonamides, zidovudine, imipenem, diacetylmorphine, and therapeutic cocaine infusions, as well as midazolam withdrawal. Van Paesschen et al. frequently found hyponatremia in their patients and reported an association between hypomagnesemia, renal failure, and status epilepticus *(92).*

There is good evidence to support a direct epileptogenic role for HIV infection of the brain. In up to half of patients with seizures and HIV infection, direct infection of the brain by the retrovirus is the presumed primary cause, there being no evidence of secondary infection or neoplasia on imaging or CSF studies *(89,92,93,95,97,103,104).* In such cases, neuropathological examination often reveals characteristic microglial nodules or multinucleated cells, or both, supporting the idea that HIV infection is the primary cause of seizures in such patients *(89).* Although neurons are not themselves infected by HIV, neuronal loss and injury do occur. The putative mechanism for such injury and loss is complex, involving HIV- or immune-related toxins, interactions between macrophages, astrocytes and neurons, increased glutamate activity, and influx of calcium into the cells leading to neuronal death. A relative imbalance of excitatory and inhibitory neurotransmitters may predispose to seizure occurrence *(17).*

Assessment and Treatment of HIV-Related Seizures

History and examination will direct investigations including neurologic imaging, lumbar puncture, microbiological cultures, serum biochemistry, and other appropriate tests. As the etiology is potentially diverse and often multifactorial, therapy should be directed specifically to the immediately identifiable cause of seizure in an HIV-infected patient. Opportunistic infections and neoplasms should be appropriately identified and treated, electrolyte and other metabolic disturbances corrected, and drugs implicated as the cause of seizures withdrawn. As seizures recur frequently in such patients, long-term treatment with antiepileptic drug therapy is indicated, even after one seizure and in the absence of an identifiable etiology. Phenytoin has been used most widely *(93,96)*. Side effects, including skin rashes, leukopenia, thrombocy-topenia, and hepatic dysfunction, occur in a significant number of patients. Other antiepileptic drugs, including both established (such as valproic acid and carbamazepine) and newer agents (such as lamotrigine), have not been studied systematically in the treatment of HIV-related seizures, although they may be as effective and acceptable as phenytoin.

The incidence of seizures directly attributable to HIV infection and HIV-related complications may be expected to decrease as the natural history of HIV infection changes. The prognosis of HIV infection in developed countries has changed dramatically over the latter part of the 1990s because of the introduction of HAART *(105,106)*. HAART consists of multidrug combinations of potent antiretroviral agents, generally three or more agents, that are capable of reducing serum concentrations of retrovirus to nearly undetectable levels and elevating CD4 lymphocyte counts significantly *(107)*. The results of widespread use of HAART have included decreases in HIV-attributable mortality, significant decreases in the incidence of opportunistic infections and hospitalization, and in some patients dramatic improvement in immune function, allowing them to clear previously untreatable opportunistic processes *(106,108–110)*. Antiretroviral agents also can have direct effects on HIV infection of the CNS. Early studies with zidovudine (AZT) alone demonstrated reversal of brain atrophy and improved cognitive function in patients with advanced HIV infection, and more potent combinations of newer drugs would be expected to have even greater effects *(111)*. Unfortunately, antiretroviral therapy is extremely expensive, and these drugs remain unavailable in many parts of the world where the rates of newly diagnosed HIV infection continue to climb.

Cerebral Abscess

The incidence of bacterial cerebral abscess has decreased in the Western world because of the availability of sensitive neurological imaging techniques that allow for early diagnosis, and the development of more effective antimicrobial agents. However, bacterial cerebral abscesses remain a problem in the less developed parts of the world. Also, the HIV infection pandemic as well as the widespread medical use of immunosuppressants and antimicrobials has resulted in the emergence of cerebral abscesses of other etiologies including nonbacterial, opportunistic, and resistant organisms.

Pathology

Cerebral abscess is defined as suppurative necrosis of the brain parenchyma. Local spread of infection from the ears or sinuses, or hematogenous spread causes a suppurative vasculitis, breakdown of the BBB, and invasion by the infecting organism leading to cerebritis, with the eventual formation of an abscess and its capsule. Most abscesses occur in the frontal and parietal lobes, and up to 75% are solitary *(112)*. However, daughter abscesses, cerebral edema, and ventriculitis can occur. Epidemiologically, young males are most commonly affected; however, all age groups and both sexes are at risk. Special at risk groups include those with congenital heart disease, middle ear and sinus infection, mastoiditis, cranial osteomyelitis, penetrating head injuries, and patients undergoing neurosurgical procedures. The location of the abscess can be a clue to its etiology, with middle ear infections localizing to cerebellum and temporal lobe, frontal sinus infections to frontal lobe, and ethmoid and sphenoid sinus infections to frontal or temporal lobe abscesses. About one-third of abscesses arise from hematogenous spread. Sources for such spread include lung abscesses and empyema, dental infection, abdominal and pelvic sepsis, distant osteomyelitis, infective endocarditis, pulmonary atrioventricular (A-V) fistulae such as those that occur in Osler–Rendu–Weber disease, and cyanotic congenital heart disease in children. These latter two conditions are associated with hypoxia and hyperviscosity, which facilitate infection. The distal territory of the middle cerebral artery (MCA) is involved most commonly in blood-borne spread affecting either the less perfused white matter or the gray/white matter junction, often with multiple abscess formation. Almost all deep cerebral abscesses have a systemic source. The source of cerebritis and cerebral abscess remains unknown in about 20% of cases. Abscesses are rare in bacterial meningitis, although they have been reported in neonates with citrobacter *(113)*. In immunosuppressed patients, abscesses are often multiple, are usually hematogenous in origin and, apart from *T. gondii,* have a predilection for MCA territory.

Etiology

Microaerophilic and anaerobic organisms are the main causes of cerebral abscesses *(112)*. Microaerophilic *Streptococcus* species, especially *Streptococcus milleri,* are found in 60–70% of cases, whereas anaerobes such as *Bacteroides* and *Propionibacterium* species are causative in another 20–40%. Aerobic Gram-negative bacilli such as *Proteus, E. coli,* and *Pseudomonas aeruginosa* are found in 25–35% of cases, with *Staphylococcus aureus* in 10–15%. *Hemophilus influenza, Streptococcus pneumoniae,* and *Neisseria meningitidis* together cause less than 1% of brain abscesses. The Gram-positive higher bacteria *Actinomyces* and *Nocardia* and certain fungi, notably *Candida, Mucor,* and *Aspergillus* have been isolated in some cases. In 30–60% of cases, there is a mixture of more than 2 organisms. The causative organism in cerebral abscess can often be deduced from the clinical circumstances, for example, *S. aureus* in penetrating head injury. In the immunosuppressed patient, yeast, fungi, nocardial, mycobacterial, and aerobic

Gram-negative bacilli organisms, as well as toxoplasmosis, are frequently responsible for abscesses. A polymicrobial brain abscess involving *Streptococcus bovis, Fusobacterium necrophorum, Peptostreptococcus,* and group G *Streptococcus* has been reported in a HIV-infected patient *(114).* Nontyphoidal *Salmonella* intracranial infections, in the form of cerebral abscess and subdural and epidural empyema, have been reported in HIV-infected patients *(115).* Diabetes mellitus patients are vulnerable to mucormycotic abscesses. In the tropics, tuberculoma and cysticercosis are common, whereas strongyloidiasis, schistosomiasis, and melioidosis rarely give rise to abscesses. The etiology of seizures in cerebral abscess may include drug toxicity, electrolyte and other metabolic abnormalities, as well as the cerebral mass lesion itself.

Clinical Features

The classical clinical triad of a cerebral abscess includes symptoms and signs of raised intracranial pressure, a focal neurologic deficit, and fever. The course of the illness is usually short and progressive. Seizures occur in 25–30% of patients, with cerebral abscesses occurring at any time in the course of the illness. Fever occurs in 45–50% of cases but is usually less than 38.6°C. Fever may normalize as the abscess encapsulates. Neck stiffness is present in about 25% of patients. Although the extracerebral signs of infection may dominate the clinical picture, systemic signs may be absent in the immunosuppressed patient.

Diagnosis, Differential Diagnosis, and Investigations

The differential diagnosis includes subdural or intracranial hemorrhage, cortical thrombophlebitis, dural sinus thrombosis, and brain tumor, as well as other infections such as meningitis, encephalitis, subdural empyema, and epidural abscess. Erythrocyte sedimentation rate (ESR) and white cell count are usually elevated. Blood cultures are positive in 10–20% of cases. Cranial CT scan may show an ill-defined hypodensity with mass effect and patchy contrast enhancement suggestive of cerebritis, or it may show a better defined mass with ring enhancement. CT may also show other features such as sinusitis, skull fracture, or osteomyelitis that may explain the source of abscess. Better definition is obtained using MRI, and gadolinium enhancement may reveal daughter abscesses. Lumbar puncture is generally contraindicated, unless it can be judged to be performed with low risk of brain herniation. If performed, CSF usually shows an elevated opening pressure, a mildly elevated protein, a normal glucose, and a modest elevation in white cells, predominantly neutrophils. Other appropriate investigations will be guided by the clinical picture, for example, dental X-rays, chest X-ray, and a HIV test. An electrolyte and metabolic profile should also be done, especially as it may help to explain the occurrence of a seizure. Definitive diagnosis is obtained by microbiological analysis and culture of the abscess material obtained neurosurgically in what is often a combined diagnostic and therapeutic procedure.

Treatment

Appropriate antibiotics given intravenously for 6–8 weeks may suffice for cerebritis alone or for a small abscess. Otherwise, surgical aspiration or drainage will also be required. Excision of the abscess may be necessary, depending on size and location, for example, a cerebellar abscess causing obstructive hydrocephalus and brainstem pressure effects. Symptomatic treatment of raised intracranial pressure using dexamethasone, mannitol, and/or hyperventilation may be necessary. If seizures have occurred, anticonvulsant medication is indicated for a minimum of 3–6 mo. Any factor contributing to seizure occurrence or recurrence, especially electrolyte disturbances or drug toxicity (e.g., penicillin or cephalosporin antibiotics) should also be addressed.

Prognosis

Modern antimicrobial therapy, as well as CT-guided aspiration, has reduced the previously dismal outcome of cerebral abscess. However, there remains a mortality of 5–15%, with an even higher morbidity *(112)*. Twenty-five to 50% of patients will have a neurological deficit, 15–30% a hemiparesis, 10–20% a speech or language disorder, and seizures persist in 30–50% of patients with cerebral abscess who develop seizures. Children are often left with intellectual impairment. Eight to 10% of abscesses recur. Seizures occurring in immunosuppressed patients with cerebral abscesses generally portend a poor prognosis. It is thus clear from these figures that cerebral abscesses still carry a high mortality and morbidity despite modern day therapy.

Infective Endocarditis

There are many reasons why infective endocarditis (IE) remains an important clinical problem. Although rheumatic heart disease has become less prevalent, IE continues to occur in a wide variety of patients including those with other congenital and acquired valvular abnormalities or prosthetic valves, intravenous drug abusers, those who develop nosocomial IE from medically invasive techniques, those with gastrointestinal and genitourinary cancer, and occasionally those with apparently normal native valves. Although the infecting organisms are still mainly bacteria, especially streptococci and staphylococci, other organisms such as fungi, rickettsiae, chlamydia, and protozoa may also cause IE in certain clinical settings such as with intravenous drug abuse and immunosuppression. History and examination are essential in directing one to the consideration of IE, although advanced microbiological methods and echocardiography (especially transesophageal) have facilitated earlier diagnosis and treatment.

The diagnosis of IE should always be considered when there is not another immediately apparent explanation for seizure, fever, and suspected infection. Neurological complications are common and protean in IE, occurring in about one-third of patients and often portending a poor prognosis *(116–118)*. For example, Pruitt et al. reported neurological complications in 39% of patients with IE, with death occurring in 58% of these *(116)*. Jones and Siekert, as well as Le Cam et al. reported similar poor prognosis for survival *(117,119)*. Kanter and Hart found that all neurological complications occurred more often with the more virulent *S. aureus* than with *Streptococcus viridans* infection *(118)*. Although focal neurological deficits, usually from stroke (embolic or hemorrhagic), altered mental state, and headache, are the most common neurological manifestations, seizures can be part of the presentation of IE *(116)* and rarely the only neurological feature *(117)*. In a retrospective study, Gergaud et al. reported neurological complications in 10 of 53 patients with IE, with seizures occurring in 2 of these *(120)*. Seizures were the most common neurological complication in children with IE *(121)*. Focal seizures occur most commonly in patients with acute embolic disease, whereas generalized seizures in IE may reflect multiple possible etiologies, including toxic and metabolic disorders such as electrolyte disturbances, uremia, hypoxia, drug toxicity (especially the use of penicillin in those with renal insufficiency), and an associated purulent meningitis *(116)*.

The management of IE consists of appropriate antimicrobial therapy and supportive treatment, sometimes including valve replacement. Drug toxicity, metabolic abnormalities, and other contributing factors should be rectified when seizures occur. Anticonvulsant drug therapy is usually indicated, the duration depending on the immediately identifiable cause(s) of seizures. The management of neurological complications such as mycotic aneurysms and stroke, as well as the use of anticoagulation in IE, remain controversial *(117,122)*.

Conclusion

The occurrence of seizures in the setting of fever and infection is a common and challenging problem. The possible causes of such seizures are numerous, their pathophysiology not completely understood, and their management guided primarily by clinical considerations. Further clinical and basic scientific research is needed to help clinicians deal effectively with the prevention and treatment of seizures in such patients.

References

1. Annegers JF, Hauser WA, Beghi E, Nicolosi A, Kurland LT. The risk of unprovoked seizures after encephalitis and meningitis. *Neurology* 1988;38:1407–1410.
2. Loiseau J, Loiseau P, Guyot M, Duche B, Dartigues J, Aublet, B. Survey of seizure disorders in the French Southwest. I. Incidence of epileptic syndromes. *Epilepsia* 1990;31:391–396.

3. Hauser WA, Annegers JF. (1997) Epidemiology of acute symptomatic seizures. In: Engel J Jr, Pedley TA (eds.), *Epilepsy: A Comprehensive Textbook,* Philadelphia, PA: Lippincott-Raven, pp 87–91.

4. Wachtel TJ, Steele GH, Day JD. Natural history of fever following seizure. *Arch Intern Med* 1987;147:1153–1155.

5. Iriki M, Saigusa T. Regional differentiation of sympathetic efferents during fever. *Prog Brain Res* 1998;115:477–497.

6. Anonymous. American College of Chest Physicians/Society of Critical Care Medicine Consensus Conference: definitions for sepsis and organ failure and guidelines for the use of innovative therapies in sepsis. *Crit. Care Med* 1992;20:864–874.

7. Anonymous. Glossary of terms for thermal physiology, 2nd ed. *Pflug* 1987; 410:567–587.

8. Sharma HS, Westman J, Nyberg F. Pathophysiology of brain edema and cell changes following hyperthermic brain injury. *Prog Brain Res* 1998;115:351–412.

9. Germano IM, Zhang YF, Sperber EF, Moshe SL. Neuronal migration disorders increase susceptibility to hyperthermia-induced seizures in developing rats. *Epilepsia* 1996;37:902–910.

10. Toth Z, Yan XX, Haftoglou S, Ribak CE, Baram TZ. Seizure-induced neuronal injury: vulnerability to febrile seizures in an immature rat model. *J Neurosci* 1998;18:4285–4294.

11. Ullal GR, Satishchandra P, Shankar SK. Hyperthermic seizures: an animal model for hot-water epilepsy. *Seizure* 1996;5:221–228.

12. Jiang W, Duong TM, de Lanerolle NC. The neuropathology of hyperthermic seizures in the rat. *Epilepsia* 1999;40:5–19.

13. Morimoto T, Kida K, Nagao H, Yoshida K, Tukuda M, Takashima, S. The pathogenic role of the NMDA receptor in hyperthermia-induced seizures in developing rats. *Brain Res Dev Brain Res* 1995;84:204–207.

14. Sharma HS, Westman J, Cervos-Navarro J, Nyberg F. Role of neurochemicals in brain edema and cell changes following hyperthermic brain injury in the rat. *Acta Neurochir Suppl (Wien).* 1997;70:269–274.

15. Dubois M, Coppola R, Buchsbaum MS, Lees DE. Somatosensory evoked potentials during whole body hyperthermia in humans. *Electroencephalogr Clin Neurophysiol* 1981;52:157–162.

16. Malamud N, Haymaker W, Custer RP. Heat stroke. Clinicopathological study of 125 fatal cases. *Milit Surg* 1946;99:397–449.

17. Delanty N, Vaughan CJ, French JA. Medical causes of seizures. *Lancet* 1998;352:383–390.

18. Kataoka K, Yanese H. Mild hypothermia—a revived countermeasure against ischemic neuronal damages. *Neurosci Res* 1998;32:103–117.

19. Kao TY, Lin MT. Brain serotonin depletion attenuates heatstroke-induced cerebral ischemia and cell death in rats. *J Appl Physiol* 1996;80:680–684.

20. Lin MT, Kao TY, Chio CC, Jin YT. Dopamine depletion protects striatal neurons from heatstroke-induced ischemia and cell death in rats. *Am J Physiol* 1995;269:H487–490.

21. Flanagan SW, Moseley PL, Buettner GR. Increased flux of free radicals in cells subjected to hyperthermia: detection by electron paramagnetic resonance spin trapping. *FEBS Lett* 1998;431:285,286.

22. Kivirante T, Tuomisto L, Airaksinen EM. Osmolality and electrolytes in cere-brospinal fluid and serum of febrile children with and without seizures. *Eur J Pediatr* 1996;155:120–125.
23. Kiviranta T, Airaksinen EM. Low sodium levels are associated with subsequent febrile seizures. *Acta Paediatr* 1995;84:1372–1374.
24. Morimoto T, Fukuda M, Aibara Y, Nagao H, Kida K. The influence of blood gas changes on hyperthermia-induced seizures in developing rats. *Brain Res Dev Brain Res* 1996;92:77–80.
25. Kivirante T, Airaksinen EM, Tuomisto L. The role of fever on cerebrospinal fluid glucose concentration with and without convulsions. *Acta Paediatr* 1995; 84:1276–1279.
26. Mistchenko AS, Diez RA, Mariani AL, et al. Cytokines in adenoviral disease in children: association of interleukin-6, interleukin-8, and tumor necrosis factor alpha levels with clinical outcome. *J Pediatr* 1994;124:714–720.
27. Yuhas Y, Weizman A, Dinari G, Ashkenazi S. An animal model for the study of neu-rotoxicity of bacterial products and application of the model to demonstrate that Shiga toxin and lipopolysaccharide cooperate in inducing neurologic disorders. *J Infect Dis* 1995;171:1244–1249.
28. Plaschke M, Strohle A, Then Bergh F, Backmund H, Trenkwalder C. Neurologic and psychiatric symptoms of legionella infection. Case report and overview of the clinical spectrum (in German). *Nervenarzt* 1997;68:342–345.
29. Johnson JD, Raff MJ, Van Arsdall JA. Neurologic manifestations of Legionnaires' disease. *Medicine* 1984;63:303–310.
30. Cimolai N, Morrison BJ, Carter JE. Risk factors for the central nervous system manifestations of gastroenteritis-associated hemolytic-uremic syndrome. *Pediatrics* 1992;90:616–621.
31. Lezama-Basulto LA, Mota-Hernandez F, Bravo-Barrios E. Cholera in children. A report of 8 cases. *Bol Med Hospital Infantil Mex* 1993;50:789–796.
32. Wallace SJ. *The Child with Febrile Seizures.* London: John Wright, 1988.
33. Commission on Epidemiology and Prognosis of the International League Against Epilepsy. Guidelines for epidemiologic studies on epilepsy. *Epilepsia* 1993;34:592–596.
34. Joint Working Group of the Research Unit of the Royal College of Physicians and the British Paediatric Association. Guidelines for the management of convulsions with fever. *Br Med J* 1991;303:634–636.
35. Hirtz DG, Camfield CS, Camfield PR. (1997) Febrile convulsions, In: Engel J Jr, Pedley, TA (eds.), *Epilepsy: A Comprehensive Textbook,* Philadelphia, PA: Lippin-cott-Raven, pp. 2483–2488.
36. Nelson KB, Ellenberg JH. Prognosis in children with febrile seizures. *Pediatrics* 1978;61:720–727.
37. Annegers JF, Hauser WA, Shirts SB, Kurland LT. Factors prognostic of unprovoked seizures after febrile convulsions. *N Engl J Med* 1987;316:493–498.
38. Verity CM, Ross EM, Golding J. Outcome of childhood status epilepticus and lengthy febrile convulsions: findings of national cohort study. *Br Med J* 1993;307:225–228.
39. Hauser WA, Kurland LT. The epidemiology of epilepsy in Rochester, Minnesota, 1935 through 1967. *Epilepsia* 1975;16:1–66.
40. Tsuboi T. Epidemiology of febrile and afebrile convulsions in children in Japan. *Neurology* 1981;34:175–181.

41. Bethune P, Gordon K, Dooley J, Camfield C, Camfield P. Which child will have a febrile seizure? *Am J Dis Child* 1993;147:35–39.
42. Berg AT. Are febrile seizures provoked by a rapid rise in temperature? *Am J Dis Child* 1993;147:1101–1103.
43. Kugler SL, Johnson WG. Genetics of the febrile seizure susceptibility trait. *Brain Dev* 1998;20:265–274.
44. Wallace RH, Wang DW, Singh R, et al. Febrile seizures and generalized epilepsy associated with a mutation in the Na^+ channel betal subunit gene SCN1B. *Nat Genet* 1998;19:366–370.
45. Wallace RH, Berkovic SF, Howell RA, Sutherland GR, Mulley JC. Suggestion of a major gene for familial febrile convulsions mapping to 8q 13-21. *J Med Genet* 1996;33:308–312.
46. Millichap JG. *Febrile Convulsions.* New York: Macmillan, 1968.
47. Barone SR, Kaplan MH, Krilov LR. Human herpesvirus-6 infection in children with first febrile seizures. *J Pediatr* 1995;127:95–97.
48. Hukin J, Farrell K, MacWilliam LM, et al. Case-control study of primary human herpesvirus 6 infection in children with febrile seizures. *Pediatrics* 1998;101:E3.
49. Gunduz Z, Yavuz I, Koparal M, Kumandas S, Sarsymen R. Serum and cerebrospinal fluid zinc levels in children with febrile convulsions. *Acta Paediatr Jpn* 1996;38:237–241.
50. Hugen CAC, Oudesluys-Murphy AM, Hop WCJ. Serum sodium levels and probability of recurrent febrile convulsions. *Eur J Pediatr* 1995;154:403–405.
51. Nagaki S, Nagaki S, Minatogawa Y, Sadmatsu M, Kato N, Osawa M, Fukuyama Y. The role of vasopressin, somatostatin and GABA in febrile convulsions in rat pups. *Life Sci* 1996;58:2233–2242.
52. Kivirante T, Tuomisto L, Airaksinen EM. Histamine in cerebrospinal fluid of children with febrile convulsions. *Epilepsia* 1995;36:276–280.
53. Kobrinsky NL, Yager JY, Cheang MS, Yatscoff RW, Tenenbein M. Does iron deficiency raise the seizure threshold? *J Child Neurol* 1995;10:105–109.
54. Fowler M. Brain damage after febrile convulsions. *Arch Dis Child* 1957;32:67–76.
55. Meldrum BS. (1976) Secondary pathology of febrile and experimental convulsions. In: Brazier MAB, Coceani F. (eds.), *Brain Dysfunction in Infantile Febrile Convulsions,* Raven, New York, pp 213–222.
56. Camfield P, Camfield C, Gordon K, Dooley J. What types of epilepsy are preceded by febrile seizures? A population-based study of children. *Dev Med Child Neurol* 1994;36:887–892.
57. van der Berg BJ, Yerushalmy J. Studies on convulsive disorders in young children. I. Incidence of febrile and nonfebrile convulsions by age and other factors. *Pediatr Res* 1969;3:298–304.
58. Nelson KB, Ellenberg JH. Predictors of epilepsy in children who have experienced febrile seizures. *N Engl J Med* 1976;295:1029–1033.
59. Annegers JF, Hauser WA, Elveback LR, Kurland LT. The risk of epilepsy following febrile convulsions. *Neurology* 1979;29:297–303.
60. Lee K, Diaz M, Melchior JC. Temporal lobe epilepsy—not a consequence of childhood febrile convulsions in Denmark. *Acta Neurol Scand* 1981;63:231–236.
61. Lennox WG. Significance of febrile convulsions. *Pediatrics* 1953;11:341–357.
62. Ellenberg JH, Nelson KB. Febrile seizures and later intellectual performance. *Arch Neurol* 1978;35:17–21.

63. Verity CM, Greenwood R., Golding J. Long-term intellectual and behavioral outcomes of children with febrile convulsions. *N Engl J Med* 1998;338:1723–1728.

64. French JA, Williamson PD, Thadani M, Darcey TM, Mattson RH, Spencer SS, Spencer DD. Characteristics of medial temporal lobe epilepsy: I. Results of history and physical examination. *Ann Neurol* 1993;34:774–780.

65. Abou-Khalil B, Andermann E, Andermann F, Olivier A, Quesney LF. Temporal lobe epilepsy after prolonged febrile convulsions: excellent outcome after surgical treatment. *Epilepsia* 1993;34:878–883.

66. Cendes F, Andermann F, Dubeau F, et al. Early childhood prolonged febrile convulsions, atrophy and sclerosis of mesial structures, and temporal lobe epilepsy: an MRI volumetric study. *Neurology* 1993;43:1083–1087.

67. Maher J, McLachlan RS. Febrile convulsions. Is seizure duration the most important predictor of temporal lobe epilepsy? *Brain* 1995;118:1521–1528.

68. Vanlandingham KE, Heinz ER, Cavazos JE, Lewis DV. MRI evidence of hippocampal injury after prolonged, focal febrile convulsions. *Ann Neurol* 1998; 43:413–426.

69. Lewis DV. Febrile convulsions and mesial temporal sclerosis. *Curr Opin Neurol* 1999;12:197–201.

70. Kuks JB, Cook MJ, Fish DR, Stevens JM, Shorvon SD. Hippocampal sclerosis in epilepsy and childhood febrile seizures. *Lancet* 1993;342:1391–1394.

71. Shinnar S. Prolonged febrile seizures and mesial temporal sclerosis. *Ann Neurol* 1998;43:411–412.

72. Mathern GW, Babb TL, Vickrey BG, Melendez M, Pretorius JK. The clinical-pathologic mechanisms of hippocampal neuronal loss and surgical outcomes in temporal lobe epilepsy. *Brain* 1995;118:105–118.

73. Mathern GW, Pretorius JK, Babb TL. Influence of the type of initial precipitating injury and at what age it occurs on course and outcome in patients with temporal lobe seizures. *J Neurosurg* 1995;82:220–227.

74. Hardiman O, Burke T, Phillips J, Murphy S, O'Moore B, Staunton H, Farrell MA. Microdysgenesis in resected temporal neocortex: incidence and clinical significance in focal epilepsy. *Neurology* 1988;38:1041–1047.

75. Berg AT, Shinnar S. Do seizures beget seizures? An assessment of the clinical evidence in humans. *J Clin Neurophysiol* 1997;14:102–110.

76. Verity CM. Do seizures damage the brain? The epidemiological evidence. *Arch Dis Child* 1998;78:78–84.

77. Sofijanov N, Emoto S, Kuturec M, et al. Febrile seizures: clinical characteristics and initial EEG. *Epilepsia* 1992;33:52–57.

78. Stores G. When does the EEG contribute to the management of febrile seizures? *Arch Dis Child* 1991;66:554–557.

79. Uhari M, Rantala H, Vainionpaa L, Kurttila R. Effect of acetaminophen and of low intermittent doses of diazepam on prevention of recurrences of febrile seizures. *J Pediatr* 1995;126:991–995.

80. Wolf SM, Carr A, Davis DC, et al. The value of phenobarbital in the child who has had a single febrile seizure: a controlled prospective study. *Pediatrics* 1977; 59:378–385.

81. Newton RW. Randomized controlled trials of phenobarbitone and valproate in febrile convulsions. *Arch Dis Child* 1988;63:1189–1191.

82. Berkovic SF, Scheffer IE. Febrile seizures: genetics and relationship to other epilepsy syndromes. *Curr Opin Neurol* 1998;11:129–134.

83. Knudsen FU, Paerregaard A, Andersen R, Andersen J. Long term outcome of prophylaxis for febrile convulsions. *Arch Dis Child* 1996;74:13–18.
84. Consensus statement. Febrile seizures: a consensus of their significance, evaluation and treatment. *Pediatrics* 1980;66:1009–1012.
85. Knudsen FU. Febrile seizures—treatment and outcome. *Brain Dev* 1996; 18:438–449.
86. Lanska DJ. Epidemiology of human immunodeficiency virus infection and associated neurologic illness. *Semin Neurol* 1999;19:105–111.
87. Levy RN, Bredesen DE, Rosenblum ML. Neurological manifestations of the acquired immunodeficiency syndrome (AIDS): experience at UCSF and review of the literature. *J Neurosurg* 1985;62:475–495.
88. Garg RK. HIV infection and seizures. *Postgrad Med J* 1999;75:387–390.
89. Wong MC, Suite NDA, Labar DR. Seizures in human immunodeficiency virus infection. *Arch Neurol* 1990;47:640–642.
90. Levy RM, Bredesen DE. Central nervous diseases in acquired immunodeficiency syndrome. *J Acquir Immune Defic Syndr Hum Retrovirol* 1988;1:41–64.
91. Pascual-Sedano B, Iranzo A, Marti-Fabregas J, et al. Prospective study of new onset seizures in patients with human immunodeficiency virus infection. *Arch Neurol* 1999;56:609–612.
92. Van Paesschen W, Bodian C, Maker H. Metabolic abnormalities and new-onset seizures in human immunodeficiency virus-seropositive patients. *Epilepsia* 1995;36:146–150.
93. Holtzman DM, Kaku DA, SoYT. New-onset seizures associated with human immunodeficiency virus infection: causation and clinical features in 100 cases. *Am J Med* 1989;87:173–177.
94. Bartolomei F, Pellegrino P, Dhiver C, Quilichini R, Gastaut JA, Gastaut JL. Crises d'epilepsie au cours de l'infection par le VIH. 52 observations. *Presse Med* 1991;20:2135–2138.
95. Dore GJ, Law MG, Brew BJ. Prospective analysis of seizures occurring in human immunodeficiency virus type-1 infection. *J Neurol AIDS* 1996;1:59–69.
96. Wong MC, Suite NDA, Labar DR. Seizures in human immunodeficiency virus infection. *Arch Neurol* 1990;47:640–642.
97. Aronow HA, Feraru ER, Lipton RB. New-onset seizures in AIDS patients: etiology, prognosis and treatment. *Neurology* 1989;39(Suppl):428.
98. Ragnaud JM, Morlat P, Dupon M, Lacoste D, Pellegrin JL, Chene G. Toxoplasmose cerebrale au cours du SIDA: 73 observations. *Presse Med* 1993;22:903–908.
99. Moulignier A, Mikol J, Pialoux G, Fenelon G, Gray F, Thiebault JB. AIDS-associated progressive multifocal leukoencephalopathy revealed by new-onset seizures. *Am J Med* 1995;99:64–68.
100. Von Einsiedel RW, Fife TD, et al. Progressive multifocal leukencephalopathy in AIDS: a clinicopathologic study and review of the literature. *J Neurol* 1993;240:391–406.
101. Koppel BS, Poon TP, Khandji A, Pavlakis SG, Pedley TA. Subacute sclerosing panencephalitis and magnetic resonance imaging. *J Neuroimaging* 1996; 6:122–125.
102. Moriarty DM, Haller JO, Loh JP, Fikrig S. Cerebral infarction in pediatric acquired immunodeficiency syndrome. *Pediatr Radiol* 1994;24:611–612.
103. Labar DR. (1992) Seizures and HIV infection. In: Pedley TA, Meldrum BS (eds.), *Recent Advances in Epilepsy,* Edinburgh: Churchill Livingstone, pp 119–126.

104. Rosenbaum GS, Klein NC, Cunba BA. Early seizures in patients with acquired immunodeficiency syndrome without mass lesion. *Heart Lung* 1989;18:526–529.

105. Update: Trends in AIDS incidence—United States, 1996. *Morbid Mortal Weekly Rep* 1997;46:861–867.

106. Palella FJ, Delaney KM, Moorman AC, et al. Declining morbidity and mortality among patients with advanced human immunodeficiency virus infection. *N Engl J Med* 1998;338:853–850.

107. Autran B, Carcelian G, Li T, et al. Positive effects of combined antiretroviral therapy on CD4+ cell homeostasis and function in advanced HIV disease. *Science* 1997;227:112–116.

108. Torres RA, Barr M. Impact of combination therapy for HIV infection on inpatient census. *N Engl J Med* 1997;336:1531–1532.

109. Teofilo E, Gouveia J, Brotas V, daCosta P. Progressive multi-focal leukoencephalopathy regression with highly active antiretroviral therapy. *AIDS* 1998;12:449.

110. Carr A, Marriot D, Field A, Vasak E, Cooper DA. Treatment of HIV-1 associated microsporidiosis and cryptosporidiosis with combination antiretroviral therapy. *Lancet* 1998;351:256–261.

111. Simpson DM. Human immunodeficiency virus-associated dementia: review of pathogenesis, prophylaxis and treatment studies of zidovudine therapy. *Clin Infect Dis* 1999;29:19–34.

112. Bharucha NE, Bharucha EP, Bhabha SK. Infections of the nervous system: Bacterial infections. In: *Neurology in Clinical Practice: The Neurological Disorders* (Bradley WG, Daroff RB, Fenichel GM, Marsden CD, eds), Butterwort–Heinemann, Boston, MA: pp 1181–1243.

113. Bruneel E, Gillis P, Raes M, et al. Radiological case of the month. Neonatal brain abscess caused by Citrobacter diversus. *Arch Pediatr Adol Med* 1998;152:297–298.

114. Maniglia RJ, Roth T, Blumberg EA. Polymicrobial brain abscess in a patient infected with human immunodeficiency virus. *Clin Infect Dis* 1997;24:449–451.

115. Aliaga L, Mediavilla JD, Lopez de la Osa A, Lopez-Gomez M, deCueto M, Miranda C. Non typhoidal salmonella intracranial infections in HIV-infected patients. *Clin Infect Dis* 1997;25:1118–1120.

116. Pruitt AA, Rubin RH, Karchmer AW, Duncan GW. Neurologic complications of bacterial endocarditis. *Medicine* 1978;57:329–343.

117. Jones HR, Siekert RG. Neurological manifestations of infective endocarditis. *Brain* 1989;112:1295–1315.

118. Kanter MC, Hart RG. Neurologic complications of infective endocarditis. *Neurology* 1991;41:1015–1020.

119. Le Cam B, Guivarch G, Boles JM, Garre M, Cartier F. Neurologic complications in a group of 86 bacterial endocarditis. *Eur Heart J* 1984;5(Suppl C):97–100.

120. Gergaud JM, Breux JP, Grollier G, Roblot P, Becq-Giraudon B. Current aspects of infectious endocarditis. Apropos of 53 cases (in French). *Ann Med Intern* 1994;145:163–167.

121. Johnson DH, Rosenthal A, Nadas AS. A forty year review of bacterial endocarditis in infancy and childhood. *Circulation* 1975;51:581–588.

122. Delahaye JP, Poncet P, Malquarti V, Beaune J, Gare JP, Mann JM. Cerebrovascular accidents in infective endocarditis: role of anticoagulation. *Eur Heart J* 1990;11:1074–1078.

9

Medication-Associated Seizures

Paul A. Garcia, MD and Brian K. Alldredge, PharmD

Introduction

Seizures are an infrequent complication of drug administration. For example, medication-associated seizures were reported in 0.08% of patients in the Boston Collaborative Surveillance Program in which 32,812 consecutive patients were monitored for medication side effects *(1)*. Nevertheless, patients with spontaneous or recurrent seizures are encountered regularly by clinicians, and these individuals are often taking medications that have been reported to cause seizures. The Physicians' Desk Reference lists seizures as a potential adverse effect for approx. 250 preparations. Establishing a causal relationship between seizures and a given medication is often difficult, however.

Because epileptic seizures are a common occurrence (with a population lifetime risk of approx. 10%) *(2)*, coincidence will account for some seizures in patients taking medication. Additionally, many patients taking medications are predisposed to seizures because of their underlying medical or neurological problems. Factors that support a causal relationship between a given medication and seizures include (1) a close temporal relationship (seizures occurring shortly after medication administration); (2) evidence for dose dependency with an increased chance for seizures occurring with increasing doses; (3) provocation of seizures in patients without predisposing medical or neurological factors, and (4) the presence of a well-defined underlying mechanism by which the medication might provoke seizures. Because the number of medications reported to cause seizures is extensive, we will only discuss medications that fulfill most of these criteria.

Based on these criteria it is often clear that an agent can provoke seizures. It is much more difficult, however, to compare the risk of the various agents.

From: *Seizures: Medical Causes and Management*
Edited by: N. Delanty © Humana Press, Inc., Totowa, NJ

Table 1
Risk of Seizures When Taken as an Overdose

Very High Risk	Intermediate Risk	Modest Risk
Cyclic antidepressants (especially amoxapine and maprotiline)	β-Lactam antibiotics	SSRIs
Theophylline	Flouroquinolones	β-Blockers
Isoniazid	Meperidine	Flumazenil
Alkylating antineoplastic agents	Tramadol	Antiviral antibiotics
Cyclosporin/FK506 (tacrolimus)	Lidocaine	
	Lithium	
	Antipsychotics	
	Anticonvulsants	

The most important consideration in this matter is that seizures are a rare complication of drug therapy. To have an 80% chance of differentiating between an incidence of 0.5% and 1.0%, a sample size of 9000 patients would be required *(3)*. Randomized, controlled studies almost never meet this requirement. Thus, comparisons are usually based on isolated case reports or small case series. This method is subject to so many potential biases that only extreme examples (such as several patients without risk factors having seizures associated with a medication) are helpful in roughly delineating the comparative risk of the agents. With the caveats noted above, **Tables 1** and **2** represent our best attempt to classify medications according to the risk for provoking seizures in overdosage and therapeutic use, respectively.

A basic understanding of medication-associated seizures enables clinicians of all specialties to make prompt, appropriate decisions. Some medication-induced seizures require a specific antidote or a preferred anticonvulsant remedy **(Table 3)**. Although drug-induced seizures are typically brief, generalized tonic-clonic convulsions, as many as 15% may present as status epilepticus *(4)*. Thus, most clinicians will face occasional seizure-related emergencies associated with medications that they prescribe.

Many factors can contribute to medication-induced seizures. These factors can be divided into those related to the medication and those intrinsic to the patient *(5)*. Often both types of factors are significant. Recognition of these factors is important in determining the risk of a medicine for any given patient.

The most important medication-related factor contributing to drug-induced seizures is the intrinsic epileptogenicity of the medication. Although the mechanism by which medications induce seizures is not always known, some medications have a well-defined mechanism for causing seizures. Some medications, such as penicillin, increase central nervous system (CNS) excitability by antagonizing the inhibitory neurotransmitter γ-amino butyric acid

Table 2
Risk of Seizures When Taken Therapeutically

Moderate Risk	Intermediate Risk	Low Risk
Chlorpromazine	Theophylline	Flouroquinolones[a]
Clozapine	Isoniazid	Antiviral antibiotics
Maprotiline	β-Lactam antibiotics	β-Blockers
Clomipramine	Cyclic antidepressants (except clomipramine and maprotiline)	Local anesthetics
Bupropion	Antipsychotic agents (except chlorpromazine and clozapine)	SSRIs
Meperidine	Contrast agents	MAO inhibitors
Anticonvulsants[b]	Tramadol	
Flumazenil[c]		

[a]Unless used with NSAIDs.
[b]When used for an inappropriate epilepsy syndrome.
[c]When used in a benzodiazepine overdose.

(GABA) *(6,7)*. Although this is an unintended coincidence with penicillin, some medications such as flumazenil, have been designed to interfere with intrinsic brain inhibition by binding to GABA-associated benzodiazepine receptors *(8)*. Medications can also cause seizures indirectly. For example, foscarnet chelates divalent cations resulting in hypocalcemia and hypomagnesemia. Either of these factors might provoke or exacerbate seizures *(9)*. Vaccines also cause seizures indirectly by provoking fevers in children *(10)*.

Other medication-related factors that increase risk of seizures include those that lead to higher serum or brain levels. Route of administration and medication dosage are the most important in this regard. Some medications, such as penicillin, are more likely to produce seizures when administered intravenously as opposed to orally. Intrinsic drug properties such as lipid solubility, molecular weight, ionization, and protein binding affect the degree of penetration into the CNS. Thus, these factors are important for any medications that produce seizures by a direct effect on the brain *(5)*.

A patient's neurological condition is probably the most important patient-related factor. Patients with epilepsy are at the highest risk for having both spontaneous and medication-associated seizures. Patients with both acute and chronic neurological conditions are also at increased risk for seizures, as most processes that injure brain tissue increase the risk for seizures. Acute neurological disorders such as meningitis also increase the risk for seizures by causing breakdown of the blood–brain barrier, thereby allowing for greater exposure to the epileptogenic agent. Patient-related medical factors can also increase the risk of seizures. Conditions that reduce drug elimination

Table 3
Specific Treatment Recommendations for Medication-Associated Seizures

Medication	Recommended Treatment
β-lactam antibiotics	Benzodiazepines, barbiturates
Flouroquinolones	Benzodiazepines, barbiturates
Isoniazid	Pyridoxine
Foscarnet	Conventional medications, Ca^{2+} or Mg^{2+} as needed
Vaccination	Treat as febrile seizure
Theophylline	May require hemodialysis
Meperidine	Naloxone may exacerbate seizures
Tramadol	Naloxone may exacerbate seizures
Local anesthetics	Benzodiazepines, barbiturates, propofol

capacity, such as hepatic or renal failure, often result in unexpectedly high serum concentrations when doses are not appropriately adjusted.

The use of penicillin in patients undergoing cardiopulmonary bypass provides an example of the interaction between patient-related and drug-related factors. In a retrospective analysis of patients in an Australian hospital, over 40% of cardiopulmonary bypass patients receiving high-dose penicillin prophylaxis suffered convulsions *(11)*. Only 3% of patients treated with low-dose prophylaxis suffered seizures. Similar results were reported in a Canadian series *(12)*. When the relationship between cardiopulmonary bypass and penicillin prophylaxis was studied in dogs, it was determined that neither high-dose penicillin nor bypass surgery alone caused seizures. The combination, however, often resulted in seizures *(13)*. The mechanism for this interaction is unclear. Perhaps microemboli breached the integrity of the blood–brain barrier during bypass procedures, thus resulting in increased brain concentrations of penicillin. Alternatively, decreased pulmonary metabolism during surgery may have led to higher serum levels. Finally, general anesthetic agents may have decreased the active transport of penicillin out of the spinal fluid resulting in high CNS concentrations *(6)*.

Medications That Commonly Cause Seizures

Anti-infectives

Antibiotics are widely used in the modern practice of medicine. Often the condition requiring treatment predisposes the person to seizures. Not surprisingly, seizures occur frequently in the setting of antibiotic use. Nevertheless, most antibiotics have not been convincingly associated with an increased risk for seizures. The most notable exceptions are the β-lactam antibiotics. The fluoroquinolones, isoniazid, and some antiviral medications can also provoke seizures.

β-*Lactam Antibiotics*

Of the antibiotic-induced seizures, penicillin-related seizures have been studied the most extensively. In fact, scientists have exploited penicillin's intrinsic epileptogenicity to produce animal models of epilepsy *(14)*. In animals, penicillin consistently causes seizures when administered intravenously in high doses or when applied directly to the brain. Studies suggest that penicillin increases brain excitability by preventing the inhibitory neurotransmitter γ-aminobutyric acid (GABA) from binding to the $GABA_A$ receptor. Additionally, penicillin seems to prevent the opening of $GABA_A$-associated chloride channels *(7)*. The net effect of this interference with GABA-related inhibitory neurotransmission is enhanced cortical excitability and spontaneous seizures.

Clinical neurotoxicity with penicillin was first described in 1945 in a baby who developed coma and myoclonic twitching after being treated with intrathecal penicillin *(15)*. Most penicillin-induced seizures occur 12 h to 3 d after initiation of treatment *(16)*. They are typically generalized tonic-clonic seizures and are usually associated with myoclonus and encephalopathy or coma *(17)*. The electroencephalogram (EEG) often shows associated generalized epileptiform discharges *(17)*.

Through the years it has become clear that the route of administration greatly influences the chance for penicillin-induced neurotoxicity. Although intrathecal dosing often causes seizures *(18)*, intravenous and oral administration is much safer *(1)*. Renal failure is probably the most important patient-related risk factor. Renal insufficiency probably predisposes to seizures in two ways: (1) Low penicillin clearance results in high serum concentrations with an increased risk for seizures; and (2) the low serum protein concentration associated with uremia probably increases the penetration of the blood–brain barrier by penicillin, thus raising the brain concentration of the medication *(19)*. Low penicillin protein binding and undeveloped renal tubular secretory function may account for the increased risk of penicillin-related seizures in babies. Similarly, increased risk for seizures in elderly patients may be the result of low plasma albumin concentrations and decreased glomerular filtration *(20)*.

Cephalosporins have also been associated with seizures in humans. Clinical and electroencephalographic features of cephalosporin-induced seizures resemble those caused by penicillin *(6)*. The carbapenem group of β-lactam antibiotics, including imipenem and meropenem, can also cause seizures. In animal models, the proconvulsant potency seems to correlate well with the affinity for $GABA_A$ receptor binding. Imipenem possesses the strongest affinity for the $GABA_A$ complex and greatest proconvulsant effect *(21)*. Risk factors for cephalosporin or carbapenem-induced seizures are much the same as for penicillin. It is thought that coadministration of cilastatin with imipenem increases the risk for seizures much as probenecid increases the risk for seizures with administration of penicillin *(6)*. However, this effect has been questioned *(22)*.

Treatment of β-lactam-induced seizures includes discontinuation of the implicated medication. Although dialysis may be effective at reducing serum levels, this intervention has never been shown to be useful in the treatment of seizures provoked by these medications. Whereas there are no head-to-head comparisons of conventional anticonvulsants in this setting, animal models suggest that anticonvulsants that enhance GABA activity are more likely to be effective than those that lack this mechanism of action. In animals, penicillin-induced seizures are terminated more effectively by diazepam than by phenytoin *(6)*. Therefore, one should probably choose diazepam, lorazepam, or barbiturates as first-line anticonvulsant treatment for seizures provoked by β-lactam antibiotics.

Flouroquinolones

Fluoroquinolones have also been associated with seizures. These medications appear to cause seizures by direct antagonism of GABA binding to the $GABA_A$ receptor *(23)*. The proconvulsant property seems to be related to the similarity in structure of the substituted seven position of the parent compound to the neurotransmitter GABA *(24)*.

Clinical experience suggests that quinolone-induced seizures are rare in patients unless associated with overdose or a predisposition to seizures. Compared to penicillin-induced seizures they typically occur after a more protracted treatment course *(6)*. The attacks consist of a single or multiple brief tonic or clonic movements and resolve quickly with the use of anticonvulsants *(25)*. In addition to the usual patient and medication-related risk factors for seizures, the risk of flouroquinolone-associated seizures is increased by concomitant use of either theophylline or nonsteroidal anti-inflammatory drugs (NSAIDs) *(5)*.

It is not surprising that the combination of theophylline and fluoroquinolones is epileptogenic, as both of these medications can cause seizures when used individually. The combination is especially epileptogenic, however, because fluoroquinolones inhibit theophylline metabolism, thus increasing serum levels of theophylline *(26)*. Additionally, animal studies suggest that $GABA_A$ receptor antagonism by fluoroquinolones is enhanced by aminophylline *(27)*. Thus, each of these medications seems to enhance the epileptogenic potential of the other.

The seizure-inducing potential of the fluoroquinolones is also enhanced by NSAIDs. Japanese physicians reported this association when patients without other risk factors developed seizures while taking both enoxacin and fenbufen

(28). Subsequent laboratory studies have demonstrated relatively weak $GABA_A$ receptor antagonism by fluoroquinolones when used alone. In fact, the effect is considerably less than would be needed to produce seizures at therapeutic serum concentrations of these medications. Coadministration of biphenyl acetic acid, an active metabolite of fenbufen, potentiated $GABA_A$ antagonism by a factor of 1000 *(28)*. The exact mechanism for the enhanced GABA antagonism is unknown. This association is particularly important, however, given the fact that several NSAIDs are available over the counter. Patients often consider these medications innocuous. Care must be taken to counsel all patients taking fluoroquinolone antibiotics to avoid the use of these compounds. Based on the mechanism of seizure provocation, benzodiazepines and barbiturates are preferred for treating seizures caused by this group of antibiotics.

Isoniazid

In recent years the incidence of isoniazid (INH)-related seizures has escalated because of the resurgence of tuberculosis in the United States. Most INH-induced seizures occur in the setting of either intentional or accidental overdosage. Acute INH-induced seizures have been an especially important medical problem for some groups of Native Americans because of the high rate of tuberculosis in this group, together with social problems leading to a high suicide rate. In the early 1970s, almost 20% of the suicide fatalities among Southwest Native Americans involved INH *(29)*. This reflects the high incidence of tuberculosis in this population, as well as the high mortality rate from INH-related neurotoxicity. Death rates from INH overdose are as high as 20% in Alaskan Native Americans *(30)*.

INH causes seizures by competing with pyridoxine for transformation to pyridoxal phosphate by the enzyme pyridoxine kinase. Pyridoxal phosphate is an essential co-factor required for the synthesis of GABA. Thus, INH inhibits production of the inhibitory neurotransmitter GABA, resulting in enhanced cortical excitability and seizures *(31)*.

Seizures have been documented in people taking less than 20 mg/kg per day of INH. The usual dosage of INH is 5 mg/kg per day in adults and 10–15 mg/kg per day in children. Thus, INH has a narrow therapeutic index *(6)*. Ingestion of >80 mg/kg typically results in severe neurotoxicity *(32)*. Renal failure and possibly slow acetylator status predispose a patient to INH-related seizures *(33,34)*.

INH-associated seizures typically begin within hours of the ingestion. They are often heralded by nausea, vomiting, and encephalopathy. Seizures are typically generalized tonic-clonic convulsions. Not infrequently, patients develop convulsive status epilepticus *(33)*. Although INH serum levels correlate with the risk for severe neurotoxicity *(35)*, these studies are of little practical use in the setting of acute INH-associated seizures. Because potentially lethal neurotoxicity can occur in patients taking doses within the usual prescribed range, it is imperative that antedotal treatment begin immediately in any patient presenting with seizures while taking INH. The treatment of choice for seizures induced by INH is intravenous pyridoxine. At least 1 g should be administered intravenously. The usual recommendation is for 5-g boluses to be repeated every 5–20 min until the seizures stop *(5,35)*. Santucci and colleagues recently found that many emergency departments are insufficiently stocked with pyridoxine to manage such an emergency *(36)*. INH-induced seizures are typically refractory to treatment with anticonvulsants such as phenytoin and barbiturates *(37)*. Benzodiazepines may be helpful in treating the seizures *(32),* especially when pyridoxine is not available.

Antiviral Agents

Antiviral agents are not commonly associated with seizures unless they are being used to treat CNS infections. Acyclovir occasionally causes acute CNS toxicity, including convulsions, when given in very high doses or when used in patients with renal failure *(38)*. Although most patients who develop seizures while taking foscarnet have underlying CNS pathology as the etiology, hypocalcemia and hypomagnesemia associated with this agent might also contribute to the risk of seizures *(9)*. When a patient taking foscarnet presents with seizures, blood work should be performed to assess for these metabolic disturbances. Although seizures are sometimes reported in patients taking antiviral therapy for HIV, it is difficult to be confident of the association given the many other risk factors for seizures in this patient population.

Vaccinations

Vaccinations are the optimum means of preventing many infections. Although children undergoing vaccinations often experience seizures shortly after their vaccination, the attacks appear to arise exclusively in the setting of fever provoked by the vaccination. Critical appraisal suggests that febrile seizures provoked by vaccination arise in patients predisposed to such attacks. Neurologic sequelae are a consequence of the underlying cerebral pathology rather than the vaccine or the vaccine-associated seizure *(10,39)*.

Antitumor Agents

Alkylating chemotherapeutic agents, including chlorambucil and busulfan, can provoke seizures. CNS toxicity is dose dependent for both of these agents. In a phase I trial with chlorambucil, 5 of 6 patients receiving a dose of 144 mg/m^2 developed CNS toxicity. Lower doses are much less likely to provoke seizures *(40)*. Vassal and colleagues found that 15% of children treated with 600 mg/m^2 busulfan suffered seizures. When dosing was based on body weight, seizures were less frequent. Pretreatment with intravenous clonazepam was effective in preventing seizures in patients at higher risk *(41)*. Other antineoplastic agents occasionally induce seizures, although usually only in acute overdosage *(5)*.

Immune System Modifying Agents

Medications Used Following Organ Transplant

Medications used for immunosuppression following organ transplant cause seizures. Cyclosporine and FK506 (tacrolimus) cause an encephalopathy associated with MRI abnormalities that involve predominantly posterior subcortical white matter. The seizures are often accompanied by acute psychosis and tremor. Wijdicks and colleagues found that over half of the seizures occurring in patients undergoing orthotopic liver transplantation occurred as a result of high levels of these immunosuppressive agents *(42)*. OKT3 caused seizures in 6% of patients with renal allografts. However, seizures only occurred when patients had nonfunctioning grafts *(43)*.

Interferons

Seizures occurred in 4 of 311 patients taking alpha interferon for chronic viral hepatitis. No other potential cause for the seizures was found. There were no seizure recurrences once the medication was withdrawn. The seizures did not occur immediately after treatment was initiated. The occurrence of seizures was delayed until after at least 2 mo of treatment *(44)*. Patients taking IFN-β1A and β1B for multiple sclerosis suffered rare convulsions. Although it is possible that the seizures were the result of the underlying condition, patients in the placebo arms did not suffer seizures during the early trial. Three percent of patients taking IFN-β1A *(45)* and 2% of patients taking IFN-β1B *(46)* suffered seizures (for a total of 6 of 282 patients, compared to 0 of 266 patients taking placebo).

Cardiovascular Agents

β-Adrenergic blocking agents may cause seizures when given in supratherapeutic doses. Cardioselective β-blockers may be less epileptogenic, although esmolol has been reported to cause seizures even in therapeutic doses. Antiarrhythmic medications such as mexiletine, tocainide, and lidocaine can cause seizures, especially in overdosage *(47,48)*. Other antiarrhythmic medications such as digoxin *(49)* and disopyramide *(50)* can cause seizures as well.

Theophylline

The incidence of theophylline-induced seizures has decreased as other treatments for asthma have become preferred. Nevertheless, it is important for clinicians to promptly recognize theophylline-induced seizures because neurotoxicity owing to theophylline is often life threatening and difficult to treat. The mechanism by which theophylline causes seizures is not known. It might antagonize the inhibitory effects of adenosine by inhibition of phosphodiesterase *(51)*. Theophylline-induced convulsions are typically unresponsive to conventional anticonvulsants, including benzodiazepines, barbiturates, and phenytoin. Hemodialysis and hemoperfusion are often used to lower serum levels acutely *(51)*. One should not rely exclusively on serum theophylline concentrations, however, as there is a poor correlation between serum and CNS concentrations *(52)*. Seizures can occur with either acute or chronic overdosage. For a given serum level of medication, however, seizures are more likely to occur in the setting of chronic overmedication *(51)*.

CNS Stimulants

Amphetamines and amphetamine derivatives are used to treat children with attention deficit disorder, patients with narcolepsy and, occasionally, patients with severe psychomotor slowing. They are also commonly abused. Although they are often associated with seizures when used illicitly *(53)*, these medications rarely cause seizures when used therapeutically. Some animal models suggest that low doses of amphetamines may even exert mild anticonvulsant effects *(54)*. Because many patients treated with amphetamines may be predisposed to seizures, it is important to recognize that therapeutic use of amphetamines is unlikely to exacerbate their condition.

Phenylpropanolamine is a common component of diet pills and decongestants. Seizures related to phenylpropanolamine have occurred most often with supratherapeutic doses. Occasional seizures have been reported with therapeutic use, however *(55)*. Hypertension typically accompanies the seizures. There are no specific antidotes for seizures elicited by stimulant medications.

Psychotropic Medications

The relationship between seizures and psychotropic medications is often difficult to assess, as many patients that require these medications are at increased risk for having seizures related to underlying brain dysfunction. Despite this confounding factor, it is clear that many psychotropic medications can cause seizures. Seizures related to specific antidepressant and antipsychotic medications are discussed below. The mechanism by which antidepressant and antipsychotic medications cause seizures is not known.

Because many patients with epilepsy suffer from depression or psychosis, the use of psychotropic drugs is often necessary in this group of patients. Although one would suspect that the risk for inducing seizures would be even greater in this group, clinical experience suggests that most patients with epilepsy will not experience a seizure exacerbation when treated with psychotropic medications *(56)*. Nevertheless, conservative clinical practice includes choosing an agent that is less likely to cause seizures and using the lowest possible dose of medication that is clinically effective.

An additional consideration in a patient with epilepsy is the potential for the psychotropic medication to interact with the patient's anticonvulsant medication. Psychotropics, especially antidepressants, tend to be inhibitors of hepatic cytochrome oxidase enzymes. Thus, it is unlikely that they will exacerbate seizures by lowering serum anticonvulsant levels. Their addition could result in anticonvulsant toxicity, however. Better predictions of this type of interaction can be made based on knowledge of the isoenzymes involved in degradation of the individual drugs *(57)*.

When seizures occur in the setting of therapeutic use of psychotropic medications, the treatment consists primarily of lowering the dose of the medication or switching to an alternate agent. When seizures occur in the setting of overdose, the primary concern is for lowering serum levels of the medication. If acute symptomatic treatment of seizures is necessary, standard anticonvulsant medications are used.

Antidepressants

The clearest relationship between antidepressant use and provoked seizures is seen in the setting of cyclic antidepressant overdose. Cyclic antidepressant overdose leads to seizures in up to 20% of patients *(58,59)*. The seizures typically occur within a few hours of ingestion and are associated with encephalopathy *(60,61)*. Amoxapine and maprotiline are particularly likely to cause seizures in the setting of overdose *(62)*. Although seizures have been reported with overdosage of serotonin-specific re-uptake inhibitors (SSRIs) such as fluoxetine, sertraline, and paroxetine, the incidence seems to be much lower than with cyclic antidepressants *(53,63)*.

Evidence for a dose-dependent seizure risk with antidepressants is apparent when considering that the incidence of seizures in patients during therapeutic use is much lower than in those taking antidepressant overdoses. In therapeutic use, some medications are much more likely than others to cause seizures. However, the low seizure incidence makes comparison between different medications very difficult. In fact, some antidepressants such as fluoxetine have an incidence of seizures no higher than placebo when used therapeutically and might even be mildly anticonvulsant *(64)*.

It is easier to compare seizure incidence in a given medication at various doses. Bupropion, a monocyclic inhibitor of dopamine re-uptake, provides an example of this type of comparison. Premarketing trials with this medication at maximal doses of 450–900 mg/d yielded an overall incidence of seizures of 1% (as high as 5% in one group of patients with bulemia) *(65)*. A subsequent analysis revealed that patients taking doses exceeding 450 mg/d had a 2.2% incidence of seizures, whereas those taking lower doses had a 0.4% incidence of seizures *(65)*. This medication was removed from the market in 1986 but was later reintroduced with the recommendation for a maximum dose of 450 mg/d. Several medications have dose-related seizure risks similar to bupropion. Imipramine, amitriptyline, and maprotiline all are more likely to provoke seizures when used therapeutically at higher doses *(66)*.

Although it is impossible to absolutely quantify the risk of individual antidepressant medications, the increased risk of seizures with some agents when used at intermediate to high doses enables us to stratify (for practical purposes) the agents as high- or low-risk agents. Bupropion and maprotiline are considered high-risk agents whereas the SSRIs and monoamine oxidase (MAO) inhibitors are low-risk agents, even when used at high doses. Tricyclic antidepressants pose an intermediate risk, especially when used at higher doses or in individuals who develop high serum levels during treatment with moderate doses *(67)*.

Antipsychotics

Antipsychotic overdosage is less likely to cause seizures when compared to overdosage with the cyclic antidepressants. A review of drug overdoses reported to the National Clearinghouse for Poison Control Centers found seizures occurring in approx. 3% of phenothiazine overdoses *(68)*. Although seizures can occur with risperidone overdose, the low potential for seizures is evidenced by a recent review of 15 patients taking risperidone overdose (as the only overdose agent). None of these patients suffered seizures *(69)*.

Whereas all phenothiazines are known to induce seizures, the aliphatic phenothiazines (especially chlorpromazine) are thought to be more epileptogenic than the piperazine (fluphenazine) or piperadine (thioridazine) derivatives. Many clinicians feel that seizures are more frequent in patients taking chlorpromazine compared to the other phenothiazines. Additionally, animal studies suggest that chlorpromazine has a greater potential for causing seizures than other antipsychotic medications *(5)*. Butyrophenones such as haloperidol can also induce seizures. The risk seems to be somewhat lower than for the phenothiazines, however *(70)*. Clozapine, a newer agent, has been reported to cause seizures in approx. 2.8% of patients *(71)*. As with antidepressants, a consistent dose-dependent risk for seizures is evident for many antipsychotic medications.

Absolute quantification of seizure risk for each antipsychotic medication is not possible to establish, as very few patients experience seizures during randomized, controlled trials. With antidepressants, however, a qualitative stratification is possible based on the frequency of reported seizures and the doses at which the seizures occurred. Clozapine and chlorpromazine seem to have the highest risk for inducing seizures. Haloperidol, fluphenazine, molindone, pimozide, trifluoperazine, and risperidone rarely cause seizures during therapeutic use in patients without underlying risk factors. Olanzapine, quetiapine, and thioridazine pose an intermediate risk.

Lithium

Lithium causes convulsions in the settings of both acute and chronic intoxication. Typically, serum levels are greater than 3 meq/L when seizures occur *(72)*. Occasionally seizures have been reported when serum levels are within the therapeutic range *(73)*. Lithium, like other psychotropic medications, can elicit paroxysmal electroencephalographic activity *(74)*. Risk factors for lithium-related seizures include a pre-existent EEG abnormality or epilepsy, acute psychotic symptoms, and decreased renal clearance *(5)*.

Anticonvulsants

Because the baseline seizure frequency fluctuates in patients with epilepsy, it is difficult to ascribe a worsening in seizures to the addition of a particular medication. A small percentage of patients enrolled in trials with the currently available anticonvulsants experienced seizure exacerbations with the addition of the study medication. In all cases, an equal or higher number of patients in the placebo arm experienced worsening of their seizures *(75)*. Thus, it seems likely that most patients undergoing seizure exacerbation after addition of a new medicine do so because of factors other than a proconvulsant response to the medication.

There are, however, two well-accepted means by which anticonvulsants exacerbate seizures. First, patients can develop neurotoxicity including seizures because of anticonvulsant overdosage *(76)*. This syndrome has been best described for phenytoin and carbamazepine. Encephalopathy and coma associated with seizures can also occur with valproic acid *(76)*. Second, anticonvulsants may exacerbate seizures when an anticonvulsant inappropriate for treating a given seizure type is selected. Patients with generalized onset seizures may have their nonconvulsive seizures worsened by the use of phenytoin or carbamazepine. This may also occur with the use of barbiturates or vigabatrin *(77)*.

Anesthetic and Analgesic Agents

Lidocaine and related local anesthetic agents rarely cause seizures unless administered intravenously either inadvertently during local anesthesia or therapeutically in the case of lidocaine being used as an antiarrhythmic drug *(78)*. Rare seizures have been reported following oral, subcutaneous, or intraurethral administration *(79,80)*. Subconvulsant levels of lidocaine are actually anticonvulsant, leading to its use in treating refractory status epilepticus *(81)*. The mechanism by which lidocaine and related compounds induce seizures is thought to be by selective blockade of inhibitory cortical synapses *(82)*. Treatment of seizures induced by local anesthetic agents includes administration of benzodiazepines, barbiturates, or propofol *(82)*.

General anesthetic agents can also induce seizures. Both clinical and electroencephalographic seizures have been induced by enflurane *(83)*. Etomidate causes severe involuntary myoclonic movements in some patients. Because these movements are not associated with ictal scalp EEG patterns and this medication is an anticonvulsant in animals *(84)*, etomidate-induced myoclonus has been considered nonepileptic. A similar phenomenon has been observed with propofol use. In epileptic patients, however, etomidate enhances epileptiform activity on the EEG and may provoke clinical seizures *(85)*.

Narcotic analgesics rarely provoke seizures when used therapeutically. Meperidine is the notable exception. It is hepatically metabolized to normeperidine, which is a potent proconvulsant *(86)*. Accumulation of normeperidine is facilitated by renal failure as well as oral administration (owing to extensive first-pass metabolism) *(87)*. There is not a specific antidote for meperidine-induced seizures. Naloxone is not beneficial, as it may exacerbate the seizures by interfering with the mild anticonvulsant effect of meperidine *(86)*.

Tramadol, a new centrally acting analgesic, has been associated with seizures in both therapeutic and toxic doses *(88,89)*. Concomitant treatment with antidepressants appears to increase this risk *(89)*. Naloxone, although potentially beneficial in the setting of tramadol overdose, may also increase the risk of spontaneous seizures *(90)*.

Flumazenil

Flumazenil is a benzodiazepine receptor antagonist that has been used to treat patients successfully in the setting of acute benzodiazepine overdose. Seizures occur occasionally. There is not a clear relationship between the dose of flumazenil and the risk of seizures. Rather, the risk for seizures with flumazenil seems to be related to a benzodiazepine withdrawal effect or unmasking of a seizure predisposition previously masked by the benzodiazepine. Patients taking multidrug overdoses, especially those taking tricyclic antidepressants in addition to benzodiazepines, seem to be especially susceptible to flumazenil-induced seizures *(91)*.

Radiographic Contrast Agents

Seizures related to contrast agents typically occur within 10 min of contrast injection. The risk is highest in patients with epilepsy or focal brain lesions.

High doses of contrast are more likely to provoke seizures. Seizures are typically self-limited, but status epilepticus can occur *(92)*. There are no specific treatments for contrast-induced seizures.

Summary

Medication-associated seizures are an uncommon but important complication of medical therapy. Clinicians of all disciplines will care for patients at risk for this dramatic medication toxicity. A working knowledge of the high-risk medications will enable clinicians to choose safer medicines for patients at risk for seizures. Furthermore, a basic understanding of these medications enables clinicians to promptly recognize medication-associated seizures and to correctly formulate an appropriate treatment plan.

References

1. Porter J, Jick H. Drug-induced anaphylaxis, convulsions, deafness, and extrapyramidal symptoms. *Lancet* 1977;1:587–588.
2. Hauser WA, Hesdorffer DC. *Epilepsy: Frequency, Causes and Consequences.* New York: Demos, 1990:11.
3. Rosenstein DL, Nelson JC, Jacobs SC. Seizures associated with antidepressants: a review. *J Clin Psychiatry* 1993;54:289–299.
4. Messing RO, Closson RG, Simon RP. Drug-induced seizures: a 10-year experience. *Neurology* 1984;34:1582–1586.
5. Garcia PA, Alldredge BK. Drug-induced seizures. *Neurol Clin* 1994;12:85–99.
6. Wallace KL. Antibiotic-induced convulsions. *Crit Care Clin* 1997;13:741–762.
7. Fujimoto M, Munakata M, Akaike N. Dual mechanisms of $GABA_A$ response inhibition by beta-lactam antibiotics in the pyramidal neurones of the rat cerebral cortex. *Br J Pharmacol* 1995;116:3014–3020.
8. Paronis CA, Bergman J. Apparent pA2 values of benzodiazepine antagonists and partial agonists in monkeys. *J Pharmacol Exp Ther* 1999;290:1222–1229.
9. Jacobson MA. Review of the toxicities of foscarnet. *J Acquir Immune Defic Syndr* 1992;5:S11–S17.
10. Griffin MR, Ray WA, Mortimer EA, Fenichel GM, Schaffner W. Risk of seizures and encephalopathy after immunization with the diphtheria-tetanus-pertussis vaccine. *JAMA* 1990;263:1641–1645.
11. Currie TT, Hayward NJ, Westlake G, Williams J. Epilepsy in cardiopulmonary bypass patients receiving large intravenous doses of penicillin. *J Thorac Cardiovasc Surg* 1971;62:1–6.
12. Dobell AR, Wyant JD, Seamans KB, Gloor P. Penicillin epilepsy. Studies on the blood-brain barrier during cardiopulmonary bypass. *J Thorac Cardiovasc Surg* 1966;52:469–475.
13. Seamans KB, Gloor P, Dobell RAR, Wyant JD. Penicillin-induced seizures during cardiopulmonary bypass. A clinical and electroencephalographic study. *N Engl J Med* 1968;278:861–868.
14. Gutnick MJ, Van Duijn H, Citri N. Relative convulsant potencies of structural analogues of penicillin. *Brain Res* 1976;114:139–143.
15. Walker AE. Convulsive factor in commercial penicillin. *Arch Surg* 1945;50:69–73.

16. Nicholls PJ. Neurotoxicity of penicillin. *J Antimicrob Chemother* 1980;6:161–165.

17. Fossieck B Jr, Parker RH. Neurotoxicity during intravenous infusion of penicillin. A review. *J Clin Pharmacol* 1974;14:504–512.

18. Edwards WM, Kellsey DC. Toxicity of intrathecal penicillin. *US Armed Forces Med J* 1950;1:806–811.

19. Schliamser SE, Cars O, Norrby SR. Neurotoxicity of beta-lactam antibiotics: predisposing factors and pathogenesis. *J Antimicrob Chemother* 1991;27:405–425.

20. Barrons RW, Murray KM, Richey RM. Populations at risk for penicillin-induced seizures. *Ann Pharmacother* 1992;26:26–29.

21. Day IP, Goudie J, Nishiki K, Williams PD. Correlation between in vitro and in vivo models of proconvulsive activity with the carbapenem antibiotics, biapenem, imipenem/cilastatin and meropenem. *Toxicol Lett* 1995;76:239–243.

22. de Sarro A, Imperatore C, Mastroeni P, de Sarro G. Comparative convulsant potencies of two carbapenem derivatives in C57 and DBA/2 mice. *J Pharm Pharmacol* 1995;47:292–296.

23. Tsuji A, Sato H, Kume Y, et al. Inhibitory effects of quinolone antibacterial agents on gamma-aminobutyric acid binding to receptor sites in rat brain membranes. *Antimicrob Agents Chemother* 1988;32:190–194.

24. Akahane K, Sekiguchi M, Une T, Osada Y. Structure-epileptogenicity relationship of quinolones with special reference to their interaction with gamma-aminobutyric acid receptor sites. *Antimicrob Agents Chemother* 1989;33:1704–1708.

25. Arcieri GM, Becker N, Esposito B, et al. Safety of intravenous ciprofloxacin. A review. *Am J Med* 1989;87:92S–97S.

26. Polk RE. Drug-drug interactions with ciprofloxacin and other fluoroquinolones. *Am J Med* 1989;87:76S–81S.

27. Segev S, Rehavi M, Rubinstein E. Quinolones, theophylline, and diclofenac interactions with the gamma-aminobutyric acid receptor. *Antimicrob Agents Chemother* 1988;32:1624–1626.

28. Halliwell RF, Davey PG, Lambert JJ. Antagonism of $GABA_A$ receptors by 4-quinolones. *J Antimicrob Chemother* 1993;31:457–462.

29. Sievers ML, Cynamon MH, Bittker TE. Intentional isoniazid overdosage among southwestern American Indians. *Am J Psychiatry* 1975;132:662–665.

30. Brown CV. Acute isoniazid poisoning. *Am Rev Respir Dis* 1972;105:206–216.

31. Gilhotra R, Malik SK, Singh S, Sharma BK. Acute isoniazid toxicity—report of 2 cases and review of literature. *Int J Clin Pharmacol Ther Toxicol* 1987;25:259–261.

32. Sievers ML, Herrier RN. Treatment of acute isoniazid toxicity. *Am J Hosp Pharm* 1975;32:202–206.

33. Miller J, Robinson A, Percy AK. Acute isoniazid poisoning in childhood. *Am J Dis Child* 1980;134:290–292.

34. Wood ER. Isoniazid toxicity. Pyridoxine controlled seizures in a dialysis patient. *J Kans Med Soc* 1981;82:551–552.

35. Wason S, Lacouture PG, Lovejoy FH Jr. Single high-dose pyridoxine treatment for isoniazid overdose. *JAMA* 1981;246:1102–1104.

36. Santucci KA, Shah BR, Linakis JG. Acute isoniazid exposures and antidote availability. *Pediatr Emerg Care* 1999;15:99–101.

37. Terman DS, Teitelbaum DT. Isoniazid self-poisoning. *Neurology* 1970;20:299–304.

38. Balfour HH. Acyclovir. In: Peterson PK, Verhoef J (eds.), *The Antimicrobial Agents Annual,* 3rd ed. Amsterdam: Elsevier Science, 1988:349.

39. American Academy of Pediatrics Committee on Infectious Diseases: The status of acellular pertussis vaccines: current perspective. *Pediatrics* 1991;88:401–405.
40. Blumenreich MS, Woodcock TM, Sherrill EJ, et al. A phase I trial of chlorambucil administered in short pulses in patients with advanced malignancies. *Cancer Invest* 1988;6:371–375.
41. Vassal G, Deroussent A, Hartmann O, et al. Dose-dependent neurotoxicity of high-dose busulfan in children: a clinical and pharmacological study. *Cancer Res* 1990;50:6203–6207.
42. Wijdicks EF, Plevak DJ, Wiesner RH, Steers JL. Causes and outcome of seizures in liver transplant recipients. *Neurology* 1996;47:1523–1525.
43. Thistlethwaite JR Jr, Stuart JK, Mayes JT, et al. Complications and monitoring of OKT3 therapy. *Am J Kidney Dis* 1988;11:112–119.
44. Shakil AO, Di Bisceglie AM, Hoofnagle JH. Seizures during alpha interferon therapy (see comments). *J Hepatol* 1996;24:48–51.
45. Munschauer FE III, Kinkel RP. Managing side effects of interferon-beta in patients with relapsing-remitting multiple sclerosis. *Clin Ther* 1997;19:883–893.
46. *Physicians Desk Reference.* Montvale: Medical Economics Company, 1999.
47. Cohen A. Accidental overdose of tocainide successfully treated. *Angiology* 1987;38:614.
48. Jequier P, Jones R, Mackintosh A. Letter: Fatal mexiletine overdose. *Lancet* 1976;1:429.
49. Douglas EF, White PT, Nelson JW. Three per second spike-wave in digitalis toxicity. Report of a case. *Arch Neurol* 1971;25:373–375.
50. Johnson N, Martin ND, Strathdee G. Epileptiform convulsion with intravenous disopyramide [letter]. *Lancet* 1978;2:848.
51. Olson KR, Benowitz NL, Woo OF, Pond SM. Theophylline overdose: acute single ingestion versus chronic repeated overmedication. *Am J Emerg Med* 1985;3:386–394.
52. Aitken ML, Martin TR. Life-threatening theophylline toxicity is not predictable by serum levels. *Chest* 1987;91:10–14.
53. Alldredge BK, Lowenstein DH, Simon RP. Seizures associated with recreational drug abuse. *Neurology* 1989;39:1037–1039.
54. Osuide G, Wambebe C, Ngur D. Studies on the pharmacology of *d*-amphetamine on maximal electroconvulsive seizure in young chicks. *Psychopharmacology* 1983;81:119–121.
55. Lake CR, Gallant S, Masson E, Miller P. Adverse drug effects attributed to phenylpropanolamine: a review of 142 case reports. *Am J Med* 1990;89:195–208.
56. Ojemann LM, Baugh-Bookman C, Dudley DL. Effect of psychotropic medications on seizure control in patients with epilepsy. *Neurology* 1987;37:1525–1527.
57. Alldredge BK. Seizure risk associated with psychotropic drugs: clinical and pharmacokinetic considerations. *Neurology* 1999;53:S68–S75.
58. Starkey IR, Lawson AA. Poisoning with tricyclic and related antidepressants—a ten-year review. *Q J Med* 1980;49:33–49.
59. Biggs JT, Spiker DG, Petit JM, Ziegler VE. Tricyclic antidepressant overdose: incidence of symptoms. *JAMA* 1977;238:135–138.
60. Ellison DW, Pentel PR. Clinical features and consequences of seizures due to cyclic antidepressant overdose. *Am J Emerg Med* 1989;7:5–10.

61. Boehnert MT, Lovejoy FH Jr. Value of the QRS duration versus the serum drug level in predicting seizures and ventricular arrhythmias after an acute overdose of tricyclic antidepressants. *N Engl J Med* 1985;313:474–479.
62. Wedin GP, Oderda GM, Klein-Schwartz W, Gorman RL. Relative toxicity of cyclic antidepressants. *Ann Emerg Med* 1986;15:797–804.
63. Phillips S, Brent J, Kulig K, Heiligenstein J, Birkett M. Fluoxetine versus tricyclic antidepressants: a prospective multicenter study of antidepressant drug overdoses. The Antidepressant Study Group. *J Emerg Med* 1997;15:439–445.
64. Favale E, Rubino V, Mainardi P, Lunardi G, Albano C. Anticonvulsant effect of fluoxetine in humans. *Neurology* 1995;45:1926–1927.
65. Davidson J. Seizures and bupropion: a review. *J Clin Psychiatry* 1989;50:256–261.
66. Skowron DM, Stimmel GL. Antidepressants and the risk of seizures. *Pharmacotherapy* 1992;12:18–22.
67. Preskorn SH, Fast GA. Tricyclic antidepressant-induced seizures and plasma drug concentration. *J Clin Psychiatry* 1992;53:160–162.
68. Cann HM, Verhulst HL. Accidental ingestion and overdosage involving psychopharmacologic drugs. *N Engl J Med* 1960;263:719–724.
69. Acri AA, Henretig FM. Effects of risperidone in overdose. *Am J Emerg Med* 1998;16:498–501.
70. Remick RA, Fine SH. Antipsychotic drugs and seizures. *J Clin Psychiatry* 1979;40:78–80.
71. Devinsky O, Honigfeld G, Patin J. Clozapine-related seizures. *Neurology* 1991;41:369–371.
72. Simard M, Gumbiner B, Lee A, Lewis H, Norman D. Lithium carbonate intoxication. A case report and review of the literature. *Arch Intern Med* 1989;149:36–46.
73. Massey EW, Folger WN. Seizures activated by therapeutic levels of lithium carbonate. *South Med J* 1984;77:1173–1175.
74. Helmchen H, Kanowski S. EEG changes under Lithium (Li) treatment. *Electroencephalogr Clin Neurophysiol* 1971;30:269.
75. Elger CE, Bauer J, Scherrmann J, Widman G. Aggravation of focal epileptic seizures by antiepileptic drugs. *Epilepsia* 1998;39:S15–S18.
76. Guerrini R, Belmonte A, Genton P. Antiepileptic drug-induced worsening of seizures in children. *Epilepsia* 1998;39:S2–S10.
77. Berkovic SF. Aggravation of generalized epilepsies. *Epilepsia* 1998;39:S11–S14.
78. Buckman K, Claiborne K, de Guzman M, Walberg CB, Haywood LJ. Lidocaine efficacy and toxicity assessed by a new, rapid method. *Clin Pharmacol Ther* 1980;28:177–181.
79. Pelter MA, Vollmer TA, Blum RL. Seizure-like reaction associated with subcutaneous lidocaine injection [letter]. *Clin Pharm* 1989;8:767–768.
80. Sundaram MB. Seizures after intraurethral instillation of lidocaine. *CMAJ.* 1987;137:219–220.
81. Pascual J, Sedano MJ, Polo JM, Berciano J. Intravenous lidocaine for status epilepticus. *Epilepsia* 1988;29:584–589.
82. Naguib M, Magboul MM, Samarkandi AH, Attia M. Adverse effects and drug interactions associated with local and regional anaesthesia. *Drug Saf* 1998;18:221–250.
83. Quail AW. Modern inhalational anaesthetic agents. A review of halothane, isoflurane and enflurane. *Med J Aust* 1989;150:95–102.

84. Ashton D. Diazepam, pentobarbital and D-etomidate produced increases in bicuculline seizure threshold; selective antagonism by RO15-1788, picrotoxin and (+/−)-DMBB. *Eur J Pharmacol* 1983;94:319–325.
85. Gancher S, Laxer KD, Krieger W. Activation of epileptogenic activity by etomidate. *Anesthesiology* 1984;61:616–618.
86. Kaiko RF, Foley KM, Grabinski PY, et al. Central nervous system excitatory effects of meperidine in cancer patients. *Ann Neurol* 1983;13:180–185.
87. Mather LE, Tucker GT. Systemic availability of orally administered meperidine. *Clin Pharmacol Ther* 1976;20:535–540.
88. Tobias JD. Seizure after overdose of tramadol. *South Med J* 1997;90:826–827.
89. Kahn LH, Alderfer RJ, Graham DJ. Seizures reported with tramadol [letter]. *JAMA* 1997;278:1661.
90. Spiller HA, Gorman SE, Villalobos D, et al. Prospective multicenter evaluation of tramadol exposure. *J Toxicol Clin Toxicol* 1997;35:361–364.
91. Spivey WH. Flumazenil and seizures: analysis of 43 cases. *Clin Ther* 1992; 14:292–305.
92. Nelson M, Bartlett RJ, Lamb JT. Seizures after intravenous contrast media for cranial computed tomography. *J Neurol Neurosurg Psychiatry* 1989;52:1170–1175.

10

Alcohol and Seizures

Gail D'Onofrio, MD, Andrew S. Ulrich, MD,
and Niels K. Rathlev, MD

Introduction

Alcohol abuse is one of the most common causes of adult-onset seizures. Earnest and Yarnell reviewed 472 adults who were admitted with seizures and found that 41% were related to alcohol abuse *(1)*. A variety of etiologies for seizures related to alcohol exist, the most frequent being the partial or absolute withdrawal of alcohol following a period of heavy use. In addition, seizures may be caused by acute head trauma or alcohol-related toxic-metabolic disorders. Other factors noted to precipitate seizures in the setting of acute and chronic alcohol abuse include pre-existing idiopathic or post-traumatic epilepsy. The term alcohol-related seizures (ARSs) has been adopted in recognition of the multifactorial origin of seizures in the setting of acute and chronic alcoholism *(2)*. Today the management of patients presenting with ARSs remains challenging, despite years of experience, observation, and study.

Historical Perspective

The observation that seizures occur as part of alcohol withdrawal was noted by Hippocrates around 400 B.C. *(3)*. As early as 1852, Huss described the relationship of seizures to the withdrawal of alcohol, often described as "rum fits" *(4)*. Victor and Adams first published clinical data in 1953 describing seizures as part of the withdrawal syndrome *(5)*.

In a classic experimental study, Isbell and colleagues *(6)* observed 10 former heroin and morphine addicts abruptly withdraw from large doses of alcohol consumed over an extended period of time. Four subjects withdrew during

From: *Seizures: Medical Causes and Management*
Edited by: N. Delanty © Humana Press, Inc., Totowa, NJ

the course of the study. The remaining 6 subjects, who consumed alcohol for 48 d or more, all experienced symptoms of withdrawal, including tremor, vomiting, diarrhea, fever, and increased blood pressure. Seizures occurred in two subjects, and two others developed delirium tremens.

Subsequently Victor and Brausch studied 241 patients with a history of drinking alcohol and experiencing seizures *(7)*. Despite such broad entrance criteria, a clinical syndrome emerged that included 90% of the patients.

The seizures, which occurred in approx. 10% of patients after the cessation of drinking, started in adulthood, following many years of heavy drinking. The seizures were noted to be generalized, tonic-clonic in type, often multiple (60%), and usually occurred 7–48 h after cessation of drinking. The interval from the first to the last seizure was 6 h or less in 85% of patients. The electroencephalograms (EEGs) were also found to be normal. A small group (7/241) had idiopathic epilepsy, and a clearly defined group (21/241) comprised patients with head trauma and alcohol dependence. The post-traumatic group frequently had focal seizures with focal EEG abnormalities. In patients with idiopathic and post-traumatic epilepsy, seizures occurred during periods of drinking but were far more frequent during periods of abstinence. The period of drinking required to precipitate seizures in both groups was brief; in some cases seizures occurred after a single evening of drinking.

Pathogenesis of Seizures Related to Alcohol

The biochemical mechanisms responsible for alcohol intoxication are complex, and no specific pathophysiologic mechanism completely explains all ARSs. Alcohol is known to be a general anesthetic with anticonvulsant properties *(8)*. Alcohol administration causes alterations in membrane receptors that may be important in the pathogenesis of seizures. Alcohol specifically potentiates the postsynaptic effect of γ-aminobutyric acid (GABA), the major inhibitory neurotransmitter in the brain *(9)*. When the blood alcohol concentration is reduced, the habituated nervous system becomes hyperexcitable and produces symptoms of tremors, seizures, and delirium. Benzodiazepines may crossreact with alcohol, substitute for the withdrawal of the GABA-enhancing effect of alcohol, and diminish the signs and symptoms of withdrawal. Modulation of G proteins *(10)* and calcium channels *(11)* are other mechanisms by which seizures can be induced in alcoholics.

Differential Diagnosis of Seizures in the Alcohol-Dependent Patient (Table 1)

Multiple possible etiologies have been postulated regarding the association between alcohol and seizure activity.

Table 1
Differential Diagnosis of Seizures in the Alcohol-Dependent Patient

Withdrawal from alcohol
Withdrawal from other drugs
  (benzodiazepines, barbiturates, narcotics)
Exacerbation of idiopathic or post-traumatic epilepsy
Acute overdose
  (alcohol, amphetamine, cocaine, anticholinergics, phenothiazines, tricyclics, isoniazid)
Metabolic disorders
  (hypoglycemia, hyponatremia, hypomagnesemia, hypocalcemia)
CNS disorders
  acute heard trauma
  infections (meningitis, encephalitis, brain abscess)
  stroke
Noncompliance with anticonvulsant medications

Partial or Complete Withdrawal of Alcohol

Clinical *(3)* and experimental *(6)* observations suggest that partial or complete abstinence in the setting of chronic alcohol dependence is the major prerequisite for alcohol withdrawal seizures. In addition to Isbell et al. *(6)* and Victor and Brausch *(7)* and as mentioned previously, other studies substantiate the withdrawal component of seizures. Hillbom *(12)* and Rathlev et al. *(13)* both reported increased seizure frequency on Sunday and Monday, 33% and 49.6%, respectively, when there was decreased access to alcohol. The frequency of seizures was evenly distributed among the other days of the week.

Alcohol as a Central Nervous System Toxin

Other studies have reported that alcohol is a central nervous system (CNS) toxin with direct epileptogenic effects. Seizures have been reported to be precipitated infrequently by high blood alcohol concentrations *(14)* and rarely by very low concentrations *(15)*. Ng and associates utilized a number of statistical analyses to argue that seizures are a direct effect of alcohol rather than of alcohol withdrawal *(14)*. They conclude that the risk of seizures increases as alcohol intake increases and that the risk is 20-fold that for nondrinkers at a daily intake of 300 g of absolute alcohol (12 g alcohol per standard drink). However, as only 16% of first seizures "fell outside the conventionally defined withdrawal period," their conclusion that withdrawal is not the primary mechanism for seizures in alcoholics appears to rely heavily on their statistical analysis and requires further confirmation.

The fact that hemodialysis in chronic alcoholics with previous history of withdrawal symptoms has resulted in improvement of the symptoms of intoxication without precipitating withdrawal signs and symptoms *(16)* also suggests that seizures may occur as a direct effect of alcohol as well as part of the withdrawal syndrome *(17)*.

Metabolic Disorders

Factors associated with early withdrawal that may contribute to seizures include metabolic disorders such as alkalosis, hypomagnesemia, and hypoglycemia.

Hyperventilation with a resultant respiratory alkalosis may produce a hyperexcitability of the CNS and contribute to lowering of the seizure threshold *(18)*. This may be attributable, in part, to lowering of ionized calcium.

Falling levels of magnesium during withdrawal have been cited as another possible precipitant of seizures. However, a randomized controlled trial studying parenteral administration of magnesium as a supplement to benzodiazepines showed no significant differences in severity of withdrawal symptoms, including the incidence of seizures and delirium *(19)*. Studies by Rathlev et al. *(20)* and D'Onofrio et al. *(21)* have also failed to show measurably low-serum magnesium levels in patients presenting with recurrent seizures related to alcohol.

Hypoglycemia related to chronic alcohol consumption has also been suggested as a cause of seizures. Several factors may contribute to the hypoglycemia. Alcohol substantially depletes liver glycogen *(22)*, and the chronic alcoholic may have poor nutritional support. In addition decreased plasma cortisol levels, hypothermia *(23)*, and sepsis may all contribute to hypoglycemia. However, several emergency department (ED)-based studies have documented that ethanol-related hypoglycemia is rare in adults. Sucov reviewed ED records of 953 consecutive patients who were evaluated for ethanol intoxication in a large urban university hospital ED over a 3-mo period. There was no correlation between ethanol and glucose concentrations in any subset of the ethanol-positive patients. Only 1 of the 584 ethanol-positive patients (0.2%) was classified as having severe hypoglycemia (< 50 mg/DL) *(24)*. There were also no reported cases of treatable hypoglycemia in the two series of patients presenting with seizures related to alcohol mentioned previously *(20,21)*.

Acute Intoxication or Poisoning

Toxic ingestions from other drugs may be potential causes of seizures in the chronic alcohol-dependent individual. The clinician should keep in mind that the chronic alcohol abuser may have other comorbid medical and psychiatric conditions and, therefore, access to a variety of drugs. Specifically, isoniazid, used for the treatment of tuberculosis, may precipitate seizures in toxic doses.

Seizures are also a complication of antidepressant overdoses such as with tri-cyclic and anti-psychotic drugs such as phenothiazines. In addition, the alcohol abuser may also utilize other drugs of abuse. Illicit drug use with cocaine, heroin, phenyclidine, and amphetamines should be considered as a cause of seizures. Seizures may also occur as a result of withdrawal from a variety of drugs such as benzodiazepines, barbiturates, and narcotics.

Preexisting Epilepsy

It is a common belief that alcohol may exacerbate seizures in patients with epilepsy, and studies have correlated alcohol abuse with poor seizure control *(25)*. Several mechanisms have been suggested to account for this increased frequency of seizures in epileptic patients who drink, including a "stimulant" effect of the alcohol, a withdrawal phenomenon, noncompliance with a pre-scribed drug regimen, an alteration of absorption of antiepileptic drugs, and enhancement of antiepileptic metabolism through hepatic enzyme induction *(14)*. However, little data support the theory that ingestion of moderate amounts of alcohol influences seizure frequency or antiepileptic drug levels. It is more likely that an altered sleep pattern or a missed dose of anticonvul-sant medication associated with drinking contributes to seizures in patients with pre-existing epilepsy *(17)*.

Lennox surveyed 361 patients with epilepsy who consumed alcohol inter-mittently and found that there was an uncommon association between seizures and alcohol intake. Seventy-nine percent reported that their seizures never occurred during or after alcohol use, 16% stated that an occasional seizure fol-lowed alcohol use, and 5% reported the frequent occurrence of seizures after alcohol ingestion *(26)*. Mattson and associates found that seizure exacerbation was reported by 5% of individuals with epilepsy who had 1–2 drinks but by 85% of those who had 5–6 drinks *(27)*. Hoppener et al. performed a double blind study of 52 patients with epilepsy. All were given 1–3 glasses of orangeade over a 2-h period daily for 16 wk. Vodka was added to the drinks of 29 patients. There was no significant change in seizure frequency, the amount of EEG epileptiform activity, or antiepileptic drug levels in patients receiving alcohol when compared to the control group *(28)*.

Structural Abnormalities

Several studies indicate that heavy alcohol consumers have an increased incidence of cerebral vascular lesions, including infarction *(29)*, hemorrhagic stroke *(30,31)*, and subarachnoid hemorrhage *(32)*, all of which may lead to an increased risk of epilepsy *(33,34)*.

Alcohol-induced spasm of cerebral blood vessels may contribute to stroke and hypertension *(35)*. Disturbances in microcirculation have been postulated to cause ARSs, possibly secondary to erythrocyte and platelet aggregation *(36)*. Changes in coagulation, fibrinolytic activity, and bleeding time secondary to alcohol may predispose to thrombus formation and ischemic brain infarction *(29)*.

Chronic alcohol-dependent individuals also have an increased incidence of head trauma *(37,38)*. They may be susceptible to brain injury as a result of cerebral atrophy related to chronic alcohol abuse *(39)*.

Kindling of the Alcohol Withdrawal Response

There is observational *(40,41)* and physiological *(42)* evidence that each episode of withdrawal has a sensitizing effect, which leads to increasingly more severe symptoms of withdrawal in the future after shorter periods of drinking, including seizures. This described phenomenon is termed kindling, which produces hyperirritability of the limbic system, increasing susceptibility to or severity of future withdrawal symptoms. Brown and colleagues *(41)* found that the number of detoxifications was an important variable in the predisposition to withdrawal seizures. They evaluated male alcoholics with and without seizures. The seizure group had 12 of 25 (25%) of patients with 5 or more previous detoxifications, compared to only 3 of 25 (12%) of the control group. It is possible that this effect is decreased by adequate treatment of each occurrence *(42,43)*.

Patient Management Involving Chronic Alcohol Abuse and Seizure

The alcohol-dependent patient with new-onset or recent seizure activity presents a difficult challenge for the physician. Management is predicated on two basic concepts: (1) treatment of convulsions and associated symptoms of withdrawal, and (2) identification and treatment of coexisting structural and/or toxic-metabolic causes of seizures.

Initial Assessment

Initial assessment is directed at ensuring appropriate "ABCs." This includes maintaining an adequate airway and assessing breathing, oxygenation, and circulation. Immobilization of the cervical spine is indicated whenever the possibility of fall and/or head trauma is entertained. Supplemental oxygen should be applied, vital signs including temperature obtained, and continuous electrocardiagraphic and oxygen-saturation monitoring initiated. Intravenous access should be obtained for fluid and drug administration. A 12-lead ECG should be obtained when possible to assess the possibility of overdose with other drugs, such as tricyclics, and identify intraventricular conduction delays and heart block, which may be problematic should treatment with phenytoin be required.

Life-threatening causes of seizures, such as head trauma and hypoglycemia, should be addressed initially with a finger stick for rapid blood sugar determination and neurological examination. Level of consciousness should be noted as well as inspection for signs of trauma, such as lacerations, ecchymosis, hematomas, Battle's sign, hemotympanum, subcutaneous emphysema, and signs of fractures. Pupil size and reaction to light should be noted, as well as the presence of any focal findings on neurologic examination.

Patients should also receive 100 mg of thiamine, particularly if receiving 5% dextrose and normal saline, to prevent Wernicke–Korsakoff syndrome. The addition of multivitamins and 2 g of magnesium to the first liter of intravenous fluids is probably warranted in chronic alcoholics. Those with glucose levels <60 mg/dL should receive glucose (50 mL of 50% dextrose).

A medical history including possible recent trauma, other medical and psychiatric problems, history of previous seizures, alcohol and other drug use, as well as medications, and compliance with the prescribed regimen should be obtained as soon as possible from the patient, family, and/or prehospital personnel.

Status epilepticus is rare in ARSs *(7,12,44,45)*. Aminoff and Simon reviewed 98 patients over 14 yr of age who presented with status epilepticus. Seizures were reported as alcohol-related in 15 patients, 11 had previous seizures, and 4 had no history of previous seizures. Many of the 15 with ARSs had other cranial pathology, including past trauma *(5)* and cerebrovascular disease *(1)*, but the "relationship of the status to alcohol was beyond question" *(44)*. Patients in status should be treated according to the algorithm published recently by Lowenstein and Alldredge *(46)*. This includes initial treatment with 0.1 mg/kg lorazepam. Isoniazid toxicity should be considered as a possible cause of status epilepticus if the patient is being actively treated for tuberculosis. Isoniazid depletes GABA in the CNS and causes seizures in overdoses. Intravenous pyridoxine should be administered at a dose equivalent to the dose of isoniazid ingested or, if unknown, a dose of 5 g *(47)*.

Laboratory Testing

The use of laboratory testing depends on the patient's known history and present physical examination. Several ED-based studies with patients presenting with ARSs and acute intoxication note that it is rare for the alcohol-dependent patient to present with life-threatening electrolyte abnormalities *(20,21)*. Without evidence of severe nutritional depletion (e.g., magnesium, phosphate, and calcium), the value of obtaining high-cost tests is suspect.

Rapid assessment of blood alcohol concentration with a breath analyzer or saliva strip test is important. A high level of alcohol may contribute to a decrease in consciousness and contraindicate the use of benzodiazepines or other drugs that may cause respiratory depression. If other drug use and/or overdose are considered, additional blood, urine, or saliva toxicologic screens may be indicated. If the patient is currently on antiepileptic drugs, blood levels should be obtained.

Urine screens for pregnancy should be obtained in all women of childbearing age.

Diagnostic Examinations

Radiographs

Chest radiographs should be considered for patients with fever, productive cough, and abnormal physical examination of the chest. Cervical spine x-rays should be ordered for patients presenting after a witnessed or suspected fall, or other evidence of trauma.

CT Examinations

Emergency noncontrast head computerized tomographic (CT) examinations of the head should be performed in all patients with evidence of head trauma, focal neurological findings, and complaints of headache, nausea, and vomiting. In addition, patients with new-onset seizures, a prolonged postictal period, or deteriorating mental status should be scanned.

The issue of whether to obtain a CT is highlighted in a study by Earnest and colleagues *(48)*. They obtained CTs in 259 patients with a first generalized, alcohol-related convulsion without evidence of major head injury or severe toxic-metabolic disorder. Sixteen patients (6.2%) had clinically significant intracranial lesions on CT, four had chronic subdural hematomas, four had subdural hygromas, two had vascular malformations, two had neurocycsticercosis, and one each showed a berry aneurysm, possible tumor, skull fracture with subarachnoid hemorrhage, and cerebral infarct. In 10 cases (3.9%), clinical management was altered as a result of the CT finding. The investigators report that there was no statistical correlation between history, signs of minor head trauma, headache, level of consciousness, or focal neurologic signs with CT findings. However, many of these parameters were present among the 16 patients. Five patients had a history of trauma, four had signs of recent head trauma, four were disoriented, thee had minor focal neurologic signs, two had depressed alertness, and two had headache. They did not report if signs and symptoms were elicited only during the initial assessment or if there were repeated assessments. Another study by Reinus et al. *(49)* retrospectively evaluated the medical records of 115 consecutive patients presenting to an ED following a seizure who underwent a noncontrast head CT. An abnormal neurologic examination predicted 19 of the 20 positive CT scans ($p < 0.001$). A history of malignancy was also found to correlate with CT findings ($p < 0.008$). Reinus suggests that patients with a history of malignancy or an abnormal neurologic examination at the time of examination in the ED benefit most from an emergency CT.

The best practice appears to be repeated neurologic assessments. If the previously mentioned signs and symptoms are observed initially or during careful observation, one should have a low threshold for ordering a noncontrast head CT, which is noninvasive and of minimal risk to the patient.

Electroencephalograms

All patients who present with new-onset seizures or presumed seizures related to alcohol without a previous workup would benefit from an electroencephalogram (EEG) to rule out all possible other etiologies of seizures and to determine if long-term treatment with drug therapy is necessary. Patients whose seizures occur only during a period of partial or complete withdrawal usually have a normal interictal EEG. Those who have had epileptic seizures before becoming alcoholic, or those with a family history of epilepsy, will often show localized or generalized abnormalities as in other epileptic conditions *(7)*.

Deisenhammer and associates *(50)* found that alcoholics without predisposing factors rarely had focal or generalized abnormalities in their EEGs before and/or after sleep deprivation. However, alcoholics with epileptic seizures for which predisposing factors could be found had focal abnormalities in 20% of their initial EEGs and spikes or spike and wave rhythms in another 20%. After sleep deprivation, epileptiform abnormalities could be provoked in an additional 10% of alcoholics. This group with epileptogenic findings would likely benefit from long-term therapy with antiepileptic drugs. This information supports Victor and Brausch's theory from 1967 that epileptic seizures during alcohol withdrawal in the absence of other epileptogenic factors "are not symptoms of a latent disorder activated by the alcoholism, but rather a transient disturbance of cerebral functioning during withdrawal" *(7)*.

Treatment of Alcohol-Related Seizures

Numerous pharmaceutical agents have been used to treat seizures related to alcohol. The pharmacologic interventions have included administration of sedative–hypnotic drugs such as benzodiazepines *(21,51–54)* and barbiturates *(55)*, as well as antiepileptic drugs such as phenytoin, carbamazepine, and valproic acid *(20,56–60)*.

The ideal agent should have properties that effectively manage all aspects of the spectrum of acute alcohol withdrawal syndrome. Treatment is directed at terminating current seizure activity while simultaneously preventing recurrent episodes. The biochemical properties of the ideal drug would include rapid and complete absorption, an intermediate elimination half-life, a wide margin of safety, an elimination process that is independent of liver or renal function, and the absence of abuse potential.

Benzodiazepines

Benzodiazepines possess many of the important properties just listed and consequently have become the mainstay of treatment for ARSs *(61,62)*. They offer excellent anticonvulsant activity with minimal respiratory and cardiac depression. They are cross-tolerant with alcohol, act at the GABA receptor site in place of alcohol, and work to abate the signs and symptoms of the alcohol withdrawal syndrome *(63)*.

Benzodiazepines have been shown to be effective in the primary prevention of seizures in patients with alcohol dependence *(64–66)*. In a retrospective series, 226 patients at risk for alcohol-related seizures received oral clorazepate administered in a tapered fashion over 5 d. Although the investigators expected the seizure rate to be 3–18% in their population, no seizures were observed during the 5-d course. Eighteen percent of the patients had a documented prior history of ARSs *(51)*. The effect of oral diazepam loading was reported in an uncontrolled study of 20 patients in acute alcohol withdrawal with a previous history of seizures. All patients received a minimum of 60 mg of diazepam for prophylaxis, and none developed seizures during their hospitalization *(52)*.

A recent prospective, randomized, controlled trial by D'Onofrio and colleagues *(21)* demonstrated lorazepam to be an extremely effective agent for the prevention of recurrent seizures in patients who presented to an urban ED following an initial seizure. A total of 186 patients over 21 yr of age with chronic alcohol abuse who presented to two inner city EDs after a witnessed, generalized seizure received either 2 mg of lorazepam or equivalent volumes of normal saline intravenously. Patients with preexisting epilepsy and known old structural lesions on head CT were included. Patients with new head trauma or other toxic-metabolic reasons for seizures were excluded. The study period ended after 6 h of observation or the development of a second generalized seizure. In the lorazepam group, 3 of 100 patients (3%) had a second seizure, as compared with 21 of 86 patients (24%) in the placebo group (10.4: 95% odds ratio for seizure with the use of placebo; 3.6–30.2 confidence interval); ($p < 0.0001$).

Lorazepam is an ideal agent to use because it has minimal depressant effects on respiration and circulation *(67,68)*, has a shorter half-life than diazepam, and has no active metabolites *(69,70)*. Because lorazepam is distributed in tissue less rapidly and less extensively than is diazepam, its ability to control seizures is prolonged *(71)*. Its half-life is not substantially prolonged in patients with liver or renal dysfunction, and parenteral administration is associated with a predictable pattern of absorption *(72,73)*.

As recurrent seizures often occur rapidly, all patients with suspected seizures related to alcohol should be treated with lorazepam as soon as possible. Patients should first be assessed rapidly for the presence of a high blood alcohol concentration with a breath analyzer or saliva testing, which may preclude the use of lorazepam because of concerns regarding respiratory depression.

Barbiturates

Barbiturates share many of the properties described earlier with regard to benzodiazepines. They are cross-tolerant with alcohol and demonstrate effective anticonvulsant activity. In an uncontrolled study, Young et al. administered phenobarbital to 38 patients who presented with an initial ARS. None of the subjects developed a recurrent seizure during a mean observation period of approx. 4 h *(55)*. However, barbiturates have a very narrow therapeutic index and are known to increase hepatic enzyme activity. Along with their high potential for abuse and possible epileptogenicity when acutely withdrawn, these properties make barbiturates a less desirable first-line agent for alcohol withdrawal treatment.

Antiepileptic Drugs

Antiepileptic drugs, specifically phenytoin, were an early mainstay of therapy for alcohol withdrawal seizures, as these seizures were equated with generalized epileptic seizures. However, phenytoin has not been demonstrated to be effective in preventing primary ARSs. Marx and colleagues randomized 831 patients admitted to a detoxification unit from the ED. Patients who received clorazepate developed significantly fewer seizures (0.7%) than patients who received phenytoin (3.0%) or placebo (6.2%) during a 96-h observation period *(53)*. Rothstein found that chlordiazepoxide plus phenytoin were no more effective than chlordiazepozide alone in the prevention of ARSs *(56)*. In another series, phenytoin plus diazepoxide were reported to be more effective than diazepoxide alone. However, patients with idiopathic epilepsy were not excluded from this study, and the mean anticonvulsant blood levels after drug administration were far below the therapeutic range in patients randomized to the phenytoin arm *(57)*.

Phenytoin has also been shown to be ineffective in preventing recurrent seizures. Alldredge et al. *(59)*, Chance *(60)* and Rathlev et al. *(20)* all documented no significant decrease in recurrent seizure rate with phenytoin compared to placebo. Patients with preexisting epilepsy and structural head abnormalities were excluded from these studies.

A randomized controlled study conducted in Finland failed to demonstrate effectiveness of either carbamazepine or valproic acid in preventing primary ARSs *(58)*.

Patients with ARSs without coexisting structural abnormalities or preexisting epilepsy do not require anticonvulsant therapy. However, patients with known CNS structural defects or positive EEGs indicating an epileptogenic focus should be treated initially, e.g., loaded with phenytoin, and placed on long-term anticonvulsant therapy and encouraged to be compliant with their medications *(37,74,75)*. Unfortunately, patients with chronic alcohol abuse who are repeatedly not compliant with their drug regimen may be at risk for further seizures *(76)*. Hillbom and Hjelm Jager *(77)* and Spencer et al. *(78)* both reported that the sudden withdrawal of phenytoin might increase seizures. When an alcohol-dependent patient with documented poor compliance with medication makes repeated visits to the ED, the primary physician and neurologist should be consulted regarding improving compliance, or discontinuing repeated, sporadic cycles of anticonvulsant loading while in the ED.

Disposition

Admission to the Hospital

Patients with new-onset seizures should be admitted to the hospital in the setting of chronic alcohol abuse. These patients often comply poorly with follow-up; therefore, it is probably prudent to have their EEGs and other possible diagnostic evaluations performed early while they are hospitalized.

Other criteria for admission to the hospital include recurrent seizure, progression to moderate or severe withdrawal symptoms, and comorbid illness requiring admission.

Discharge and Referral

Most patients with ARSs who have been treated with lorazepam and have had all other possible causes of seizures ruled out by history, physical examination, and/or diagnostic tests can be safely discharged after a period of observation. Vital signs should all be normal, and the patient should be fully awake and ambulatory. Although it is possible that discharge can occur several hours after drug administration, no studies to date have reported observation periods less than 6 h.

Ideally the patient should be referred to a detoxification unit and be treated with longer-acting benzodiazepines to prevent further sequellae of alcohol withdrawal. Unfortunately, this does not often occur, as either the provider fails to refer patients for counseling and substance abuse treatment or the patient is not ready to accept abstinence. However, the occurrence of a seizure can be viewed as a major negative consequence of alcohol dependence and presents an opportunity for the physician to assess the patient's readiness to change and successfully link them to a treatment center *(79)*.

References

1. Ernest MP, Yarnell PR. Seizure admissions to a city hospital: the role of alcohol. *Epilepsia* 1976;17:387–393.
2. Freedland ES, McMicken DB. Alcohol-related seizures, Part 1: pathophysiology, differential diagnosis, and evaluation. *J Emerg Med* 1993;11:463–473.
3. Hippocrates: *Hippocrates, with an English translation by WHS Jones,* 4 vols. The Loeb Classical Library, 1923–1931.
4. Jellinek EM. Classics of the alcohol literature: Magnus Huss Alcoholismus chronicus. *Q J Stud Alcohol* 1943;4:85–92.
5. Victor M, Adams RD. The effect of alcohol on the nervous system. *Res Publ Ass Nervment Dis* 1953;32:526–573.
6. Isbell H. Fraser HF, Wikler A, et al. An experimental study of rum fits and delirium tremens. *Q J Stud Alcohol* 1955;16:1–33.
7. Victor M, Brausch CC. The role of abstinence in the genesis of alcoholic epilepsy. *Epilepsia* 1967;8:1–20.
8. Morris JC, Victor M. Alcohol withdrawal seizures. *Emerg Clin North Am* 1987;5:827–839.
9. Hunt WA. The effect of ethanol on GABAergic transmission. *Neurosci Biobehav Rev* 1983;7:87–95.
10. Charness ME, Querimit LA, Henteleff M. Ethanol differentially regulates G proteins in neuronal cells. *Biochem Biophys Res Commun* 1988;155:138–143.
11. Greenberg DA, Darpenter CL, Messing RO. Ethanol-induced component of $^{45}Ca^{2+}$ uptake in PC12 cells is sensitive to Ca^{2+} channel modulating drugs. *Brain Res* 1987;410:143–146.
12. Hillbom ME. Occurrence of cerebral seizures provoked by alcohol abuse. *Epilepsia* 1980;21:459–466.
13. Rathlev NK, Shieh T, Callum M. Etiology of alcohol withdrawal seizures and their occurrence in relation to decreased availability of alcohol. *Ann Emerg Med* 1992;21:663 (abstract).
14. Hauser W, Ng S, Brust J. Alcohol, seizures and epilepsy. *Epilepsia* 1988;29(Suppl 2):566–578.
15. Marinacci A. A special type of temporal lobe (psychomotor) seizures following ingestion of alcohol. *Bull L A Neurol Soc* 1963;27:241–245.
16. Walder A, Redding J, Faillace L, and Steenberg RW. Rapid detoxification of the acute alcoholic with hemodialysis. *Surgery* 1969;66:201–207.
17. Simon R. Alcohol and seizures. *N Engl J Med* 1988;319:715–716.
18. Victor M. The role of hypomagnesemia and respiratory alkalosis in the genesis of alcohol-withdrawal symptoms. *Ann N Y Acad Sci* 1973;215:235–248.
19. Wilson A, Vulcano B. A double-blind, placebo-controlled trial of magnesium sulfate in the ethanol withdrawal syndrome. *Alcohol Clin Exp Res* 1984;8:542–545.
20. Rathlev NK, D'Onofrio G, Fish SS, et al: The efficacy of phenytoin in the prevention or recurrent alcohol withdrawal seizures. *Ann Emerg Med* 1994;23:513–518.
21. D'Onofrio G, Rathlev NK, Ulrich AS, Fish SS, Freedland ES. Lorazepam for the prevention of recurrent seizures related to alcohol. *N Engl J Med* 1999;340:915–919.
22. Isslbacher K. Metabolic and hepatic effects of alcohol. *N Engl J Med* 1077; 296:612–616.
23. Fitgerald FT. Hypoglycemia and accidental hypothermia in an alcoholic population. *West J Med* 1980;113:105–107.

24. Sucov A, Woolard RH. Ethanol-associated hypoglycemia is uncommon. *Acad Emerg Med* 1995;2:185–189.
25. Lambie DG, Stanway L, Johnson RH. Factors which influence the effectiveness of treatment of epilepsy. *Aust NZ J Med* 1986;16:779–784.
26. Lennox WG. Alcohol and epilepsy. *Q J Stud Alcohol* 1941;2:1–11.
27. Mattson RH, Sturman JK, Gronowski ML, Goico H. Effect of alcohol intake in non-alcoholic epileptics. *Neurology* 1975;25:361–362.
28. Hoppener RJ, Kuyer A, van der Lugt PJM. Epilepsy and alcohol: the influence of social alcohol intake on seizures and treatment in epilepsy. *Epilepsia* 1983; 24:459–471.
29. Hillbom M, Kaste M, Rasi V. Can ethanol intoxication affect hemocoagulation to increase the risk of brain infarction in young adults? *Neurology* 1983;33:381–384.
30. Gill JS, Shipley MJ, Tsementzis SA, et al. Alcohol consumption—a risk factor for hemorrhagic and non-hemorrhagic stroke. *Am J Med* 1991;90:489–497.
31. Weisber LA. Alcoholic intracerebral hemorrhage. *Stroke* 1988;19:1565–1569.
32. Hillbom M, Kaste M. Alcohol intoxication: a risk for primary subarachnoid hemor-rhage. *Neurology* 1982;32:706–711.
33. Hauser W, Hesdorffer D. *Epilepsy: Frequency, Causes , and Consequences.* New York: Demos, 1990.
34. Yamane H, Kiatoh N. Alcoholic epilepsy: a definition and a description of other con-vulsions related to alcoholism. *Eur Neurol* 1981;20:17–24.
35. Altura B, Gebrewold A. Alcohol-induced spasms of cerebral blood vessels: relation to cerebrovascular accidents and sudden death. *Science* 1983;720:331–333.
36. Larkin E, Watson-Williams E. Alcohol and the blood. *Med Clin North Am* 1984;68:105–120.
37. Annegers J, Grabow J, Groover RV, Laws ER Jr, Elveback LR, Kurland LT. Seizures after head trauma: a population study. *Neurology* 1980;30:683–689.
38. McMicken D, Freedland E, D'Onofrio G. Alcohol and trauma. *Emerg Med Clin North Am* 1993;11:225–239.
39. Pfefferbaum A, Rosenbloom M, Crusan K, and Jernigan TL. Brain CT changes in alcoholics: effects of age and alcohol consumption. *Alcoholism* 1988;12:81–87.
40. Ballenger JC, Post RM. Kindling as a model for the alcohol withdrawal syndromes. *Br J Psychiatry* 1078;133:1–14.
41. Brown ME, Anton RF, Malcolm R, Ballenger JC. Alcohol detoxification and with-drawal seizures: Clinical support for a kindling hypothesis. *Biol Psychiatry* 1988; 23:507–514.
42. Linnoila M, Mefford I, Nutt D, and Adinoff. Alcohol withdrawal and noradrenergic function: NIH Conference. *Ann Intern Med* 1987;107:875–889.
43. Rosenblood A. Emerging treatment options in the alcohol withdrawal syndrome. *J Clin Psychiatry* 1988;49(Suppl):28–31.
44. Aminoff M, Simon R. Status epilepticus: causes, clinical features and consequences in 98 patients. *Am J Med* 1988;68:657–666.
45. Pilke A, Partinen M, Kovanen J. Status epileptiacus and alcohol abuse: an analysis of 82f status epileptiacus admissions. *Acta Neurol Scand* 1984;70:443–450.
46. Lowenstein DH, Alldredge BK. Status epilepticus. *N Eng J Med* 1998;338:970–977.
47. Wason S, Lacouture PG, Lovejosy FH Jr. Single high-dose pyridoxine treatment for isoniazid overdose. *JAMA* 1981;246:1102–1104.

48. Earnest MP, Feldman H, Marx JA, Harris BS, Biletch M, Sullivan LP. Intracranial lesions shown by CT scans in 259 cases of first alcohol-related seizures. *Neurology* 1988;38:1561–1565.

49. Reinus WR, Wippold FJ II, Erickson KK: Seizure patient selection for emergency computed tomography. *Ann Emerg Med* 1993;22:1298–1303.

50. Deisenhammer E, Klingler D, Tragner H. Epileptic seizures in alcoholism and the diagnostic value of EEG after sleep deprivation. *Epilepsia* 1984;25:526–530.

51. Haddox VG, Bidder TG, Waldron LE, Derby P, and Achen SM. Chlorazepate use may prevent alcohol withdrawal convulsions. *West J Med* 1987;146:695–696.

52. Devenyi P, Harrison ML. Prevention of alcohol withdrawal seizures with oral diazepam loading. *Can Med Assoc J* 1985;132:798–800.

53. Marx JA, Berner J, Bar-Or D, et al. Prophylaxis of alcohol withdrawal seizures: a prospective study. *Ann Emerg Med* 1986;15:637 (abstract).

54. Browne TR, Penry JK. Benzodiazepines in the treatment of epilepsy: a review. *Epilepsia* 1973;14:277–310.

55. Young G, Rores C, Murphy C, Dailey RH. Intravenous phenobarb for alcohol withdrawal and convulsions. *Ann Emerg Med* 1987;16:847–850.

56. Rothstein E. Prevention of alcohol withdrawal seizures: the roles of diphenylhydantoin and chloridazepoxide. *Am J Psychiatry* 1973;130:1381–1382.

57. Sampliner R, Iber FL. Diphenylhydantoin control of alcohol withdrawal seizures: results of a controlled study. *JAMA* 1974;20:1430–1432.

58. Hillbom M, Tokola R, Kuusela V, et al. Prevention of alcohol withdrawal seizures with carbamazepine and valproic acid. *Alcohol* 1989;6:223–226.

59. Alldredge B, Lowenstein D, Simon R. Placebo-controlled trial of intravenous diphenylhydantoin for short-term treatment of alcohol withdrawal seizures. *Am J Med* 1989;87:645–648.

60. Chance J. Emergency department treatment of alcohol withdrawal seizures with phenytoin. *Ann Emerg Med* 1991;20:520–522.

61. Litten RZ, Allen JP. Pharmacotherapies for alcoholism: promising agents and clinical issues. *Alcohol Clin Exp Res* 1991;15:620–633.

62. Seller EM. Alcohol, barbiturate and benzodiazepine withdrawal syndromes: clinical management. *Can Med Assoc J* 1988;139:113–120.

63. Greenblatt DJ, Shader RI. *Benzodiazepines in Clinical Practice.* New York: Raven 1974.

64. Kaim SC, Klett CJ, Rothfeld B. Treatment of the cute alcohol withdrawal state: a comparison of four drugs. *Am J Psychiatry* 1969;125:1640–1646.

65. Sellers EM, Naranjo CA, Harrison M, Devenyi P, Roach C, Sykora K. Diazepam loading: simplified treatment of alcohol withdrawal. *Clin Pharmacol Ther* 1983; 34:822–826.

66. Naranjo CA, Sellers EM, Chater K, Iversen P, Roach C, Sykora K. Nonpharmacologic intervention in acute alcohol withdrawal. *Clin Pharmacol Ther* 1983; 34:214–219.

67. Elliot HW, Nomof N, Navarro G, Ruelius HW, Knowles JA, Comer WH. Central nervous system and cardiovascular effects of lorazepam in man. *Clin Pharmacol Ther* 1971;12:468–481.

68. Greenblatt DJ, Shader RI. Prazepam and lorazepam, two new benzodiazepines. *N Engl J Med* 1978;299:1342–1344.

69. Miller WC Jr, McCurdy L. A double-blind comparison of the efficacy and safety of lorazepam and diazepam in the treatment of the acute alcohol withdrawal syndrome. *Clin Ther* 1984;6:364–371.

70. O'Brien J, Meyer R, Thomas D. Double-blind comparison of lorazepam and diazepam in the treatment of the acute alcohol abstinence syndrome. *Curr Ther Res* 1983;34:825–831.

71. Brown TR. The pharmacokinetics of agents used to treat status epilepticus. *Neurology* 1990;40(Suppl 2):28–32.

72. Hoyumpa AM Jr. Disposition and elimination of minor tranquilizers in the aged and in patients with liver disease. *South Med J* 1978;71(Suppl 2)23–28.

73. Kraus JW, Desmond PV, Marshall JP, Johnson RF, Schenker S, Wilkinson GR. Effects of aging and liver disease on disposition of lorazepam. *Clin Pharmacol Ther* 1978;24:411–419.

74. Temkin NR, Dikmen SS, Wilesndky AJ, Keihm J, Chabal S, Winn HR. A randomized, double-blind study of phenytoin for the prevention of post-traumatic seizures. *N Engl J Med* 1990;323:497–502.

75. Hauser WA, Ramirez-Lassepas M, Rosenstein R. Risk for seizures and epilepsy following cerebrovascular insults. *Epilepsia* 1984;25:666 (abstract).

76. Pinel JP. Alcohol withdrawal seizures: implications of kindling. *Pharmacol Biochem Behav* 1980;13(Suppl 1):225–231.

77. Hillbom M, Hjelm-Jager M. Should alcohol withdrawal seizures be treated with antiepileptic drugs? *Acta Neurol Scand* 1984;69:39–42.

78. Spencer SS, Spencer DD, Williamson PD, Mattson RH. Ictal effects of anticonvulsant medication withdrawal in epileptiac patients. *Epilepsia* 1981;22:297–307.

79. Bernstein E, Bernstein J, Levenson S. Project ASSERT: An ED-based intervention to increase access to primary care, preventive services and the substance abuse treatment system. *Ann Emerg Med* 1997;30:181–189.

11

Seizures and Illicit Drug Use

John C. M. Brust, MD

Introduction

Drug dependence is of two types. Psychic dependence is a psychic drive to use a drug periodically or continuously, i.e., addiction. Physical dependence is an adaptive state in which cessation of drug use or administration of an antagonist produces physical withdrawal signs. Psychic and physical dependence can exist together or independently. Tolerance refers to the need to take an ever-increasing dose of a drug to achieve the desired effect or to prevent craving or physical withdrawal *(1)*.

Different kinds of drugs are used recreationally around the world, and the ability to produce psychic or physical dependence varies among different agents. This chapter addresses those drugs most often used in North America and Europe, exclusive of ethanol, tobacco, and caffeine.

Illicit Drugs and Seizures: Indirect Mechanisms

Parenteral drug users are subject to systemic and central nervous system (CNS) infection and thus indirectly to seizures. Endocarditis causes cerebral infarction, intracranial hemorrhage, cerebral abscess, and meningitis. Seizures in AIDS can be the result of either opportunistic infections and neoplasms or direct infection of the brain by human immunodeficiency virus (HIV). Like alcoholics, illicit drug users are often immunocompromised in the absence of HIV infection.

In addition to endocarditis, illicit drug users are at risk for ischemic or hemorrhagic stroke secondary to embolization of foreign material, vasculitis, or coagulopathy. Psychostimulant drugs, especially cocaine, cause hemorrhagic stroke, probably secondary to acute hypertension, and ischemic stroke, probably secondary to cerebral vasospasm.

From: *Seizures: Medical Causes and Management*
Edited by: N. Delanty © Humana Press, Inc., Totowa, NJ

183

Illicit drug use also predisposes to metabolic derangement such as hypo-glycemia or renal failure. Drug users also are frequent victims of cerebral trauma, which can cause acute seizures or chronic epilepsy. Many illicit drug users also abuse ethanol.

Direct Mechanisms: Toxicity vs Withdrawal

In addition to such diverse indirect mechanisms, illicit drugs cause seizures by direct actions. With some drugs, seizures are a manifestation of direct tox-icity, and with others, of physical dependence and withdrawal. It is important to keep in mind that many drug abusers use multiple agents, including ethanol, and that a user simultaneously may be acutely toxic from one drug while physically withdrawing from another.

Individual Agents

Opiates

Opiate drugs include a large number of agonists (e.g., morphine, methadone, meperidine, fentanyl, codeine), antagonists (e.g., naloxone), and mixed agonists/antagonists (e.g., pentazocine). The most widely abused opi-ate is the agonist heroin, which is most often injected intravenously or subcu-taneously. The AIDS epidemic, as well as plentiful supplies of cheap potent heroin, have increased the popularity of nonparenteral routes of administra-tion (e.g., snorting or smoking). Commercial street heroin contains a variety of pharmacologically active and inactive adulterants, often including quinine.

Except possibly in neonates, seizures are not a feature of pure opiate with-drawal, which in adults produces flu-like symptoms and intense craving. Meperidine causes seizures and myoclonus as an acute neurotoxic side effect of its metabolite, normeperidine (which also causes delirium and hallucina-tions) (2,3). Seizures have also been anecdotally reported as a direct toxic effect of fentanyl, propoxyphene, or pentazocine. Overdose with heroin or methadone can also cause seizures, but the appearance of seizures in such patients is so unusual that alternative explanations, e.g., other drugs, ethanol, CNS infection, cerebral trauma, or metabolic derangement, should always be sought (4,5).

In a case-control study at Harlem Hospital in New York, it was found that heroin use, both past and current, was a risk factor for new-onset seizures independent of overdose, infection, head trauma, stroke, ethanol, or other drugs (6). The odds ratio (OR) was 2.57 for unprovoked seizures (no under-lying precipitant such as stroke, infection, or trauma) and 3.65 for provoked seizures. It was highest if heroin had been used on the day of the seizure (OR = 6.61), but in no patient did the seizure occur in the setting of obvious overdose, and risk persisted even in those abstinent for a year.

The pharmacological basis of this risk is not known. In animal studies opiates are variably proconvulsant *(7,8)*, anticonvulsant *(9,10)*, or both *(11,12)*, with such actions either blocked or not blocked by naloxone. Different effects depend on animal species, seizure model, agent used (e.g., μ, δ, or κ agonists), dose, and rate of administration. For example, morphine's proconvulsant actions have been variably attributed to μ receptor agonism, δ receptor agonism, and nonopiate receptor-mediated GABA antagonism *(13–15)*.

In newborns of opiate-dependent mothers, a withdrawal syndrome can be severe or even fatal, with tremor, screaming, sweating, fever, tachypnea, tachycardia, vomiting, and explosive diarrhea. Seizures and myoclonus are described in such infants but can be difficult to distinguish from jitteriness *(16)*. Moreover, neonatal seizures should not be attributed to opiate withdrawal unless hypoglycemia, hypocalcemia, intracranial hemorrhage, meningitis, sepsis, and other drug (or ethanol) withdrawal have been excluded.

Psychostimulants

Psychostimulant drugs include a large number of amphetamine-like agents (e.g., dextroamphetamine, methamphetamine, methylphenidate, ephedrine, phenylpropanolamine), which act by releasing monoamines at synaptic nerve endings. Cocaine produces similar subjective effects, but it acts by blocking re-uptake of monoamines at synaptic nerve endings, and, unlike amphetamine, cocaine has local anesthetic properties. Used recreationally, amphetamine-like drugs are taken orally or parenterally; methamphetamine ("ice") is sometimes smoked. Cocaine hydrochloride is either snorted intranasally or injected parenterally; alkaloidal "crack" cocaine is smoked.

Psychostimulant overdose causes various combinations of fever, hypertension, cardiac arrhythmia, delirium, or coma. Seizures are a frequent accompaniment and carry a poor prognosis.

Seizures can occur as a direct toxic effect of psychostimulant use in the absence of other signs of overdose. They are particularly common with cocaine, perhaps because of the drug's local anesthetic properties *(17–23)*. Seizures occur immediately or within a few hours of cocaine administration and are usually generalized; focality might reflect a cocaine-induced ischemic or hemorrhagic stroke. Status epilepticus, when it occurs, tends to be refractory to conventional anticonvulsant treatment *(21)*.

In a report from Minneapolis, of 474 patients treated for acute cocaine intoxication, 44 (9.3%) had seizures within 30 min of drug use *(24)*. In 32, seizures were of new onset, and most of these were precipitated by intravenous use of cocaine hydrochloride or smoking of crack cocaine. In 12, seizures occurred in patients who had had earlier seizures unrelated to cocaine, and most of these were precipitated by intranasal use of cocaine hydrochloride. In both groups 40% of seizures followed first-time use of cocaine. In a later report, the same investigators reported that seizures associated with cocaine use were three times more common in women (18.4%) than in men (6.2%) *(25)*.

A lower prevalence of seizures among cocaine-intoxicated patients has been reported by others: 4 of 283 (1.4%) in New York *(26)* and 29 of 1275 (2.3%) in San Francisco *(19)*. Phone surveys suggest much higher seizure prevalences, especially in crack smokers *(27)*. A large survey in Virginia found that seizures occurred in none of the intranasal cocaine users, in 1% of "experimental" crack smokers, and in 9% of heavy crack smokers *(28)*.

Bizarre behavior developed in a woman who had smoked crack over a 3-d period; what was initially considered cocaine-induced psychosis turned out to be complex partial status epilepticus *(29)*.

Seizures sometimes occur several hours or more after cocaine use. Studies with rats reveal epileptogenicity of the cocaine metabolite benzoylecgonine *(30)*.

Animal studies also have shown that repeated administration of cocaine eventually produces seizures at what were originally subthreshold doses (kindling, sensitization, reverse tolerance) *(31)*. Kindled seizures also occur with other local anesthetics that lack cocaine's behavioral effects *(32)*.

Seizures are described in association with phenylpropanolamine, an amphetamine-like drug available over the counter in decongestant and appetite-suppressant remedies *(33,34)*. Seizures were a late development in a chronic methylphenidate abuser, suggesting kindling. Methylenedioxymethamphetamine (MDMA, "ecstasy"), which has properties of both psychostimulant and hallucinogenic drugs, is popular on American college campuses. It is usually taken orally in groups. Overdose can result in delirium, seizures, coma, and death *(35)*.

Sedatives and Hypnotics

Recreational use of barbiturates can be either oral or parenteral; short-acting agents (e.g., secobarbital, pentobarbital, amobarbital) are most popular. Benzodiazepine drugs (e.g., diazepam, chlordiazepoxide, lorazepam, triazolam) have considerably less abuse potential. Among other nonbarbiturate, nonbenzodiazepine sedatives, some (e.g., glutethimide) are well-recognized street drugs, and others (e.g., buspirone) seem to have little or no addiction liability. Barbiturates, benzodiazepines, and many nonbarbiturate and nonbenzodiazepine sedatives produce both psychic and physical dependence, with withdrawal symptoms—including seizures—similar to those encountered in alcoholics.

With short-acting barbiturates, seizures are most likely to occur on the second or third day of abstinence; full-blown delirium tremens sometimes follows *(36)*. In a study of human volunteers, abrupt withdrawal from secobarbital or pentobarbital after several months of a daily dose of 400 mg produced paroxysmal electroencephalographic (EEG) changes without symptoms in one-third of the subjects. Withdrawal from 600 mg daily caused minor symptoms in half the subjects and a seizure in 10%. Of those taking 900 mg or more daily, three-fourths had seizures and two-thirds developed delirium tremens *(37)*.

Withdrawal symptoms associated with benzodiazepines—anxiety, tremor—can be difficult to distinguish from the symptoms that the drug was being taken for in the first place. Seizures, hallucinations, and delirium tremens do occur, however *(38,39)*. Withdrawal symptoms usually begin 3–10 d after stopping long-acting agents and within 24 h of stopping short-acting agents *(40)*. As with barbiturates, seizures are dose related; in a placebo-controlled study of patients taking therapeutic doses of benzodiazepines for at least 9 mo, withdrawal symptoms included tinnitus, muscle twitching, and confusion but not seizures *(41)*.

Barbiturates and benzodiazepines potentiate GABA neurotransmission through stereospecific receptors on the supramolecular GABA–chloride channel complex *(42)*. Barbiturates also have direct actions on chloride channels and antagonize glutamate excitatory neurotransmission. Differences in these actions probably explain why some barbiturates (e.g., phenobarbital) but not others (e.g., secobarbital) can prevent seizures without producing coma *(43)*. Downregulation of GABA receptors probably contributes to seizures induced by barbiturate or benzodiazepine withdrawal.

Some nonbarbiturate, nonbenzodiazepine sedatives, for example, chloral hydrate and meprobamate, also produce seizures on withdrawal. In contrast, glutethimide (which as a street drug is often combined with codeine—"hits," "loads") reportedly can cause seizures as an acute toxic effect. The mechanism is probably its anticholinergic properties *(44)*.

Seizures also affect recreational users of antihistamines. During the 1980s pentazocine combined with tripelennamine was a popular form of parenteral drug abuse ("Ts and blues"), and seizures were a frequent complication *(45)*.

Cannabis

Marijuana is made from cut tops and leaves of the hemp plant *Cannabis sativa.* A more potent preparation, hashish, is made from resin covering the flowers and leaves. Either preparation can be smoked or eaten. Among the plant's many cannabinoid compounds (cannabinoids), Δ-9-tetrahydrocannabinol (Δ-9-THC) is the principal psychoactive ingredient. Mammalian brain contains stereospecific cannabinoid receptors as well as an endogenous ligand, anandamide.

In a case-control study from Harlem Hospital Center, marijuana use was protective against new onset seizures in men; 29% of patients with seizures used marijuana, compared to 41% of controls (OR = 0.42) *(6)*. For provoked seizures marijuana was protective only in those who had never used heroin. Among women, a trend toward risk reduction did not achieve statistical significance.

Cannabinoid compounds vary in their proconvulsant and anticonvulsant properties, and particular compounds have different effects depending on species and seizure model *(46,47)*. For example, Δ-9-THC has been described as epileptogenic *(48)*, anticonvulsant *(49)*, or without effect *(50)*. The nonpsychoactive cannabinoid, cannabidiol, is more consistently anticonvulsant *(51)*. The relationship of this property to cannabinoid receptors is unclear *(52,53)*. Electrophysiological studies suggest that cannabidiol and phenytoin, although effective against similar types of seizures, have different mechanisms of action *(54)*.

Human experience with anticonvulsant cannabinoids is limited. In a single case report, marijuana smoking was necessary for seizure control *(55)*. A survey of 12 young epileptics who used marijuana found 1 subject whose seizure frequency decreased with use and another whose seizure frequency increased *(56)*. In another report intravenous cannabidiol did not alter (and maybe even increased) the EEG epileptiform abnormalities of a young epileptic *(57)*. In a placebo-controlled study of 16 epileptics refractory to other drugs, cannabidiol exacerbated EEG acutely but not behavioral seizures; after several months, however, 7 of 8 patients receiving cannabidiol were seizure-free compared to 1 of 8 controls *(58)*.

Hallucinogens

A large number of hallucinogenic plants are used recreationally (and ritualistically) worldwide. In North America the most popular agents are peyote cactus containing mescaline, mushrooms containing psilocybin and psilocin, and the synthetic ergot drug lysergic acid diethylamide (LSD). The perceptual alterations induced by these substances are not considered epileptic in nature. True seizures can follow very high doses, however *(59)*.

Inhalants

Recreational inhalation of volatile substances is especially popular among children and adolescents. Numerous products are used, including aerosols, cleaning fluids, glues, paint thinners, petroleum, lighter fluid, anesthetics, and nitrites, and the intoxicating compounds include aliphatic, aromatic, and halogenated hydrocarbons, esters, ketones, and ethers. Desired effects resemble those produced by ethanol, but large doses can be hallucinogenic, and seizures have been described in severely intoxicated subjects *(60,61)*. Withdrawal symptoms are mild and do not include seizures *(62)*.

Phencyclidine

Classified as a dissociative anesthetic, phencyclidine (PCP, "angel dust") can be eaten, snorted, or injected but is most often smoked. As a noncompetitive inhibitor at glutamate NMDA receptors, PCP should have anticonvulsant properties. As with other anticonvulsant drugs, however, overdose can cause myoclonus and seizures, including status epilepticus *(63–65)*.

Anticholinergics

A number of plants contain atropine and scopolamine, and in North America *Datura stramonium* (jimsonweed) is a popular recreational agent among adolescents. Seeds, leaves, or roots are ingested orally. Pharmaceuticals with anticholinergic properties, e.g., amitriptyline, are also available as street drugs. Overdose causes fever, dilated unreactive pupils, dry flushed skin, delirium, hallucinations, myoclonus, and seizures *(66)*.

References

1. Brust JCM. *Medical Aspects of Substance Abuse.* Boston, MA: Butterworth-Heinemann, 1993.
2. Kaiko RF, Foley K, Grabinski PY, et al. Central nervous system excitatory effects of meperidine in cancer patients. *Ann Neurol* 1983;13:180–185.
3. Hershey LA. Meperidine and central neurotoxicity. *Ann Intern Med* 1983; 98:548–549.
4. Volavka J, Zaks A, Roubicek J, Fink M. Electroencephalographic effects of diacetyl-morphine (heroine) and naloxone in man. *Neuropharmacology* 1970;9:587–593.
5. Landow L. An apparent seizure following inadvertent intrathecal morphine. *Anesthesiology* 1985;62:545–546.
6. Ng SKC, Brust JCM, Hauser WA, Susser M. Illicit drug use and the risk of new onset seizures. *Am J Epidemiol* 1990;132:47–57.
7. Walker GE, Yaksh TL. Studies on the effects of intrathecally injected DADL and morphine on nociceptive thresholds and electroencephalographic activity: a thalamic delta receptor syndrome. *Brain Res* 1986;383:1–14.
8. Sztriha L, Lelkes Z, Benedek G, et al. Potentiating effect of morphine on seizures induced by kainic acid in rats: an electroenephalographic study. *Naunyn Schmiedbergs Arch Pathol* 1986;333:47–51.
9. Bohme GA, Stutzmann JM, Rouges BP, et al. Effects of selective mu- and delta-opioid peptides on kindled amygdaloid seizures in rats. *Neurosci Lett* 1987; 74:227–231.
10. Czuczwar SJ, Frey HH. Effect of morphine and morphine-like analgesics on susceptibility to seizures in mice. *Neuropharmacology* 1986;25:465–469.
11. Tortella FC, Robles L, Holaday JW. 050488, a highly selective kappa opioid; anticonvulsant profile in rats. *J Pharmacol Exp Ther* 1986;237:49–53.
12. Frey HH. Anticonvulsant effect of morphine and morphine-like analgesics in Mongolian gerbils. *Pharmacology* 1986;32:335–339.
13. Puglisi-Alegra S, Cabib S, Oliyerio A. Pharmacological evidence for a protective role of the endogenous opioid system on electroshock-induced seizures in the mouse. *Neurosci Lett* 1985;62:241–247.

14. Aleman V, deMunoz DM. Effect of different convulsant drugs on some seizure parameters in morphine-dependent mice. *Exp Neurol* 1983;80:451–456.
15. Tortella FC. Endogenous opioid peptides and epilepsy: quieting the seizing brain? *Trends Pharmacol Sci* 1988;9:366–372.
16. Fulroth R, Phillips B, Durand DJ. Perinatal outcome of infants exposed to cocaine and/or heroin in utero. *Am J Dis Child* 1989;143:905–910.
17. Alldredge BK, Lowenstein DH, Simon RP. Seizures associated with recreational drug abuse. *Neurology* 1989;39:1037–1039.
18. Johnson S, O'Meara M, Young JB. Acute cocaine poisoning. Importance of treating seizures and acidosis. *Am J Med* 1983;75:1061–1064.
19. Lowenstein DA, Masse SM, Rowbotham MC, et al. Acute neurologic and psychiatric complications associated with cocaine. *Am J Med* 1987;83:841–846.
20. Myers JA, Earnest MP. Generalized seizures and cocaine abuse. *Neurology* 1984;34:675-676.
21. Schwartz RH, Estroff T, Hoffman NG. Seizures and syncope in adolescent cocaine abusers. *Am J Med* 1988;85:462.
22. Harden CL, Montjo RE, Tuchman AJ, Daras M. Seizures provoked by cocaine use. *Ann Neurol* 1990;28:263–264.
23. Kramer LD, Locke GE, Ogunyemi A, Nelson L. Cocaine-related seizures in adults. *Am J Drug Alcohol Abuse* 1990;16:307–317.
24. Pascuale-Leone A, Dhuna A, Altafullah I, Anderson DC. Cocaine-induced seizures. *Neurology* 1990;40:404–407.
25. Dhuna A, Pascual-Leone H, Langendorf F, Anderson DC. Epileptogenic properties of cocaine in humans. *Neurotoxicology* 1991;12:621–626.
26. Choy-Kwong M, Lipton RB: Seizures in hospitalized cocaine users. *Neurology* 1989;39:425–427.
27. Washton AM, Tatarsky A. Adverse effects of cocaine abuse. In: Harris L (ed), *Problems of Drug Dependence*. NIDA Research Monograph 49, Washington, D.C.: DHHS, 1983, pp 247–254.
28. Schwartz RH, Luxenberg MG, Hoffman NG. Crack use by American middle-class adolescent polydrug abusers. *J Pediatr* 1991;118:150–155.
29. Ogunyemi AO, Locke GE, Kramer LD, Nelson L. Complex partial status epilepticus provoked by "crack" cocaine. *Ann Neurol* 1989;26:785–786.
30. Konkol RJ, Erickson BA, Doerr JK, et al. Seizures induced by the cocaine metabolite benzoylecgonine in rats. *Epilepsia* 1992;33:420.
31. Post RM, Rose H. Increasing effects of repetitive cocaine administration in the rat. *Nature* 1976;260:731–732.
32. Reith MEA, Meisler BE, Lajtha A. Locomotor effects of cocaine, cocaine congeners and local anesthetics in mice. *Pharmacol Biochem Behav* 1985;23:831–836.
33. Mueller SM, Solow EB. Seizures associated with a new combination "pick-me-up" pill. *Ann Neurol* 1982;11:322.
34. Cornelius JR, Soloff PH, Reynolds CF. Paranoia, homicidal behavior and seizures associated with phenylpropanolamine. *Am J Psychiatry* 1984;141:120–121.
35. Henry JA, Jeffreys KJ, Dawling S. Toxicity and deaths from 3,4-methylenedioxymethamphetamine ("ecstasy"). *Lancet* 1992;340:384–387.
36. Wulff MH. The barbiturate withdrawal syndrome: a clinical and electrophysiologic study. *Electroencephalogr Clin Neurophysiol* 1959;14(Suppl):1–173.
37. Fraser HF, Wikler A, Essig EF, Isbell H. Degree of physical dependence induced by secobarbital or pentobarbital. *JAMA* 1958;166:126–129.

38. DuPont RL. A practical approach to benzodiazepine discontinuation. *J Psychiatr Res* 1990;24(Suppl 2):81–90.

39. Nutt D. Benzodiazepine dependence in the clinic: reason for anxiety? *Trends Pharmacol Sci* 1986;7:457–460.

40. Committee on the Review of Medicines. Systematic review of the benzodiazepines. *Br Med J* 1980;1:910–912.

41. Busto U, Sellers EM, Naranjo CA, et al. Withdrawal reaction after long-term therapeutic use of benzodiazepines. *N Engl J Med* 1986;315:854–859.

42. Schofield PR. The GABA-A receptor: molecular biology reveals a complex. *Trends Pharmacol Sci* 1989;10:476–478.

43. MacDonald RL, McLain MJ: Anticonvulsant drugs: mechanisms of action. *Adv Neurol* 1986;44:713.

44. Myers RR, Stockard JJ. Neurologic and electroencephalographic correlates in glutethimide intoxication. *Clin Pharmacol Ther* 1975;17:212–220.

45. Caplan LR, Thomas C, Banks G. Central nervous system complications of addiction to "T's and Blues." *Neurology* 1982;32:623–628.

46. Pertwee RG. The central neuropharmacology of psychotropic cannabinoids. *Pharmacol Ther* 1988;36:189–261.

47. Seth R, Sinha S. Chemistry and pharmacology of cannabis. *Prog Drug Res* 1991; 36:71–115.

48. Turkanis SA, Karler R: Central excitatory properties of delta-9-tetrahydrocannabinol and its metabolites in iron-induced epileptic rats. *Neuropharmacology* 1982;21:7–13.

49. Wada JA, Oswa T, Corcoran ME. Effects of tetrahydrocannabinols on kindled amygdaloid seizures in Senegalese baboons, *Papio papio. Epilepsia* 1975;16:439–448.

50. Meldrum BS, Fariello RG, Puil EA, et al. Delta-9-tetrahydrocannabinol and epilepsy in the photosensitive baboon, *Papio papio. Epilepsia* 1974;15:255–264.

51. Consroe P, Benedito MA, Leite JR, et al. Effects of cannabidiol on behavioral seizures caused by convulsant drugs or current in mice. *Eur J Pharmacol* 1982; 83:293–298.

52. Howlett AC, Bidaut-Russell M, Devane WA, et al. The cannabinoid receptor: biochemical, anatomical, and behavioral characterization. *Trends Neurosci* 1990; 13:420–423.

53. Devane WA, Hanus L, Breuer A, et al. Isolation and structure of a constituent that binds to the cannabinoid receptor. *Science* 1992;258:1946–1949.

54. Karler R, Turkanis SA. The cannabinoids as potential antiepileptics. *J Clin Pharmacol* 1981;21:437S–448S.

55. Consroe PF, Wood GC, Buchsbaum A. Anticonvulsant nature of marijuana smoking. *JAMA* 1975;234:306–307.

56. Feeney DM: Marijuana use among epileptics. *JAMA* 1976;235:1105.

57. Perez-Reyes M, Wingfield M. Cannabidiol and electroencephalographic epileptic activity. *JAMA* 1974;230:1635.

58. Cunha JM, Carlini EA, Periera AE, et al. Chronic administration of cannabidiol to healthy volunteers and epileptic patients. *Pharmacology* 1980;21:175–185.

59. Fisher D, Underleider J. Grand mal seizures following ingestion of LSD. *Calif Med* 1976;106:210–212.

60. Meredith TJ, Ruprah M, Little A, Flanagan RJ. Diagnosis and treatment of acute poisoning with volatile substances. *Hum Toxicol* 1989;8:277–286.

61. Watson JM. Solvent abuse and adolescents. *Practitioner* 1984;228:487–490.

62. Skuse D, Burrell S. A review of solvent abusers and their management by a child-psychiatric outpatient service. *Hum Toxicol* 1982;1:321–329.

63. McCarron MM, Schulze BW, Thompson GA, et al: Acute phencyclidine intoxication: clinical patterns, complications, and treatment. *Ann Emerg Med* 1981; 10:290–297.

64. Stockard JJ, Werner SS, Albers JA, Chippa KH. Electroencephalographic findings in phencyclidine intoxication. *Arch Neurol* 1976;33:200–203.

65. Kessler GF, Demers LM, Brennan RW. Phencyclidine and fatal status epilepticus. *N Engl J Med* 1974;291:979.

66. Mickolich JR, Paulson GW, Cross CJ, Calhoun R: Neurologic and electroencephalographic effects of jimson weed intoxication. *Clin Electroencephalogr* 1976; 7:49–57.

12

Seizures Attributable to Environmental Toxins

Fernando Cendes, MD, PhD

Introduction

General Management

Seizures induced by toxins most often present as generalized tonic-clonic convulsions of acute onset, either recurrent frequent seizures or consisting of status epilepticus. However, in some circumstances, poisons and toxins can induce partial seizures of different types, including complex partial status, which may be difficult to identify promptly *(1–4)*.

The standard approach of acute anticonvulsant therapy, including benzodiazepines and phenytoin, is usually effective, independent of the agent responsible for toxin-induced seizures, but sometimes the early identification of the toxin may modify the treatment and prognosis *(3,4)*.

For poisoned patients with seizures, the general principles of poison management still apply. Although seizures need to be treated aggressively, one should not forget the basic principles of poisoning and overdose management. The "ABCs" (airways, breathing, and circulation) of resuscitation are of foremost concern and should be addressed immediately.

Part of the initial management of all poisoned patients is decontamination. The method of decontamination depends on the route of exposure of the toxin. With inhalation exposures of chemicals, such as carbon monoxide, the patient needs to be removed immediately from the toxic environment and supplemented with high-flow oxygen. With dermal exposures, the patient's clothing should be removed and discarded immediately followed by washing the skin. Most toxic exposures occur by ingestion, and aggressive gastrointestinal decontamination should be initiated as soon as possible. Gastric lavage followed by activated charcoal with a cathartic, such as sorbitol, is commonly performed in the initial management.

From: *Seizures: Medical Causes and Management*
Edited by: N. Delanty © Humana Press, Inc., Totowa, NJ

Marine Neurotoxic Syndromes

The classic marine neurotoxic syndromes include shellfish poisonings, pufferfish *(Fugu)* poisoning, and ciguatera. The symptoms of ciguatera and neurotoxic shellfish poisoning are often similar. The diagnosis is made by a high index of suspicion and a specific history of fish ingestion.

Shellfish

Shellfish poisoning is attributable to tetrodotoxin and saxitoxin, two of the most potent poisons known *(5,6)*. Tetrodotoxin is found in the gonads and other visceral tissues of some fish of the order *Tetraodontiformes* (to which the Japanese *Fugu,* or pufferfish, belongs); it also occurs in the skin of some newts of the family Salamandridae and of the Costa Rican frog *Atelopus.* Saxitoxin, and possibly some related toxins, are elaborated by the dinoflagellates *Gonyaulax catanella* and *Gonyaulax tamerensis* and are retained in the tissues of clams and other shellfish that eat these organisms. Given the right conditions of temperature and light, the *Gonyaulax* may multiply so rapidly as to discolor the ocean; hence, the term red tide. Shellfish feeding on *Gonyaulax* at this time become extremely toxic to human beings and are responsible for periodic outbreaks of paralytic shellfish poisoning *(5)*. Both toxins, in nanomolar concentrations, specifically block the outer mouth of the pore of Na^+ channels in the membranes of excitable cells. Both toxins cause death by paralysis of the respiratory muscles; therefore, the treatment in severe cases of poisoning requires artificial ventilation. Early gastric lavage and therapy to support blood pressure also are indicated. If the patient survives paralytic shellfish poisoning for 24 h, the prognosis is good *(5,6)*. Seizures may occur in some patients with paralytic shellfish poisoning, most likely not as consequence of a single neurotoxin but as suggested by the study of Novelli et al. *(7)*, because of a possible potentiation of the excitotoxic effect of glutamic acid and aspartic acid also present in high concentrations in mussel tissue. This, in association with other factors, such as old age, amount of sea food ingested, and reduced renal clearance, helps to explain why all individuals do not develop an overt neurotoxicity; these factors also explain the variation in the severity of toxicity in the affected patients.

Domoic Acid

Domoic acid is a neuroexcitotoxic compound and analog of kainic acid that can be considered a conformationally restricted form of glutamic acid. Domoic acid binds to the non-methyl-*N*-D-aspartate (MNDA) kainate receptors resulting in a nonphysiologic activation of neurons and their processes, ultimately leading to neuronal disruption and cellular death *(8–14)*.

Domoic acid is found in the environment as a contaminant of some sea organisms and was first chemically identified following its isolation in 1957 from the seaweed *Chondria armata* found off the coast of Japan *(15)*.

In late November 1987, reports of individuals who developed acute gastrointestinal symptoms, confusion, memory loss, and motor symptoms were received by the Canadian Department of National Health and Welfare. Patients in 4 index cases had eaten mussels cultured in eastern Prince Edward Island within 24 h before symptom onset. Additional patients were identified rapidly throughout Canada by an active search, and the distribution of mussels was immediately suspended *(2,16)*. The causative agent of toxicity in cultured mussels from a localized area of eastern Prince Edward Islands was isolated by a number of different techniques *(17)*. The mussels feeding response is controlled by algal density *(18)*. During the chemical search for the source of domoic acid, investigators in the field found that over 90% of the algae available to these mussels were *Nitzschia pungens,* the major constituent of a plankton bloom at the time of the outbreak. Later, *N. pungens* was proven to be the source of domoic acid *(19)*.

A major central nervous system (CNS) manifestation of the 1987 domoic acid intoxication were seizures, both acute and chronic. The convulsive potential of domoic acid is attributable to its action as a potent glutamate agonist *(8,11,12)*. Experimental data indicate that domoic acid produces neuronal damage both by direct excitation of kainate receptors and by inducing acute recurrent seizures throughout limbic circuits *(10–13,20,22)*. Moreover, neuronal death induced by domoic acid excitotoxicity in the hippocampus and related structures resulted in the delayed onset of complex partial seizures, consistent with the latency of other hippocampal injuries *(1,23,24)*.

Acute seizures were observed in 5 of the 14 patients studied by Teitlebaum et al. *(2)*. Three had generalized seizures, two had complex partial, and 1 had focal motor seizures. It is likely that limbic ictal manifestations were not recognized in some subjects; indeed, the acute intoxication was characterized by unusual motor activity reminiscent of grimacing or chewing. Recognized seizure activity was relatively resistant to intravenous (IV) infusion of phenytoin and required high doses of IV diazepam and phenobarbital for control during the acute illness. Seven patients had electroencephalograms (EEGs) during the acute phase. Moderate-to-severe generalized disturbance of background activity was seen in all seven patients. Only one patient had clear epileptiform EEG activity. Eight weeks after mussel ingestion the seizures became progressively less frequent and ceased within 4 mo in all subjects. Thus, the acute domoic acid intoxication syndrome behaved as an excitatory insult to limbic structures, producing clinical seizure activity mimicking naturally occurring temporal lobe epilepsy with damage of the hippocampus and related structures *(1)*.

Long after complete cessation of convulsive activity of the acute phase of the intoxication, two patients developed temporal lobe epilepsy. One of these patients was reported in detail *(1)*. Following the intoxication, an 84-yr-old man had nausea, vomiting, and confusion, progressively developed coma, generalized convulsions, and complex partial status epilepticus. After 3 weeks he improved and was seizure free with severe residual memory deficit. EEGs initially showed periodic epileptiform discharges, later evolving to epileptiform abnormalities over frontotemporal regions with diffuse slowing. Eight months after the intoxication the EEG was normal. One year after the acute episode he developed complex partial seizures. EEGs at that time showed epileptic discharges independently over both temporal lobes, with left-sided predominance. Magnetic resonance imagery (MRI) revealed hyperintense T2-weighted signal and severe atrophy of both hippocampi; a positron emission tomography (PET) scan showed bitemporal decreased glucose metabolism. The patient developed pneumonia and died $3\frac{1}{4}$ yr after the intoxication. Autopsy disclosed severe bilateral hippocampal sclerosis. Microscopically, the hippocampi showed complete neuronal loss in CA1 and CA3, almost total loss in CA4, and moderate loss in CA2. Dentate cells were focally diminished in numbers. The amygdala showed patchy neuronal loss in medial and basal portions, with neuronal loss and gliosis in the overlying cortex *(1)*.

Another four victims of the mussel poisoning who died and were autopsied had acute lesions in the hippocampi and related limbic structures, and persistent convulsions were a typical feature of the acute intoxication *(2,16)*.

Only limited data on previous human exposure to domoic acid are available. In Japan, domoic acid, contained in seaweed extracts, was used as a home remedy to treat intestinal parasites, and as an insecticide *(15,25,26)*. Presumably, the insecticidal activity prompted use as an antihelminthic in humans. Studies of seaweed extracts given as an antihelminthic to children were reported as showing no side effects. Domoic acid, purified from the seaweed, was also given orally to children in Japan (0.5 mg/kg), and no ill effects were reported *(26)*. It is possible that there was no CNS toxicity in those children because of age specificity, and because of poor gastrointestinal absorption *(22,27)*. The amount of domoic acid consumed by victims of mussel poisoning in Canada was calculated to be as much as 5–6 mg/kg, which is 10 times higher than the amounts administered as an antihelminthic in Japan *(2,10,16)*.

Ciguatera

Ciguatera is a serious although rarely fatal human food poisoning related to the consumption of tropical reef fish. Contained in the muscles, head, viscera, and roe of the fish is one or more toxins acquired in the food chain. Ciguatera is one of the most common nonbacterial form of food poisoning related to seafood ingestion in the United States, Canada *(28)*, and, more recently, Europe *(29)*. The problem is endemic in certain areas of the Caribbean (especially the Virgin Islands and Puerto Rico) *(30)*. Ciguatera is caused by ingestion of multiple toxins found in benthic dinoflagellates. Several toxins have been identified including ciguatoxin, scaritoxin, maitotoxin, palytoxin, okadaic acid, and multiple subvarieties *(29,31)*.

Neurologic manifestations include dysesthesias of the extremities and temperature reversal (where cold objects feel hot or, occasionally, vice versa: "hot–cold inversion"). This inverted sensory phenomenon is considered by some to be typical of intoxication by marine toxins *(32)*. Headaches, vertigo, dizziness, metallic taste, dry mouth, carpopedal spasm, trismus, meningismus, and cranial nerve palsies may occur. Rarely, a patient will develop stupor, peripheral flaccid paralysis, respiratory muscle paralysis with respiratory failure, generalized tonic-clonic seizures, or death *(29,30,32)*.

Treatment is symptomatic and supportive. IV mannitol is the first drug of choice for acute situations, especially within the first 24 hr.

Muscarine Mushroom-Induced Seizures

Mushroom poisoning has been known for centuries. In recent years the number of cases of mushroom poisoning has increased as a result of the current popularity of the consumption of wild mushrooms *(33)*. Various species of mushrooms contain many toxins, and species within the same genus may contain distinct toxins *(34)*.

Intoxication produced by *Amanita muscaria* and related *Amanita* species arises from the neurologic and hallucinogenic properties of muscimol, ibotenic acid, and other isoxazole derivatives. These agents stimulate excitatory and inhibitory amino acid receptors. Symptoms range from irritability, restlessness, ataxia, hallucinations, and delirium to drowsiness, and sedation and may include generalized seizures as well *(33,35–37)*.

Benjamin *(35)* described the clinical features and management of nine patients with mushroom poisoning attributable to *Amanita pantherina* (eight patients) and *A. muscaria* (one patient). Most ingestions were in the toddler age group. Symptoms occurred between 30 and 180 min after ingestion, with the onset of CNS depression, waxing and waning torpor, ataxia, hallucinations, and hyperkinetic behavior. Vomiting was rare. Seizures or myoclonic twitching occurred in four of nine patients but was controlled with standard anticonvulsant therapy. No other anticholinergic or cholinergic signs were prominent. Recovery was rapid and complete in all nine patients *(35)*.

Treatment is mainly supportive; benzodiazepines are indicated when excitation predominates, whereas atropine often exacerbates the delirium. Because the severity of toxicity and treatment strategies for mushroom poisoning depend on the species ingested, their identification should be sought. Often symptomatology is delayed; therefore, gastric lavage and administration of activated charcoal may be of limited value *(34)*.

Toxic Plant Ingestions

Accidental hemlock poisoning (cicutoxin poisoning) is probably the most common cause of seizures induced by poisonous plant ingestion *(38–46)*. Water hemlock, beaver poison, cowbane, five-finger root, wild carrot, wild parsnip, and false parsley are some of the popular common names of the several toxic members of the genus *Cicuta (42,44,45,47)*. Water hemlock is probably the most poisonous plant that grows in North America and is known to be extremely toxic to livestock and humans, with an overall mortality of about 70% *(42,44,45,47)*. Water hemlock grows in moist ground along rivers or ditches and can be easily confused with celery, artichokes, sweet potatoes, or sweet anise.

The most important symptoms of cicutoxin poisoning include nausea, abdominal cramps followed by unconsciousness, generalized convulsions, reddish-tinted cyanosis, dilated pupils, and marked metabolic acidosis. In one report of a severe intoxication, the patient survived because of treatment with hemodialysis, hemoperfusion, forced diuresis, and artificial ventilation *(44)*. The cicutoxin molecule size was calculated, and it was found to be dialyzable *(44)*.

Jimsonweed (*Datura stramonium,* a member of the belladonna alkyloid family) is a plant growing naturally in West Virginia and has been used as a home remedy since colonial times. Because of its easy availability and strong anticholinergic properties, teenagers use jimsonweed as a drug. Plant parts can be brewed as a tea or chewed, and seed pods can be eaten. The anticholinergic side effects of ingestion of jimsonweed include tachycardia, dry mouth, dilated pupils, blurred vision, hallucinations, confusion, combative behavior, and difficulty urinating. Severe toxicity has been associated with coma and seizures, although death is rare *(38)*.

Other toxic plants that can cause seizures include *Phoradendron (39)*, nightshade *(Atropa belladonna)* berries *(43)*, *Urginea maritime* (squill) plant (a folk remedy) *(40)*, azalea (grayanotoxin), bleeding hearts (isoquinoline alkaloids), and Christmas rose (glycosides) *(3)*.

Carbon Monoxide

Clinical diagnosis of carbon monoxide poisoning is based more on the history of exposure than on the findings of the clinical examination. The classic cherry-red color of the skin is seen rarely in nonfatal cases. Carbon monoxide is a colorless, odorless, and tasteless gas; therefore, the only evidence of exposure may be an elevated carboxyhemoglobin (COHb) level in the blood, but the severity of signs and symptoms does not always correspond to this. In cases with delayed manifestations, COHb level may no longer be elevated *(3,48,49)*.

The major property of carbon monoxide is its affinity to bind hemoglobin to form COHb. Other undesirable effects of carbon monoxide are the shifting of the oxyhemoglobin dissociation curve to the left and the inhibition of the cytochrome oxidase system. Overall, these effects result in the lowering of tissue oxygen partial pressure and increasing cellular hypoxia *(49)*.

Carbon monoxide can produce several nonspecific symptoms and can mimic several diseases. Most of the signs and symptoms are the result of hypoxia, which affects mainly the brain, but other vital organs such as the heart may also be involved. The onset may be acute or it may be insidious if it is caused by chronic, low-grade carbon monoxide poisoning *(48),* and partial epileptic seizures have been reported in chronic carbon monoxide poisoning *(50)*.

The severity of symptoms is related to blood COHb level, but there are frequent disparities. The most frequent neurologic manifestations of mild acute carbon monoxide poisoning (10–20% COHb) are headache (90%), dizziness (82%), and visual disturbances. Such manifestations may be accompanied by impairment of higher cerebral function, nausea, weakness, and abdominal pain. With a moderate degree of poisoning (20–40% COHb), the patient may present with cardiac disturbances, dyspnea, vomiting, and loss of consciousness. Severe poisoning (40–60% COHb) may lead to coma, generalized convulsions, and respiratory impairment. Recovery from coma may be followed by a vegetative state, extrapyramidal rigidity and involuntary movement disorders, or severe memory deficits *(49,51)*.

The most important diagnostic test for carbon monoxide poisoning is the direct spectroscopic measurement of COHb level in the blood. An indirect way to estimate this is to measure carbon monoxide content of the exhaled breath. In severely ill patients with suspicion of exposure to carbon monoxide, oxygen therapy should not be delayed pending COHb estimation even though oxygen, by lowering COHb, may remove the evidence of carbon monoxide exposure. Hyperbaric oxygen therapy is mandatory when available. Computerized tomography (CT) is the neuroimaging method used most widely for patients with carbon monoxide poisoning. Common CT findings are symmetrical, low-density basal ganglia abnormalities and diffuse low-density lesions of white matter. Globus pallidus lucencies may be unilateral, and white matter involvement may show marked asymmetry *(49)*. The mortality of acute carbon monoxide poisoning is about 30%. It is reduced to 1.7–9.6% in series of patients treated by hyperbaric oxygen therapy *(3,49,51)*.

Heavy Metals

People always have been exposed to heavy metals in the environment, and in areas with high concentrations, metallic contamination of food and water probably led to the first poisonings. Metals leached from eating utensils and cookware also have contributed to inadvertent poisonings. The emergence of the industrial age and large-scale mining brought occupational diseases caused by various toxic metals. Metallic constituents of pesticides and therapeutic agents (e.g., antimicrobials) have been additional sources of hazardous exposure. The burning of fossil fuels containing heavy metals, the addition of tetraethyllead to gasoline, and the increase in industrial applications of metals have now made environmental pollution the major source of heavy-metal poisoning.

Heavy metals exert their toxic effects by combining with one or more reactive groups (ligands) essential for normal physiological functions. Heavy-metal antagonists (chelating agents) are designed specifically to compete with these groups for the metals and thereby prevent or reverse toxic effects and enhance the excretion of metals. Heavy metals, particularly those in the transition series, may react in the body with ligands containing oxygen, sulfur, and nitrogen, resulting in a metal complex.

Lead

Lead is found in food, water, air, dust, and soil. Children ingest lead in the form of lead paint chips, wood painted with lead paint, and lead-contaminated soil *(52–56)*. Adolescents become encephalopathic because of organic lead poisoning from gasoline sniffing. Occupational exposure to lead may occur in the manufacture of metal products, such as solder, pipes, and storage battery components. Lead is used in the synthesis of fuel additives and in the preparation of paints and pigments. Exposure to lead is also a principal hazard in stained glass work, jewelry making, ceramic painting, and lead paint removal *(55,56)*.

Signs and symptoms of chronic lead poisoning (plumbism) can be divided into six categories: gastrointestinal, neuromuscular, CNS, hematological, renal, and other. They may occur separately or in combination. The neuromuscular and CNS syndromes usually result from acute exposure, whereas the abdominal syndrome is a more common manifestation of a chronic insidious intoxication. This gastrointestinal syndrome is more prevalent in adults (colic, vomiting, diarrhea, jaundice, gingival blue lines, weight loss, and constipation) *(57)*. In chronic lead poisoning, concentrations of lead in blood exceed 60 µg/dL (2.9 µmol) of whole blood, and X-rays may show heavy, multiple bands of increased density in the growing long bones.

The CNS syndrome is the most serious manifestation of lead poisoning and is much more common in children than in adults. The early signs of the syndrome are clumsiness, vertigo, ataxia, falling, headache, insomnia, restlessness, irritability, and vomiting. The patient may first become excited and confused and later present with delirium and repetitive tonic-clonic convulsions, followed by lethargy and coma. Visual disturbances may also be present *(52–54,57,58)*.

Initial treatment of the acute phase of lead intoxication involves supportive measures. Prevention of further exposure is important. Seizures are treated with benzodiazepines and phenytoin. Fluid and electrolyte balances must be maintained. Cerebral edema is treated with mannitol and dexamethasone. The concentration of lead in blood should be determined, or at least a blood sample for subsequent analysis obtained, prior to initiation of chelation therapy. Chelation therapy is indicated in symptomatic patients or in patients with a blood lead concentration in excess of 50–60 μg/dL (about 2.5 μmol). Four chelators have been used: edetate calcium disodium (CaNa^2 EDTA), dimercaprol, D-penicillamine, and succimer (2,3-dimercaptosuccinic acid). CaNa^2 EDTA and dimercaprol usually are used in combination for lead encephalopathy.

Mercury

Mercury was an important constituent of drugs for centuries as an ingredient in many diuretics, antibacterials, antiseptics, skin ointments, and laxatives. More specific, effective, and safer modes of therapy have largely replaced the mercurials in recent decades, and drug-induced mercury poisoning has become rare. However, mercury has a number of important industrial uses, and poisoning from occupational exposure and environmental pollution continues to be an area of concern.

Three major chemical forms of the metal must be distinguished: mercury vapor (elemental mercury), salts of mercury, and organic mercurials. Short-term exposure to vapor of elemental mercury may produce symptoms within several hours, which include weakness, chills, metallic taste, nausea, vomiting, diarrhea, dyspnea, cough, and a feeling of tightness in the chest. Generalized tonic-clonic seizures may occur. Chronic exposure to mercury vapor produces a more insidious form of toxicity that is dominated by neurological effects and a severe form of gingivitis. Most human toxicological data about organic mercury concern methylmercury and have been collected as the unfortunate result of several large-scale accidental exposures. Symptoms of exposure to methylmercury are also mainly neurological and include hyperexcitability, ataxia, tremors, choreoathetosis, action myoclonus, deafness, and blindness *(57)*.

Tin

Organic tin compounds are used as heat stabilizers and in the production of silicone rubber. Organotins are used as preservatives for wood, textiles, leather, paper, and glass. The organotin compounds, particularly triethyltin and trimethyltin (TMT) are highly neurotoxic. TMT is a neurotoxin that damages the limbic system, cerebral cortex, and brainstem. Bilateral symmetrical neuronal damage of the hippocampi, pyriform cortex, amygdala, and neocortex was documented after administration of TMT chloride to rats *(59)*. An acute limbic–cerebellar syndrome was seen in six industrial workers who inhaled TMT *(60)*. Clinical features included hearing loss, disorientation, confabulation, amnesia, aggressiveness, hyperphagia, disturbed sexual behavior, complex partial and tonic-clonic seizures, nystagmus, ataxia, and mild sensory neuropathy. Severity paralleled maximal urinary organotin levels *(60)*. Long-term sequelae of TMT poisoning include memory impairment and temporal lobe complex partial seizures.

Other Metals

Seizures may occur after intoxication by a number of other heavy metals, although they are less frequent than those outlined above. Such seizures are usually associated with isolated accidents in work environments that utilize high concentrations of metals or with contamination of food. These include arsenic *(61)*, manganese *(62)*, tungsten *(63,64)*, and cadmium *(65)*, among others.

Solvents and Vapors

Organic solvents and their vapors are a common part of our environment. Short, incidental exposure to low concentrations of solvent vapors, such as gasoline, lighter fluids, aerosol sprays, and spot removers, may be relatively harmless; however, exposure to paint removers, floor and tile cleaners, and other solvents in the home or industry may be quite dangerous. In addition, disposal of many of these chemicals has been improper; as a result, there is leakage from toxic dump sites and contamination of drinking water. Because so many industrial workers are exposed to toxic solvents and vapors, considerable effort has gone into determining safe levels of exposure. A variety of anesthetic gases, solvents, and fluorohydrocarbons (used as propellants in aerosol products) cause subjective effects when inhaled and frequently are abused in this way, resulting in many deaths.

Intoxication by ingestion of gasoline and kerosene resembles that of ethyl alcohol. Signs and symptoms include incoordination, restlessness, excitement, confusion, disorientation, ataxia, delirium, generalized tonic-clonic seizures and, finally, coma, which may last a few hours or several days. Inhalation of high concentrations of gasoline vapors, as by workmen cleaning storage tanks, can cause immediate death *(57)*.

The neurotoxicity of organic solvents is well known, although there is controversy about the chronic neurologic effects, in particular with regard to risk of seizures *(66–68)*. Case reports suggest that generalized, as well as partial, seizures might be associated with both acute and chronic solvent exposure *(66,67,69)*. A case report of a 58-yr-old sign writer with lifelong exposure to a mixture of organic solvents (mainly cyclohexanone, white spirit, and isopropanol) suggests that temporal lobe seizures may occur in relation to chronic solvent exposure. His seizures disappeared shortly after stopping exposure but returned just after a short-term re-exposure to cyclohexanone *(67)*.

References

1. Cendes F, Andermann F, Carpenter S, Zatorre RJ, Cashman NR. Temporal lobe epilepsy caused by domoic acid intoxication: evidence for glutamate receptor-mediated excitotoxicity in humans. *Ann Neurol* 1995;37:123–126.
2. Teitelbaum JS, Zatorre RJ, Carpenter S, et al. Neurologic sequelae of domoic acid intoxication due to the ingestion of contaminated mussels. *N Engl J Med* 1990;322:1781–1787.
3. Kunisaki TA, Augenstein WL. Drug- and toxin-induced seizures. *Emerg Med Clin North Am* 1994;12:1027–1056.
4. Delanty N, Vaughan CJ, French JA. Medical causes of seizures. *Lancet* 1998;352:383–390.
5. Ritchie JM. Tetrodotoxin and saxitoxin and the sodium channels of excitable tissues. *Trends Pharmacol Sci* 1980;1:275–279.
6. Catterall W, Mackie K. Local anesthetics: Tetrodotoxin and saxitoxin. In: Hardman JG, Limbrird LE, Molinoff PB, Ruddon RW, Gilman AG (eds.), *Goodman & Gilman's the Pharmacological Basis of Therapeutics,* 9th ed. New York: McGraw-Hill, 1996, CD-Rom.
7. Novelli A, Kispert J, Fernandez-Sanchez MT, Torreblanca A, Zitko V. Domoic acid-containing toxic mussels produce neurotoxicity in neuronal cultures through a synergism between excitatory amino acids. *Brain Res* 1992;577:41–48.
8. Wright JL, Bird CJ, de Freitas AS, Hampson D, McDonald J, Quilliam MA. Chemistry, biology, and toxicology of domoic acid and its isomers. *Can Dis Wkly Rep* 1990;16(Suppl 1E):21–26.
9. Shinozaki H. Discovery of novel actions of kainic acid and related compounds. In: McGeer EG, Olney JW, McGeer PL (eds.), *Kainic Acid as a Tool in Neurobiology.* New York: Raven, 1978, pp 17–35.
10. Debonnel G, Weiss M, de Montigny C. Neurotoxic effect of domoic acid: mediation by kainate receptor electrophysiological studies in the rat. *Can Dis Wkly Rep* 1990;16(Suppl 1E):59–68.
11. Tryphonas L, Iverson F. Neuropathology of excitatory neurotoxins: the domoic acid model. *Toxicol Pathol* 1990;18:165–169.
12. Takeuchi H, Watanabe K, Nomoto K, Ohfune Y, Takemoto T. Effects of alpha-kainic acid, domoic acid and their derivatives on a molluscan giant neuron sensitive to beta-hydroxy-L-glutamic acid. *Eur J Pharmacol* 1984;102:325–332.
13. Debonnel G, Weiss M, de Montigny C. Reduced neuroexcitatory effect of domoic acid following mossy fiber denervation of the rat dorsal hippocampus: further evidence that toxicity of domoic acid involves kainate receptor activation. *Can J Physiol Pharmacol* 1989;67:904–908.
14. Strain SM, Tasker RA. Hippocampal damage produced by systemic injections of domoic acid in mice. *Neuroscience* 1991;44:343–352.

15. Takemoto T. *Kainic Acid as a Tool in Neurobiology.* New York: Raven, 1978.
16. Perl TM, Bedard L, Kosatsky T, Hockin JC, Todd EC, Remis RS. An outbreak of toxic encephalopathy caused by eating mussels contaminated with domoic acid. *N Engl J Med* 1990;322:1775–1780.
17. Wright JL, Boyd RK, de Freitas AS, et al. Identification of domoic acid, a neuroexcitatory amino acid, in toxic mussels from eastern Prince Edward Island. *Can J Chem* 1989;481–490.
18. Bayne BL, Widdows J, Thompson RJ. Physiology of marine mussels. In: Bayne BL (ed.), *Marine Mussels: Their Ecology and Physiology.* London: Cambridge University Press, 1976, pp 207–260.
19. Bates SS, Bird CJ, de Freitas ASW, et al. Pennate diaton *Nitzschia pungens* as the primary source of domoic acid, a toxin in shellfish from eastern Prince Edward Island, Canada. *Can J Fish Aquat Sci* 1989;46:1203–1215.
20. Debonnel G, Beauchesne L, de Montigny C. Domoic acid, the alleged "mussel toxin," might produce its neurotoxic effect through kainate receptor activation: an electrophysiological study in the dorsal hippocampus. *Can J Physiol Pharmacol* 1989;67:29–33.
21. Glavin GB, Pinsky C, Bose R. Domoic acid-induced neurovisceral toxic syndrome: characterization of an animal model and putative antidotes. *Brain Res Bull* 1990; 24:701–703.
22. Iverson F, Truelove J, Tryphonas L, Nera EA. The toxicology of domoic acid administered systemically to rodents and primates. *Can Dis Wkly Rep* 1990;16(Suppl 1E):15–18.
23. Cavazos JE, Golarai G, Sutula TP. Mossy fiber reorganization induced by kindling: time course of development, progression and permanence. *J Neurosci* 1991; 11:2795–2803.
24. Sutula TP. Experimental models of temporal lobe epilepsy: new insights from the study of kindling and synaptic reorganization. *Epilepsia* 1990;31:S45–S54.
25. Maeda M, Kodama T, Tanaka T, et al. Insecticidal and neuromuscular activities of domoic acid and its related compounds. *J Pesticide Sci* 1984;9:27–32.
26. Daigo K. Studies on the constituents of chondria armata. II, Isolation of an antihelmintical constituent. *J Jpn Pharmacol Assoc* 1959;79:353.
27. Tryphonas L, Truelove J, Todd E, Nera E, Iverson F. Experimental oral toxicity of domoic acid in cynomolgus monkeys *(Macaca fascicularis)* and rats. Preliminary investigations. *Food Chem Toxicol* 1990;28:707–715.
28. Centers for Disease Control. *Fish Borne Disease Outbreaks: Annual Summary* 1982, 1985.
29. Lange WR. Ciguatera fish poisoning. *Am Fam Physician* 1994;50:579–584.
30. Payne CA, Payne SN. Ciguatera in Puerto Rico and the Virgin Islands. *N Engl J Med* 1977;296:949–950.
31. Yasumoto T, Satake M. Chemistry, etiology and determination methods of ciguatera toxins. *J Toxicol Toxin Rev* 1996;15:91–107.
32. Bagnis R, Kiberski T, Lauguer S. Clinical observation on 3009 cases of ciguatera (fish poisoning) in the South Pacific. *Am J Trop Med Hyg* 1979;28:1067–1073.
33. Goldfrank LR. Mushrooms: toxic and hallucinogenic. In: Goldfrank LR, Flomenbaum NE, Lewin NA, Weisman RS, Howland MA, Hoffman RS (eds.), *Toxicologic emergencies.* Norwalk, CT: Appleton and Lange, 1994.
34. Brown JH, Taylor P. Muscarinic receptor agonists and antagonists. In: Hardman JG,

Limbrird LE, Molinoff PB, Ruddon RW, Gilman AG (eds.), *Goodman & Gilman's the Pharmacological Basis of Therapeutics,* 9th ed. New York: MGraw-Hill, 1996, CD-Rom.

35. Benjamin DR. Mushroom poisoning in infants and children: the Amanita pantherina/muscaria group. *J Toxicol Clin Toxicol* 1992;30:13–22.
36. Buck RW. Mycetism. *N Engl J Med* 1969;280:1363.
37. Hanrahan JP, Gordon MA. Mushroom poisoning. Case reports and a review of therapy. *JAMA* 1984;251:1057–1061.
38. Dewitt MS, Swain R, Gibson LB Jr. The dangers of jimson weed and its abuse by teenagers in the Kanawha Valley of West Virginia. *W V Med J* 1997;93:182–185.
39. Spiller HA, Willias DB, Gorman SE, Sanftleban J. Retrospective study of mistletoe ingestion. *J Toxicol Clin Toxicol* 1996;34:405–408.
40. Tuncok Y, Kozan O, Cavdar C, Guven H, Fowler J. *Urginea maritima* (squill) toxicity. *J Toxicol Clin Toxicol* 1995;33:83–86.
41. Fitzgerald P, Moss N, O'Mahony S, Whelton MJ. Accidental hemlock poisoning. *Br Med J* (Clin Res Ed) 1987;295:1657.
42. Landers D, Seppi K, Blauer W. Seizures and death on a white river float trip. Report of water hemlock poisoning. *West J Med* 1985;142:637–640.
43. Trabattoni G, Visintini D, Terzano GM, Lechi A. Accidental poisoning with deadly nightshade berries: a case report. *Hum Toxicol* 1984;3:513–516.
44. Knutsen OH, Paszkowski P. New aspects in the treatment of water hemlock poisoning. *J Toxicol Clin Toxicol* 1984;22:157–166.
45. Starreveld E, Hope E. Cicutoxin poisoning (water hemlock). *Neurology* 1975;25:730–734.
46. Withers LM, Cole FR, Nelson RB. Water-hemlock poisoning. *N Engl J Med* 1969;281:566–567.
47. Centers for Disease Control and Prevention. Water hemlock poisoning—Maine, 1992. *JAMA* 1994;271:1475.
48. Theuma A, Vassallo MT. Occult CO poisoning presenting as an epileptic fit. *Postgrad Med J* 1997;73:448.
49. Jain KK. Neurologic aspects of carbon monoxide poisoning. In: Gilman S, Goldstein GW, Waxman SG (eds), *Neurobase,* 2nd ed. San Diego, CA: Arbor Publishing, 1999, CD-Rom.
50. Durnin C. Carbon monoxide poisoning presenting with focal epileptiform seizures. *Lancet* 1987;1:1319.
51. Mathieu D, Nolf M, Durocher A, et al. Acute carbon monoxide poisoning risk of late sequelae and treatment by hyperbaric oxygen. *Clin Toxicol* 1985;23:315–324.
52. Kumar A, Dey PK, Singla PN, Ambasht RS, Upadhyay SK. Blood lead levels in children with neurological disorders. *J Trop Pediatr* 1998;44:320–322.
53. Yu EC, Yeung CY. Lead encephalopathy due to herbal medicine. *Chin Med J* (English) 1987;100:915–917.
54. Selbst SM, Henretig FM, Pearce J. Lead encephalopathy. A case report and review of management. *Clin Pediatr* 1985;24:280–282, 285.
55. Whitfield CL, Ch'ien LT, Whitehead JD. Lead encephalopathy in adults. *Am J Med* 1972;52:289–298.
56. Feldman RG. Urban lead mining—lead intoxication among de-leaders. *N Engl J Med* 1978;298:1143–1145.

57. Feldman RG. Effects of toxins and physical agents on the nervous system. In: Bradley WG, Daroff RB, Fenichel GM, Marsden CD (eds.), *Neurology in Clinical Practice*. Boston, MA: Butterworth-Heinemann, 1991, pp 1185–1209.

58. Mirando EH, Ranasinghe L. Lead encephalopathy in children. Uncommon clinical aspects. *Med J Aust* 1970;2:966–968.

59. Brown AW, Aldridge WN, Street BW, Verschoyle RD. The behavioral and neuropathologic sequelae of intoxication by trimethyltin compounds in the rat. *Am J Pathol* 1979;97:59–82.

60. Besser R, Kramer G, Thumler R, Bohl J, Gutmann L, Hopf HC. Acute trimethyltin limbic-cerebellar syndrome. *Neurology* 1987;37:945–950.

61. Ortel TL, Bedrosian CL, Simel DL. Arsenic poisoning and seizures. *N C Med J* 1987;48:627–630.

62. Komaki H, Maisawa S, Sugai K, Kobayashi Y, Hashimoto T. Tremor and seizures associated with chronic manganese intoxication. *Brain Dev* 1999;21:122–124.

63. Marquet P, Francois B, Vignon P, Lachatre G. A soldier who had seizures after drinking quarter of a litre of wine. *Lancet* 1996;348:1070.

64. Marquet P, Francois B, Lotfi H, et al. Tungsten determination in biological fluids, hair and nails by plasma emission spectrometry in a case of severe acute intoxication in man. *J Forens Sci* 1997;42:527–530.

65. Friberg L, Piscator M, Nordberg GF, Kjellstrom T. *Cadmium in the Environment*, 2nd ed. Cleveland, OH: CRC Press, 1974.

66. Littorin ME, Fehling C, Attewell RG, Skerfving S. Focal epilepsy and exposure to organic solvents: a case-referent study. *J Occup Med* 1988;30:805–808.

67. Jacobsen M, Baelum J, Bonde JP. Temporal epileptic seizures and occupational exposure to solvents. *Occup Environ Med* 1994;51:429–430.

68. Silva-Filho AR, Pires ML, Shiotsuki N. Anticonvulsant and convulsant effects of organic solvents. *Pharmacol Biochem Behav* 1992;41:79–82.

69. Allister C, Lush M, Oliver JS, Watson JM. Status epilepticus caused by solvent abuse. *Br Med J* (Clin Res Ed) 1981;283:1156.

13

Seizures in Cancer Patients

Myrna R. Rosenfeld, MD, PhD and Josep Dalmau, MD, PhD

Introduction

It is estimated that at least 15% of all cancer patients will have a symptomatic neurologic complication during the course of their disease *(1)*. With 1 million new cases of cancer diagnosed in the United States each year, neurologic complications of cancer are therefore a relatively common medical problem *(2)*.

Cancer may affect the nervous system at any level of the neuraxis through either direct (metastatic) or indirect (nonmetastatic or paraneoplastic) mechanisms. Direct effects of cancer on the nervous system are due to primary nervous system tumors or metastatic deposits of cancer in the brain, spine, leptomeninges, nerves and, most rarely, muscle. In these cases, nervous system function is affected because of compression or destruction of normal structures. Indirect effects of cancer on the nervous system are nonmetastatic complications, which affect the nervous system through a variety of mechanisms, including side effects of treatment, vascular disorders, metabolic and nutritional deficits, infections, and paraneoplastic or remote effects.

This chapter will focus on the etiology of seizures in patients with cancer. In this population, seizures are the result of many different pathological processes but are most commonly attributable to metastasis and vascular events **(Table 1)** *(3)*. For cancer patients, seizure etiology is not always obvious, and metabolic abnormalities, infections, and toxic side effects of treatment are among other pathogenetic mechanisms to be considered *(4)*. Clinical clues can be helpful; generalized or multifocal motor seizures are more likely to occur in association with systemic problems such as metabolic disturbances, infections, and toxic effects of therapy, whereas focal seizures are often the result of an underlying structural brain abnormality such as a metastasis *(5)*.

From: *Seizures: Medical Causes and Management*
Edited by: N. Delanty © Humana Press, Inc., Totowa, NJ

Table 1
Causes of Seizures in Cancer Patients[a]

Direct (metastatic)
  Primary brain tumors
  Metastasis
    parenchyma
    calvarium
    dura
    leptomeninges
Indirect (nonmetastatic)
  Cerebrovascular Disorders
    infarction
    hemorrhage
  Metabolic Abnormalities
    electrolyte disturbances
    endocrine abnormalities
    organ failure
  Infections
    bacterial
    viral
    fungal
    parasitic
  Treatment-Related
    chemotherapy
    radiation
    supportive medications
    biologic response modifiers
    antibiotics
  Paraneoplastic
    paraneoplastic limbic encephalitis

[a]Adapted from Stein and Chamberlain *(146)*.

Seizures Resulting from Direct Effects of Cancer

Primary Brain Tumors

Primary brain tumors are the most frequent cause of new-onset seizures in adults between the ages of 35 and 55 yr and are a major cause of seizures in the elderly *(6)*. Approximately 30–60% of all patients with primary brain tumors have seizures during the course of their illness *(7–9)*. About half will have focal seizures (either simple or complex partial), and the rest, secondarily generalized seizures *(10,11);* primary generalized seizures are rare with brain tumors. For up to one-third of patients, seizures may be the initial and often only manifestation of the underlying tumor. Patients whose brain tumors present with seizures almost always have recurrent seizures. These patients are also at a higher risk of developing status epilepticus than patients who have seizures late in the course of their illness *(11)*. Because primary brain tumors in children are more often infratentorial, brain tumors are uncommon causes of seizures in this population *(10)*.

For seizures associated with primary brain tumors, there is an inverse correlation between tumor grade and seizure frequency. Slow-growing, indolent tumors such as low-grade gliomas, gangliogliomas, and oligodendrogliomas are often associated with seizures *(7,12)*. Approximately 10–15% of patients undergoing surgery for chronic, intractable seizures have an associated tumor, usually a low-grade glioma *(13,14)*. Some series report that at least 90% of patients with cerebral hemispheric low-grade glial tumors present with seizures and have a normal neurological examination *(15,16)*. Faster-growing, more aggressive tumors such as anaplastic astrocytomas and glioblastoma multiforme are less often associated with seizures. It is not clear whether this is attributable to the shorter life span of patients with aggressive tumors, therefore allowing less time for a seizure focus to develop.

The epileptic phenomenology of seizures associated with tumors reflects the location of the lesion and does not differ from seizures caused by other mechanisms such as temporal sclerosis. Temporal lobe tumors often cause simple partial seizures characterized by olfactory and gustatory hallucinations or feelings of fear, pleasure, or *déjà vu,* or complex partial seizures with impairment of consciousness or repetitive psychomotor movements. Tumors of the parietal lobe can result in sensory seizures, whereas occipital lobe tumors may lead to visual seizures characterized by lights, colors, and formed geometric patterns *(17)*.

The pathogenic mechanisms behind epileptogenesis in patients with brain tumors are not fully known. It is likely that the location and the infiltrative properties of the tumor are at least as important in the development of the seizures as the histopathology of the lesion *(6)*. Lesions that involve gray matter are associated most often with seizures, whereas tumors in subcortical areas such as the thalamus and posterior fossa are rarely associated with seizures. White-matter lesions, even when associated with edema, disrupt projections that likely interfere with the spread of epileptic discharges, accounting in part for the lesser association of these lesions with seizure activity *(10,18–20)*. Hemorrhage, necrosis, inflammation, and ischemia related to the tumor also contribute to epileptogenesis. Although mass effect may result in neuronal injury or irritation of adjacent normal brain, studies have demonstrated little correlation between the degree of mass effect and the incidence of seizures *(12,21)*. Local decreases in inhibitory transmitters leading to hyperexcitability of the tissues surrounding the tumor have also been postulated to be another epileptogenic mechanism *(22,23)*.

Seizures associated with primary brain tumors are often reduced or eliminated by surgical resection. For example, one study reported that 82% of patients with low-grade glial tumors and intractable seizures became seizure free after resection *(18)*. Continued seizures were associated with incomplete resection. Of these patients, 63% had temporal tumors and 18% occipital lobe tumors. Almost all tumors involved the limbic and perilimbic neocortical gray matter *(14)*. Other studies have shown similar benefits of resection for patients with intractable seizures attributable to low-grade glial tumors *(24,25)*. For some patients seizures previously refractory to anticonvulsants may become responsive after resection *(26,27)*. Others may become seizure free on medication after resection, but at lower doses, whereas some patients continue to have seizures but at reduced frequency and with less severity. When surgical resection is not complete or contraindicated, irradiation may reduce seizure frequency markedly *(28)*.

For most patients who become seizure free after resection, tumor progression is a common cause of seizure recurrence. However, there are patients who after becoming seizure free develop recurrent seizures months to years afterward in the absence of tumor regrowth *(26,29)*. It is speculated that these seizures are the result of secondary epileptogenesis as a result of kindling in tissue near the original lesion site or in the contralateral cortex *(29)*.

The use of prophylactic anticonvulsants for patients with brain tumors who have not had a seizure is controversial. It is accepted that patients with multifocal or hemorrhagic tumors are at increased risk for seizures and should be given prophylactic anticonvulsants. Some studies suggest that the use of prophylactic anticonvulsants after surgical resection and irradiation reduces seizure frequency *(30)*. However, in several other studies, anticonvulsants did not reduce the frequency of first-time seizures, arguing against the use of long-term seizure prophylaxis for patients who are seizure free at presentation *(11,31)*. Furthermore, although a generalized seizure may be life threatening if prolonged, or if the patient does not recover consciousness, the potential benefit of anticonvulsants must be compared to the morbidity associated with their use. Anticonvulsants may cause unacceptable toxicity, including death, and can have troublesome interactions with other drugs *(32,33)*. About 15% of brain tumor patients who receive phenytoin while undergoing cranial irradiation develop a rash that in a small percentage progresses to a Stevens–Johnson syndrome *(34)*. This has also been reported with the concurrent use of other anticonvulsants and cranial irradiation *(35)*. There is also evidence suggesting that some anticonvulsants possess adverse immunosuppressive effects *(36)*.

Intracranial Metastasis

Metastases to the base of the skull and brain parenchyma are the most frequent neurologic complication in cancer patients and occur in approximately 25–30% of all patients *(6)*. There are some systemic cancers such as melanoma *(37)*, choriocarcinoma *(38)*, and lung cancers *(39)* that have a predilection for metastasizing to the brain, whereas others such as prostate *(40)*, ovarian *(41)*, and Hodgkin's lymphoma *(42)* rarely do so.

Brain metastases may occur early in the course of the systemic disease, as is seen with lung cancer, in which 10–20% of patients present with symptoms of brain metastases before the systemic disease has even been diagnosed *(1)*. For some tumors such as breast cancer or sarcoma, which are often systemically controlled with chemotherapy, the incidence of cerebral metastases appears to be increasing *(43,44)*. This is likely attributable to improvements in diagnosis and treatment that have resulted in prolonged survival for some patients and the presence of the blood–brain barrier that isolates the nervous system and neoplastic cells from the effects of systemic treatments *(45,46)*.

The signs and symptoms of brain metastases are highly dependent on the location of the metastasis. The majority of brain metastases originate by embolization of neoplastic cells to the brain and, similar to emboli of other origins, lodge in the terminal ends of the arterial supply, at the gray/white-matter junction *(47)*. The relative distribution of brain metastases is a function of the volume of blood flow to each cerebral region *(47)*. The main exceptions are tumors that are localized to the pelvis (prostate, uterine) and the digestive tract, which for reasons that are not fully clear, tend to metastasize to the posterior fossa.

The most frequent presenting signs and symptoms of brain metastases are headache (50%), alteration of mental status (33%), and weakness (30%). Seizures are a presenting complaint in approx. 20% of patients and occur in almost 40% of all patients with brain metastases at some point during their disease *(48,49)* **(Fig. 1)**. Seizures due to brain metastases most commonly are attributable to compression of the brain parenchyma, and because they originate in the region of the tumor, are most often focal with or without secondary generalization. Even when scalp electroencephalography has demonstrated bilateral sharp waves or a contralateral onset, invasive electrode studies of patients with seizures secondary to metastasis reveal the focal onset *(13,50)*.

Seizures attributable to metastases (and other mass lesions) are dangerous for several reasons. Seizures raise cerebral blood flow and increase cerebral blood volume and intracranial pressure, which can lead to cerebral herniation. The seizures may also progress to status epilepticus, which can be lethal, and repetitive seizures secondary to metastasis may result in permanent neurologic damage *(51)*.

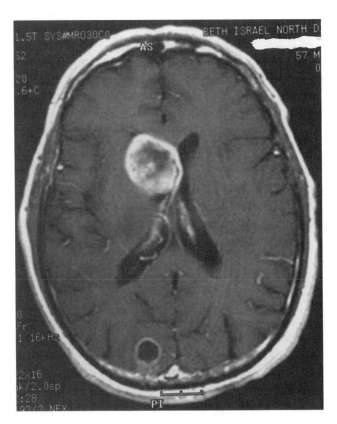

Fig. 1. Brain metastases in a patient with renal cell carcinoma. The presenting symptoms were focal seizures involving the left lower extremity.

In addition to metastases to the brain parenchyma, metastases to other intracranial sites can occur and produce seizures. For example, calvarial metastases are usually asymptomatic but can grow to such a size that they cause compression of the dural sinuses and brain *(52,53)*. Metastases to the dura may result in focal deficits or seizures resulting from focal invasion of the brain parenchyma, venous obstruction, or subdural hemorrhage *(54–56)*.

Patients with brain metastasis may also develop intracranial hypertension and "plateau waves" *(57)*. These are intermittent, abrupt rises of intracranial pressure, resulting in transitory symptoms such as worsening headache, diplopia, visual obscurations, fluctuating mental status, and motor deficits. These transient symptoms may often be confused with episodes of seizures or transient ischemic attacks.

The treatment of brain metastases depends on the size, number, location of the lesions, and the general clinical status of the patient. Both surgical resection and/or irradiation of the metastasis have been shown to decrease or eliminate seizures *(58–60)*. Unlike primary brain tumors, brain metastases are usually well demarcated from the surrounding brain, making them susceptible to complete surgical removal. Surgery is considered for patients with a limited number of accessible lesions, particularly if no primary tumor has been identified, or for patients with large metastases, which may cause severe edema during irradiation *(60,61)*. For multiple brain metastases, whole brain irradiation is used. Focal treatment with radiation (gamma knife or stereotactic radiosurgery) is often considered if there are three or fewer lesions of the appropriate size.

Retrospective studies of patients with brain metastases have shown an equal incidence of seizures with or without anticonvulsant prophylaxis *(48,62,63)*. These studies do not support initiating these medications unless patients have had a seizure. In some institutions, all patients undergoing craniotomy for removal of one or more brain metastases are started on anticonvulsants prior to surgery, regardless of their seizure history. However, there have not been any conclusive prospective studies evaluating the effectiveness of anticonvulsant therapy in preventing postcraniotomy seizures in this population.

Based on retrospective studies that have found an equal incidence of seizures with or without anticonvulsant prophylaxis, it appears safe to avoid anticonvulsants in patients with brain metastases unless they have already had a seizure. Exceptions to this are patients with metastasis who are considered at high risk for seizures. These exceptions include patients with metastases attributable to melanoma in which the incidence of seizures is as high as 50% because of the predilection of this tumor to involve gray matter *(37)*, as well as those with hemorrhagic metastases *(37)*.

The use of iodinated contrast dye, such as that used for computerized tomography (CT) scanning has been shown to provoke seizures in patients with previously asymptomatic brain metastases *(64,65)*. This is likely the result of breakdown of the blood–brain barrier and direct toxicity of the high osmolarity contrast dye. In these cases, a one-time oral dose of 5–10 mg of diazepam, 30 min prior to contrast administration, will substantially reduce the risk of a seizure *(66)*. For unknown reasons, the risk of seizures after iodinated contrast dye administration is greater for patients with metastasis than those with primary brain tumors.

Leptomeningeal Metastasis

When neoplastic cells enter the cerebrospinal fluid (CSF) they may spread to any area of the nervous system in contact with it. These cells seed the meninges in discrete clumps or become widely disseminated, resulting in what is called leptomeningeal metastasis (known previously as carcinomatous meningitis) *(67)*.

It is estimated that approx. 5–10% of all cancer patients will develop leptomeningeal metastases and about 30% of these will have concurrent intraparenchymal metastases *(68)*. The incidence of leptomeningeal metastases is rising because of improved control of systemic disease and increased life expectancy, combined with the inability of many chemotherapeutic agents to enter the nervous system at therapeutic doses *(69)*. Whereas any tumor may be associated with leptomeningeal seeding, the solid tumors most frequently involved are lung, breast, melanoma, and adenocarcinomas of the digestive system *(70)*. Non-Hodgkin's lymphoma and lymphoblastic leukemias appear to have higher incidences of leptomeningeal seeding than other types of lymphoma and leukemia *(71–73)*. Primary tumors of the central nervous system (CNS) such as medulloblastomas, pineoblastomas, germinomas, ependymomas and, less commonly, glioblastoma multiforme can also spread through the leptomeninges.

The signs and symptoms of leptomeningeal metastases are often attributable to obstruction of CSF flow producing hydrocephalus, infiltration of cranial and peripheral nerve roots, and neoplastic infiltration of the nervous system parenchyma. Leptomeningeal metastases have been reported in association with seizures in 6–14% of patients *(74,75)*. Seizures occur when there is parenchymal invasion and must be differentiated from episodic loss of consciousness attributable to increased intracranial pressure and plateau waves *(69,76)*. Patients with leptomeningeal disease can develop nonconvulsive status epilepticus that may be misdiagnosed as a confusional state or psychosis.

The prognosis for patients with leptomeningeal metastases is poor, and treatment regimens are variable. Some patients respond to irradiation of symptomatic regions, although most patients with seizures require whole brain irradiation. The use of intrathecal chemotherapy may prove beneficial for some patients but can produce seizures as a side effect *(68)*.

Seizures Attributable to Indirect Effects of Cancer

Cerebrovascular Disorders

After metastatic disease, cerebrovascular disease is the second most common neuropathological finding in patients dying from systemic cancer *(77,78)*. Although cancer patients are at risk for atherosclerotic events, in these patients symptoms of cerebral infarcts are often caused by other mechanisms such as nonbacterial thrombotic endocarditis (NBTE) or disseminated intravascular coagulation (DIC) **(Table 2)** *(79)*. Other mechanisms such as direct effects of the tumor, side effects of treatment, and other types of coagulopathies are also important causes of vascular events in the cancer patient *(77)*. In all of these settings, seizures are usually the result of ischemic brain infarction or intracerebral hemorrhage.

Table 2
Cerebrovascular Complications in Cancer Patients[a]

Mechanism	Neurologic Complication
Direct Effects of the Tumor	
Tumor emboli	Embolic infarct
(myxoma, choriocarcinoma)	Oncotic aneurysm
Dural metastasis	Sagittal sinus thrombosis
(neuroblastoma, adenocarcinoma)	Subdural hematoma
Infiltration of vasculature	Hemorrhage
(melanoma, choriocarcinoma, lung)	
Leukostasis	Cerebral hemorrhage
(leukemia)	
Related to Sepsis	
Septic emboli	Embolic infarct
(leukemia, lymphoma)	
Vasculitis (varicella-zoster)	Thrombotic infarct
Related to Coagulopathy	
Disseminated intravascular cogulation	Thrombotic infarct
(mainly leukemias, lymphomas, and	Venous sinus thrombosis
solid tumors)	Intracranial hemorrhage
Nonbacterial thrombotic endocarditis	Embolic infarct
(solid tumors)	
Thrombocytopenia	Hemorrhage
(advanced leukemias)	
Thrombocytosis	Thrombotic infarct
Hyperviscosity syndrome	Cerebral hemorrhage
(lymphoma, macroglobulinemia)	Thrombotic infarct
Thrombotic microangiopathy	Cerebral infarct
(lung)	
Related to Diagnostic Studies or Treatment	
Lumbar puncture	Subdural or epidural hematoma
Radiotherapy	Carotid atherosclerosis or thrombosis
	Ischemic infarct (secondary to
	Moyamoya-like changes)
Chemotherapy	
L-asparaginase	Sagittal sinus thrombosis
Suramin	Intracranial hemorrhage
Mitomycin, *cis*-platinum	Thrombotic microangiopathy

[a]Adapted from Graus et al. *(77)*.

Simple partial and complex partial seizures account for 80% of seizures after stroke of either etiology. The seizure phenomenology depends on the site of cerebral injury. Lobar hemorrhages are associated with the highest rate of early seizures. Generalized convulsive seizures are relatively uncommon during the evolving phases of stroke, although an acute embolus may cause a focal seizure. Thrombotic events are rarely convulsive at onset but may later cause seizures if they involve the cortex.

Hemorrhage into a metastatic tumor is the most common cause of intracranial hemorrhage in cancer patients with nonhematological malignancies. Invasion of cerebral blood vessels by metastatic disease leads to hemorrhage. The most common cause is metastasis from lung cancer because this tumor has the highest incidence of brain metastasis *(80)*. However the likelihood of a hemorrhage into any metastasis is greater for malignant melanoma, germ-cell tumors, and renal-cell carcinomas *(81)*. Symptoms of hemorrhage into a brain metastasis are the sudden onset of headache and focal neurologic signs, such as hemiparesis or seizures *(82)*.

Almost all cancer patients will develop evidence of coagulopathy during the course of their disease *(83)*. These hemostatic abnormalities can be divided into deficiencies of coagulation or the existence of a hypercoagulable state. Hemorrhage is most often attributable to thrombocytopenia as a result of bone marrow replacement by the cancer, bone marrow damage by chemotherapy or irradiation, or platelet consumption caused by DIC. Destruction of the liver by metastatic disease can result in decreased production of clotting proteins. Spontaneous intracerebral hemorrhages usually occur only when the platelet count is less than 10,000 platelets/mm^3 *(77)*. Intracranial hemorrhage is more common in patients with hematological malignancies than in those with solid tumors. In general, the onset of symptoms is slower than in the case of hemorrhage into a metastasis, suggesting that the hemorrhage is the result of involvement of veins or arterioles rather than a large vessel.

Disseminated intravascular coagulation is a hypercoagulable state that often presents with mental confusion and, in one-third of the cases, generalized seizures *(84)*. Although DIC can occur at any time during the cancer course, it is seen more commonly in patients with advanced leukemias and lymphomas and often in association with sepsis. If there is an underlying focal brain abnormality, focal seizures may also occur.

Excessive coagulation can lead to nervous system infarction and is most often seen in patients with widespread systemic cancers. L-asparaginase is well known for causing cerebral sinus thrombosis with associated seizures *(85,86)*. The sagittal sinus is commonly most involved. The mechanism appears to be interference with antithrombin III production *(87,88)*.

Spontaneous venous sinus thrombosis secondary to hypercoagulopathy can complicate hematological malignancies but has also been reported with solid tumors such as carcinomas of the breast and lung. Patients present with the sudden onset of headache and focal seizures. This may progress to stupor, coma, and death as a result of cerebral herniation. In some patients the process is more benign and symptoms resolve.

Emboli from a variety of sources are a common cause of cerebral infarction in patients with cancer *(89–91)*. Nonbacterial thrombotic endocarditis affects about 1% of all cancer patients *(92,93)*. Most patients with NBTE also have an associated coagulopathy. In one series, 13% of patients with NBTE and cerebral infarction presented with seizures *(94)*. Other sources of emboli include infectious material, tumor, fat, mucin, and air.

Radiation of the neck for head and neck carcinomas or lymphoma can result in extracranial carotid stenosis or occlusion *(95)*. Symptoms can include transient ischemic attacks or infarcts, which may be associated with seizures.

Metabolic Disturbances

Cancer patients frequently suffer from metabolic and nutritional disorders. The most common neurologic presentation is diffuse encephalopathy, characterized by confusion, disorientation, and lethargy. In addition to cognitive and behavioral changes, about 10% of patients will have seizures. Seizures secondary to metabolic disturbances are usually generalized but may be focal because of the presence of a structural brain lesion such as metastasis or the presence of vascular disease.

The causes of metabolic encephalopathy in cancer patients are similar to that in noncancer patients and include drugs, organ failure, electrolyte disturbances, endocrine disorders, and infection. For almost two-thirds of cancer patients there will be multifactorial causes.

Patients undergoing surgery or radiation for carcinoma of the thyroid, larynx, or pharynx are prone to develop hypoparathyroidism with hypocalcemia, often associated with hypomagnesemia and hypokalemia *(4,96)*. Seizures secondary to hypocalcemia and hypomagnesemia may be focal but are most often generalized *(97,98)*. Hypocalcemic-related seizures are difficult to control, can occur in the absence of tetany, and their presence is a poor prognostic factor for recovery.

Hyponatremia is a relatively common problem in many cancer patients and may be accompanied by seizures. Neurologic signs are more frequent when the hyponatremia is acute rather than chronic *(99)*. Seizures, which can be focal or generalized, usually occur at serum sodium levels of <115 meq/L but can occur at normal serum levels if the decrease in serum sodium is rapid *(4)*. For 2% of all cancer patients, hyponatremia is attributable to the syndrome of inappropriate secretion of antidiuretic hormone (SIADH) *(100,101)*. Approximately 70% will have neurologic manifestations, including seizures *(102)*. The most frequently associated tumor is small cell lung cancer (SCLC), with 15% of patients developing SIADH *(103,104)*. A variety of other tumors have also been reported including primary brain tumors, carcinomas of the breast, prostate, head and neck, and gastrointestinal tract and with hematological malignancies *(105,106)*. It also has been reported that drugs such as vincristine and cyclophosphamide may produce SIADH *(107–110)*. In addition to SIADH, hyponatremia may be the result of extensive liver metastases or mineralcorticoid deficiency secondary to adrenal metastases *(101)*.

Fluid restriction and successful treatment of the underlying tumor often results in resolution of the SIADH *(111,112)*. If the patient is actively having seizures, hypertonic saline with a diuretic may be needed to correct the hyponatremia *(113)*. Care must be taken to limit the rate of rise of the serum sodium to 0.5 meq/L per hour to avoid the risk of central pontine myelinolysis.

Seizures are a rare complication of hypercalcemia *(114)*. This may be seen with renal cell carcinomas that secrete erythropoietin and parathyroid-like hormones *(115)*. It is often found in patients with multiple myeloma as a result of an increase in bone resorption and a decrease in bone formation and in patients with widespread bone metastases from solid tumors such as breast, prostate, and lung carcinomas.

Infections

Patients with cancer are at increased risk for systemic and CNS infections. Such infections can be attributable to neutropenia, immunological defects resulting from the cancer or treatment. Seizures occur most often with meningoencephalitis and brain abscess *(4,116)*. When seizures occur early in the course of infectious meningitis, they are likely attributable to direct invasion of the brain parenchyma by the organism. When seizures occur late, they are related more often to vasculitis with thrombosis and infarction. Septic infarction is commonly associated with seizures and occurs more often in patients with leukemia and fungal sepsis *(77,117)*.

The site of the infection impacts on seizure development and is often agent related. *Nocardia* and *Toxoplasma* most often infect the brain parenchyma producing focal encephalitis or abscesses, both having the potential for inducing seizures. Seizures are often associated with varicella-zoster viral infection, which produces a diffuse encephalitis or vasculitis. Some organisms, such as *Aspergillus,* cause thrombosis of blood vessels, resulting in septic infarction or hemorrhage often in association with seizures *(118,119)*. In contrast, *Listeria* and *Cryptococcus* usually only infect the leptomeninges and do not often cause seizures; rarely, they cause encephalitis, cerebritis, or brain abscess in which case, seizures may occur *(120–122)*.

In the past, granulocytopenia resulting from cytotoxic chemotherapy or post-bone marrow transplantation was associated with an increased risk of bacterial meningitis *(123)*. Seizures were reported in almost 40% of these patients.The use of granulocyte and granulocyte macrophage colony-stimulating factors has markedly decreased this and other neutropenia-associated infections *(124,125)*.

Treatment is based on the drug sensitivities of the offending organism. Cerebral abscess usually requires surgical intervention, and infected shunts and Ommaya reservoirs often need to be removed. The continued use of anticonvulsants after successful treatment is case dependent. For patients with permanent damage to the nervous system, long-term anticonvulsants may be needed.

Chemotherapy and Radiation-Related Seizures

For the physician approaching a cancer patient with new-onset or recurrent seizures, treatment-related toxicity must always be kept in the differential diagnosis. Cancer patients take many medications that produce toxic side effects directly or through interactions with other drugs *(126,127)*. Some chemotherapeutic drugs produce an acute encephalopathy characterized by confusion and seizures that cannot be differentiated from an acute encephalopathy because of metabolic or endocrine disturbances. Other agents are associated more often with the development of a subacute or chronic encephalopathy characterized by dementia with or without seizures.

As noted, the use of chemotherapy has been associated with the development of SIADH, which can be complicated by seizures *(128–130)*. The use of high-dose intravenous methotrexate is associated with an acute stroke-like syndrome characterized by seizures, confusion, and hemiparesis *(131–133)*. Symptoms occur acutely, often several days after the drug has been administered, and usually resolve spontaneously. There are reports of a similar syndrome occurring in patients receiving moderate doses of methotrexate *(134)*. Systemic or intrathecal methotrexate can also produce a chronic delayed leukoencephalopathy that begins months to years after the drug use and can present with focal seizures *(135,136)*. Drugs used for supportive or palliative care also should be considered such as opiates, which at high doses can result in seizures both during use and during drug withdrawal *(137–139)*. Ifosfamide therapy may be associated with an encephalopathy accompanied by seizures *(140,141)*.

For some agents, the mode of administration will affect the toxicity profile. *Cis*-platinum rarely produces encephalopathy when given intravenously unless accompanied by hyponatremia resulting from the extensive hydration that accompanies its use *(142)*. An acute encephalopathy with seizures is seen more commonly with intra-arterial *cis*-platinum *(143)*. Similarly, intravenous carmustine is rarely associated with neurotoxic side effects, whereas intra-arterial carmustine can produce a necrotizing encephalopathy with seizures, especially in patients who have been irradiated previously *(144,145)*.

Brain irradiation invariably produces some form of neurotoxicity, depending on the underlying disease, the total irradiation dose, the number of radiation treatments, and the radiation dose per treatment. Seizures associated with acute radiation toxicity are thought to be secondary to edema, whereas late-occurring seizures are associated with tissue necrosis *(146,147)*.

In general, seizures rarely result from conventional external beam brain irradiation. Seizures are more common after the use of stereotactic radiation (stereotactic radiosurgery) and the gamma knife. Studies have reported seizures in 8–21% of patients within weeks of stereotactic radiosurgery for brain metastasis *(148,149)*. Seizures were focal, and the symptomatology was related to the location of the lesion. Patients with lesions in or adjacent to the motor strip were at increased risk of developing post-treatment seizures *(149)*. Pretreatment edema and the size of the lesion were not related to the seizure risk.

Bone Marrow and Peripheral Stem Cell Transplantation

Allogenic and autologous bone marrow transplantation with intensive or high-dose chemotherapy are used widely for treatment of several types of neoplasm *(150)*. Allogeneic bone marrow transplantation involves the use of hematopoietic stem cells from a human leukocyte antigen (HLA)-matched donor, whereas autologous bone marrow transplantation uses the patient's own bone marrow or peripheral stem cells. Recipients of allogeneic transplants must remain on life-long immunosuppression to avoid rejection, and to decrease the frequency and severity of graft versus host disease.

Neurologic complications of bone marrow transplantation are the result of the underlying disease, prolonged myelosuppression, and the use of immuno-suppressive drugs *(151,152)*. Neurologic complications occurring soon after transplant have been reported in 40–60% of patients undergoing autologous bone marrow transplantation. Such complications include encephalopathy, seizures, and cerebral hemorrhage *(153)*. Seizures, most often generalized, may occur in association with sepsis or metabolic abnormalities attributable to electrolyte disturbances or organ failure *(154)*. Opportunistic infections usually occur within 2–4 wk after transplantation, and new-onset seizures in this time period should prompt the search for a CNS infection, in particular, *Aspergillus* and *Toxoplasma (4)*. Generalized seizures also have been reported in the absence of obvious metabolic disturbances and without underlying structural abnormalities. It is likely that these seizures are iatrogenic and related to one or a combination of drugs (i.e., cyclosporine, imipenem, busulfan) *(155,156)*. Seizures presumed secondary to medication usually do not recur if the drug is discontinued or the dose is decreased.

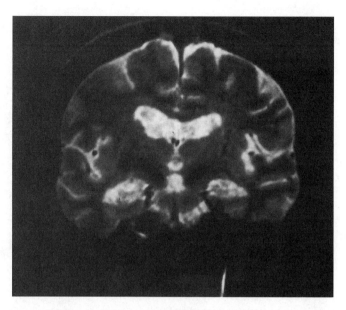

Fig. 2. MRI of a patient with paraneoplastic limbic encephalitis associated with SCLC. Note the T2-weighted abnormalities in the medial aspect of the temporal lobes.

Paraneoplastic Disorders

Paraneoplastic neurologic syndromes may affect any part of the nervous system. These syndromes are defined as neurologic disorders pathogenetically related to cancer but not ascribable to nervous system metastases or any cancer-related mechanism, such as coagulopathy and vascular disorders, infections, metabolic and nutritional deficits, and toxic effects of treatment *(1,157)*.

The pathogenesis of most paraneoplastic syndromes is unknown. However, for many of these disorders, immunological responses against the nervous system have been identified *(158)*. These immunological responses are characterized by the presence of antibodies that react with neurons or other parts of the nervous system (neuromuscular junction, peripheral nerve) and with the causal tumor *(159,160)*. Paraneoplastic antibodies are detected in serum and CSF of patients with paraneoplastic syndromes and are highly specific for one or a restricted group of syndromes and types of tumors *(161,162)*.

Paraneoplastic limbic encephalitis is the only paraneoplastic neurologic syndrome in which seizures occur as a direct result of the paraneoplastic process. Paraneoplastic limbic encephalitis is a rare disorder that presents with a diversity of symptoms including personality changes, irritability, depression, seizures, memory problems, and sometimes dementia *(163)* **(Fig. 2).** The typical clinical picture is characterized by the subacute onset of confusion with marked reduction of short-term memory. Seizures, both generalized and

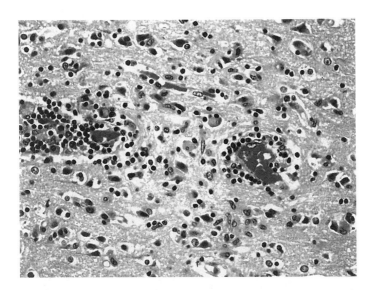

Fig. 3.   Inflammatory infiltrates of T cells in the hippocampus of a patient with para-neoplastic limbic encephalitis associated with SCLC.

partial, are not uncommon, and they may precede the onset of cognitive deficits by months *(164)*.

The more frequently associated cancers are lung (usually SCLC), testicular, Hodgkin's lymphoma, thymoma, and breast *(164–166)* **(Fig. 3).** For more than half of the patients, the neurological symptoms occur following the cancer diagnosis. This makes recognition of the disorder difficult, as similar symptoms (seizures, memory problems, irritability, depression, confusion, and dementia) can be caused by many other cancer-related complications, including brain metastases, toxic and metabolic encephalopathies, infections, and side effects of cancer therapy *(1)*. Of course, diagnosis may also be difficult when symptoms precede the diagnosis of cancer.

About two-thirds of patients with paraneoplastic limbic encephalitis develop symptoms of multifocal involvement of the nervous system. For these patients the limbic encephalitis is part of a larger clinical syndrome known as paraneoplastic encephalomyelitis *(166)*. In a recent study of a large series of patients with paraneoplastic limbic encephalitis, 12% presented with seizures, with 50% ultimately having seizures at some point in their illness *(167)*. Depending on the type of tumor, several antineuronal antibodies have been identified in the serum and CNS of patients with paraneoplastic limbic encephalitis including anti-Hu (SCLC) and anti-Ta (testicular tumors) anti-bodies *(167,168)*. In general, there is a relentless progression or, less frequently, intermittent progression of symptoms until stabilization. Spontaneous improvement is rare but has been described.

Biologic Response Modifiers

The use of biologic response modifiers has become the fourth line of cancer treatment after surgery, irradiation, and standard chemotherapy. These agents have no known direct antitumor activity; rather, they mediate cytotoxicity through the activation of immune effector cells such as T cells, natural killer cells, and lymphokine-activated killer cells. The most commonly used biologic response modifiers are interferons. Seizures have been reported infrequently with alpha interferon (IFN-α) treatment, more commonly in patients with cerebral metastasis, possibly caused by the transient increase in edema and intracranial pressure *(169–171)*. The intraperitoneal administration of lymphokine-activated killer cells and interleukin-2 was associated with unexplained seizures in one patient *(172)*.

Other new agents such as monoclonal antibodies and immunotoxins have been reported to produce seizures in individual case reports or small clinical trials, but the number of patients treated is low and further evaluations are needed *(173)*.

Summary

Cancer patients often have multiple concurrent medical problems, and seizures may result from many conditions. The prompt diagnosis and treatment of seizures in cancer patients results in decreased morbidity and improved quality of life. Appropriate diagnosis of the seizure etiology may obviate the need for long-term anticonvulsant use and help prevent seizure recurrence.

References

1. Posner JB. *Neurologic Complication of Cancer.* Philadelphia, PA: FA Davis, 1995.
2. Boring CC, Squires TS, Tong T, Montgomery S. Cancer statistics. *CA Cancer J Clin* 1994;44:7–26.
3. Gilbert MR, Grossman SA. Incidence and nature of neurologic problems in patients with solid tumors. *Am J Med* 1986;81:951–954.
4. Boggs JG. Seizures in medically complex patients. *Epilepsia* 1997;38(Suppl 4):S55–S59.
5. Miller RB. Central nervous system manifestations of fluid and electrolyte disturbances. *Surg Clin North Am* 1968;48:381–393.
6. Ettinger AB. Structural causes of epilepsy. Tumors, cysts, stroke, and vascular malformations. *Neurol Clin* 1994;12:41–56.
7. LeBlanc FE. Cerebral seizures and brain tumors. In: Vinken PJ, Bruyn GW (eds.), *Handbook of Clinical Neurology.* Amsterdam: North Holland, 1974, pp 295–301.
8. Cascino GD. Epilepsy and brain tumors: implications for treatment. *Epilepsia* 1990;31(Suppl 3):S37–S44.
9. Bartolomei JC, Christopher S, Vives K, Spencer DD, Piepmeier JM. Low-grade gliomas of chronic epilepsy: a distinct clinical and pathological entity. *J Neurooncol* 1997;34:79–84.

10. Ketz E. Brain Tumors and Epilepsy. In: Vinken PJ, Bruyn GW, editors: Handbook of Clinical Neurology. Amsterdam: North Holland, 1974:254–269.

11. Moots PL, Maciunas RJ, Eisert DR, Parker RA, Laporte K, Abou-Khalil B. The course of seizure disorders in patients with malignant gliomas. *Arch Neurol* 1995;52:717–724.

12. Berger MS, Ghatan S, Geyer JR, Keles GE, Ojemann GA. Seizure outcome in children with hemispheric tumors and associated intractable epilepsy: the role of tumor removal combined with seizure foci resection. *Pediatr Neurosurg* 1991;17:185–191.

13. Morris HH, Estes ML. In: Wyllie E (ed.), *The Treatment of Epilepsy: Principles and Practice.* Philadelphia, PA: Leas and Febiger, 1993, pp 659–666.

14. Spencer DD, Spencer SS, Mattson RH, Williamson PD. Intracerebral masses in patients with intractable partial epilepsy. *Neurology* 1984;34:432–436.

15. Vertosick FT, Jr., Selker RG, Arena VC. Survival of patients with well-differentiated astrocytomas diagnosed in the era of computed tomography. *Neurosurgery* 1991;28:496–501.

16. Piepmeier JM. Observations on the current treatment of low-grade astrocytic tumors of the cerebral hemispheres. *J Neurosurg* 1987;67:177–181.

17. Adams RD, Victor M. *Principles of Neurology,* 3rd ed. New York: McGraw-Hill, 1985.

18. Fried I, Kim JH, Spencer DD. Limbic and neocortical gliomas associated with intractable seizures: a distinct clinicopathological group. *Neurosurgery* 1994; 34:815–823.

19. Berger MS, Ojemann GA, Lettich E. Neurophysiological monitoring during astrocytoma surgery. *Neurosurg Clin N Am* 1990;1:65–80.

20. Grisar TM. Neuron-glia relationships in human and experimental epilepsy: a biochemical point of view. *Adv Neurol* 1986;44:1045–1073.

21. Strowbridge BW, Masukawa LM, Spencer DD, Shepherd GM. Hyperexcitability associated with localizable lesions in epileptic patients. *Brain Res* 1992; 587:158–163.

22. Haglund MM, Berger MS, Kunkel DD, Franck JE, Ghatan S, Ojemann GA. Changes in gamma-aminobutyric acid and somatostatin in epileptic cortex associated with low-grade gliomas. *J Neurosurg* 1992;77:209–216.

23. Bateman DE, Hardy JA, McDermott JR, Parker DS, Edwardson JA. Amino acid neurotransmitter levels in gliomas and their relationship to the incidence of epilepsy. *Neurol Res* 1988;10:112–114.

24. Eliashiv SD, Dewar S, Wainwright I, Engel J Jr., Fried I. Long-term follow-up after temporal lobe resection for lesions associated with chronic seizures. *Neurology* 1997;48:621–626.

25. Kirkpatrick PJ, Honavar M, Janota I, Polkey CE. Control of temporal lobe epilepsy following en bloc resection of low-grade tumors. *J Neurosurg* 1993;78:19–25.

26. Berger MS, Ghatan S, Haglund MM, Dobbins J, Ojemann GA. Low-grade gliomas associated with intractable epilepsy: seizure outcome utilizing electrocorticography during tumor resection. *J Neurosurg* 1993;79:62–69.

27. Whittle IR, Beaumont A. Seizures in patients with supratentorial oligodendroglial tumours. Clinicopathological features and management considerations. *Acta Neurochir (Wien)* 1995;135:19–24.

28. Rogers LR, Morris HH, Lupica K. Effect of cranial irradiation on seizure frequency in adults with low-grade astrocytoma and medically intractable epilepsy. *Neurology* 1993;43:1599–1601.

29. Morrell F. Secondary epileptogenesis in man. *Arch Neurol* 1985;42:318–335.
30. Boarini DJ, Beck DW, VanGilder JC. Postoperative prophylactic anticonvulsant therapy in cerebral gliomas. *Neurosurgery* 1985;16:290–292.
31. Glantz MJ, Cole BF, Friedberg MH, et al. A randomized, blinded, placebo-controlled trial of divalproex sodium prophylaxis in adults with newly diagnosed brain tumors. *Neurology* 1996;46:985–991.
32. Chalk JB, Ridgeway K, Brophy T, Yelland JD, Eadie MJ. Phenytoin impairs the bioavailability of dexamethasone in neurological and neurosurgical patients. *J Neurol Neurosurg Psychiatry* 1984;47:1087–1090.
33. Haque N, Thrasher K, Werk EE Jr., Knowles HC Jr., Sholiton LJ. Studies on dexamethasone metabolism in man: effect of diphenylhydantoin. *J Clin Endocrinol Metab* 1972;34:44–50.
34. Delattre JY, Safai B, Posner JB. Erythema multiforme and Stevens-Johnson syndrome in patients receiving cranial irradiation and phenytoin. *Neurology* 1988;38:194–198.
35. Khe HX, Delattre JY, Poisson M. Stevens-Johnson syndrome in a patient receiving cranial irradiation and carbamazepine. *Neurology* 1990;40:1144–1145.
36. Kikuchi K, McCormick CI, Neuwelt EA. Immunosuppression by phenytoin: implication for altered immune competence in brain-tumor patients. *J Neurosurg* 1984;61:1085–1090.
37. Byrne TN, Cascino TL, Posner JB. Brain metastasis from melanoma. *J Neurooncol* 1983;1:313–317.
38. Kobayashi T, Kida Y, Yoshida J, Shibuya N, Kageyama N. Brain metastasis of choriocarcinoma. *Surg Neurol* 1982;17:395–403.
39. Sorensen JB, Hansen HH, Hansen M, Dombernowsky P. Brain metastases in adenocarcinoma of the lung: frequency, risk groups, and prognosis. *J Clin Oncol* 1988;6:1474–1480.
40. Sarma DP, Godeau L. Brain metastasis from prostatic cancer. *J Surg Oncol* 1983;23:173–174.
41. Abrey LE, Dalmau JO. Neurologic complications of ovarian carcinoma. *Cancer* 1999;85:127–133.
42. Sapozink MD, Kaplan HS. Intracranial Hodgkin's disease. A report of 12 cases and review of the literature. *Cancer* 1983;52:1301–1307.
43. Gerl A, Clemm C, Kohl P, Schalhorn A, Wilmanns W. Central nervous system as sanctuary site of relapse in patients treated with chemotherapy for metastatic testicular cancer. *Clin Exp Metastasis* 1994;12:226–230.
44. Boogerd W. Central nervous system metastasis in breast cancer. *Radiother Oncol* 1996;40:5–22.
45. Baethmann A, Maier-Hauff K, Kempski O, Unterberg A, Wahl M. Therapeutic considerations in blood-brain barrier disturbances. *Acta Neuropathol Suppl (Berlin)* 1983;8:119–128.
46. Delattre J-Y, Posner JB. The blood-brain barrier: Morphology, physiology and its change in cancer patients. In: Hildebrand J (ed.), *Neurological Adverse Reactions to Anticancer Drugs*. Berlin: Springer-Verlag, 1990, pp 3–24.
47. Delattre JY, Krol G, Thaler HT, Posner JB. Distribution of brain metastases. *Arch Neurol* 1988;45:741–744.
48. Cohen N, Strauss G, Lew R, Silver D, Recht L. Should prophylactic anticonvulsants be administered to patients with newly-diagnosed cerebral metastases? A retrospective analysis. *J Clin Oncol* 1988;6:1621–1624.

49. Simonescu ME. Metastatic tumors of the brain. A follow-up study of 195 patients with neurosurgical considerations. *J Neurosurg* 1960;17:361–373.

50. Sammaritano M, de Lotbiniere A, Andermann F, Olivier A, Gloor P, Quesney LF. False lateralization by surface EEG of seizure onset in patients with temporal lobe epilepsy and gross focal cerebral lesions. *Ann Neurol* 1987;21:361–369.

51. Mathern GW, Babb TL, Vickrey BG, Melendez M, Pretorius JK. The clinical-pathogenic mechanisms of hippocampal neuron loss and surgical outcomes in temporal lobe epilepsy. *Brain* 1995;118:105–118.

52. Mones RJ. Increased intracranial pressure due to metastatic disease of venous sinuses. A report of six cases. *Neurology* 1965;15:1000–1007.

53. Stark RJ, Henson RA. Cerebral compression by myeloma. *J Neurol Neurosurg Psychiatry* 1981;44:833–836.

54. Perry JR, Bilbao JM. Metastatic alveolar soft part sarcoma presenting as a dural-based cerebral mass. *Neurosurgery* 1994;34:168–170.

55. Hiraki A, Tabata M, Ueoka H, et al. Direct intracerebral invasion from skull metastasis of large cell lung cancer. *Intern Med* 1997;36:720–723.

56. Nagayama I, Katoh H, Sakumoto M, Itoh M, Yoshida K. Subdural hematoma associated with dural metastasis from paranasal sinus cancer: a case report and review of the literature. ORL *J Otorhinolaryngol Relat Spec* 1993;55:240–243.

57. Hayashi M, Handa Y, Kobayashi H, Kawano H, Ishii H, Hirose S. Plateau-wave phenomenon (I). Correlation between the appearance of plateau waves and CSF circulation in patients with intracranial hypertension. *Brain* 1991;114:2681–2691.

58. Boogerd W, Vos VW, Hart AAM, et al. Brain metastases in breast cancer; natural history, prognostic factors and outcome. *J Neurooncol* 1993;15:165–174.

59. Patchell RA, Tibbs PA, Regine WF, et al. Postoperative radiotherapy in the treatment of single metastases to the brain: a randomized trial. *JAMA* 1998;280:1485–1489.

60. Breneman JC, Warnick RE, Albright REJ, Kukiatinant N, Shaw J, Armin D, et al. Stereotactic radiosurgery for the treatment of brain metastases. Results of a single institution series. *Cancer* 1997;79:551–557.

61. Sampson JH, Carter JHJ, Friedman AH, Seigler HF. Demographics, prognosis, and therapy in 702 patients with brain metastases from malignant melanoma. *J Neurosurg* 1998;88:11–20.

62. Hung S, Hilsenbeck S, Feun L. Seizure prophylaxis with phenytoin in patients with brain metastasis. *Proc Am Soc Clin Oncol* 1991;10:327.

63. Weaver S, Forsyth P, Fulton D. A prospective randomized study of prophylactic anticonvulsants in patients with primary brain tumors or metastatic brain tumors and without prior seizures. *Neurology* 1995;45:A263.

64. Avrahami E, Weiss-Peretz J, Cohn DF. Epilepsy in patients with brain metastases triggered by intravenous contrast medium. *Clin Radiol* 1989;40:422–423.

65. Scott WR. Seizures: a reaction to contrast media for computed tomography of the brain. *Radiology* 1980;137:359–361.

66. Pagani JJ, Hayman LA, Bigelow RH, Libshitz HI, Lepke RA, Wallace S. Diazepam prophylaxis of contrast media-induced seizures during computed tomography of patients with brain metastases. *Am J Roentgenol* 1983;140:787–792.

67. Gasecki AP, Bashir RM, Foley J. Leptomeningeal carcinomatosis: A report of 3 cases and review of the literature. *Eur Neurol* 1992;32:74–78.

68. Balm M, Hammack J. Leptomeningeal carcinomatosis. Presenting features and prognostic factors. *Arch Neurol* 1996;53:626–632.

69. Kaplan JG, DeSouza TG, et al. Leptomeningeal metastases: comparison of clinical features and laboratory data of solid tumors, lymphomas and leukemias. *J Neurooncol* 1990;9:225–229.
70. Posner JB, Chernik NL. Intracranial metastases from systemic cancer. *Adv Neurol* 1978;19:575–587.
71. Ersboll J, Schultz HB, Thomsen BL, Keiding N, Nissen NI. Meningeal involvement in non-Hodgkin's lymphoma: symptoms, incidence, risk factors and treatment. *Scand J Haematol* 1985;35:487–496.
72. Dekker AW, Elderson A, Punt K, Sixma JJ. Meningeal involvement in patients with acute nonlymphocytic leukemia. Incidence, management, and predictive factors. *Cancer* 1985;56:2078–2082.
73. Hoerni-Simon G, Suchaud JP, Eghbali H, Coindre JM, Hoerni B. Secondary involvement of the central nervous system in malignant non-Hodgkin's lymphoma. A study of 30 cases in a series of 498 patients. *Oncology* 1987;44:98–101.
74. Little JR, Dale AJ, Okazaki H. Meningeal carcinomatosis. Clinical manifestations. *Arch Neurol* 1974;30:138–143.
75. Olson ME, Chernik NL, Posner JB. Infiltration of the leptomeninges by systemic cancer. A clinical and pathologic study. *Arch Neurol* 1974;30:122–137.
76. Broderick JP, Cascino TL. Nonconvulsive status epilepticus in a patient with leptomeningeal cancer. *Mayo Clin Proc* 1987;62:835–837.
77. Graus F, Rogers LR, Posner JB. Cerebrovascular complications in patients with cancer. *Medicine* 1985;64:16–35.
78. Rogers LR. Cerebrovascular complications in cancer patients. *Oncology* 1994;8:23–30.
79. Rogers LR, Cho ES, Kempin S, Posner JB. Cerebral infarction from non-bacterial thrombotic endocarditis. Clinical and pathological study including the effects of anticoagulation. *Am J Med* 1987;83:746–756.
80. Mandybur TI. Intracranial hemorrhage caused by metastatic tumors. *Neurology* 1977;27:650–655.
81. Wakai S, Yamakawa K, Manaka S, Takakura K. Spontaneous intracranial hemorrhage caused by brain tumor: its incidence and clinical significance. *Neurosurgery* 1982;10:437–444.
82. Paillas JE, Pellet W. Brain Metastasis. In: Vinken PJ, Bruyn GW (eds.), *Handbook of Clinical Neurology.* New York: Elsevier, 1975, pp 201–232.
83. Bick RL. Coagulation abnormalities in malignancy: a review. *Semin Thromb Hemost* 1992;18:353–372.
84. Collins RC, Al Mondhiry H, Chernik NL, Posner JB. Neurologic manifestations of intravascular coagulation in patients with cancer. A clinicopathologic analysis of 12 cases. *Neurology* 1975;25:795–806.
85. Packer RJ, Rorke LB, Lange BJ, Siegel KR, Evans AE. Cerebrovascular accidents in children with cancer. *Pediatrics* 1985;76:194–201.
86. Reddingius RE, Patte C, Couanet D, Kalifa C, Lemerle J. Dural sinus thrombosis in children with cancer. *Med Pediatr Oncol* 1997;29:296–302.
87. Liebman HA, Wada JK, Patch MJ, McGehee W. Depression of functional and antigenic plasma antithrombin III (AT-III) due to therapy with L-asparaginase. *Cancer* 1982;50:451–456.
88. Andrew M, Brooker L, Mitchell L. Acquired antithrombin III deficiency secondary to asparaginase therapy in childhood acute lymphoblastic leukaemia. *Blood Coagul Fibrinolysis* 1994;5(Suppl 1):S24–S36.

89. Biller J, Challa VR, Toole JF, Howard VJ. Nonbacterial thrombotic endocarditis. A neurologic perspective of clinicopathologic correlations of 99 patients. *Arch Neurol* 1982;39:95–98.

90. Bedikian A, Valdivieso M, Luna M, Bodey GP. Nonbacterial thrombotic endocarditis in cancer patients: comparison of characteristics of patients with and without concomitant disseminated intravascular coagulation. *Med Pediatr Oncol* 1978;4:149–157.

91. Rosen P, Armstrong D. Nonbacterial thrombotic endocarditis in patients with malignant neoplastic diseases. *Am J Med* 1973;54:23–29.

92. Deppisch LM, Fayemi AO. Non-bacterial thrombotic endocarditis: clinicopathologic correlations. *Am Heart J* 1976;92:723–729.

93. Biller J, Challa VR, Toole JF, Howard VJ. Nonbacterial thrombotic endocarditis. A neurologic perspective of clinicopathologic correlations of 99 patients. *Arch Neurol* 1982;39:95–98.

94. Rogers LR, Cho ES, Kempin S, Posner JB. Cerebral infarction from non-bacterial thrombotic endocarditis. Clinical and pathological study including the effects of anticoagulation. *Am J Med* 1987;83:746–756.

95. Atkinson JL, Sundt TM, Jr., Dale AJ, Cascino TL, Nichols DA. Radiation-associated atheromatous disease of the cervical carotid artery: report of seven cases and review of the literature. *Neurosurgery* 1989;24:171–178.

96. Wingert DJ, Friesen SR, Iliopoulos JI, Pierce GE, Thomas JH, Hermreck AS. Post-thyroidectomy hypocalcemia. Incidence and risk factors. *Am J Surg* 1986; 152:606–610.

97. Isaacson SR. Hypocalcemia in surgery for carcinoma of the pharynx and larynx. *Otolaryngol Clin North Am* 1980;13:181–191.

98. Fonseca OA, Calverley JR. Neurological manifestations of hypoparathyroidism. *Arch Intern Med* 1967;120:202–206.

99. Riggs JE. Neurologic manifestations of fluid and electrolyte disturbances. *Neurol Clin* 1989;7:509–523.

100. Markman M. Common complications and emergencies associated with cancer and its therapy. *Cleve Clin J Med* 1994;61:105–114.

101. Sorensen JB, Andersen MK, Hansen HH. Syndrome of inappropriate secretion of antidiuretic hormone (SIADH) in malignant disease. *J Intern Med* 1995; 238:97–110.

102. De Troyer A, Demanet JC. Clinical, biological and pathogenic features of the syndrome of inappropriate secretion of antidiuretic hormone. A review of 26 cases with marked hyponatraemia. *Q J Med* 1976;45:521–531.

103. Lokich JJ. Plasma CEA levels in small cell lung cancer. Correlation with stage, distribution of metastases, and survival. *Cancer* 1982;50:2154–2156.

104. List AF, Hainsworth JD, Davis BW, Hande KR, Greco FA, Johnson DH. The syndrome of inappropriate secretion of antidiuretic hormone (SIADH) in small-cell lung cancer. *J Clin Oncol* 1986;4:1191–1198.

105. Eliakim R, Vertman E, Shinhar E. Syndrome of inappropriate secretion of antidiuretic hormone in Hodgkin's disease. *Am J Med Sci* 1986;291:126–127.

106. Kefford RF, Milton GW. Fatal inappropriate ADH secretion in melanoma. *Med J Aust* 1986;144:333–334.

107. Kosmidis HV, Bouhoutsou DO, Varvoutsi MC, et al. Vincristine overdose: experience with 3 patients. *Pediatr Hematol Oncol* 1991;8:171–178.

108. Stahel RA, Oelz O. Syndrome of inappropriate ADH secretion secondary to vinblastine. *Cancer Chemother Pharmacol* 1982;8:253–254.
109. Levin L, Sealy R, Barron J. Syndrome of inappropriate antidiuretic hormone secretion following dis-dichlorodiammineplatinum II in a patient with malignant thymoma. *Cancer* 1982;50:2279–2282.
110. Tweedy CR, Silverberg DA, Scott L. Levamisole-induced syndrome of inappropriate antidiuretic hormone. *N Engl J Med* 1992;326:1164.
111. Hansen M, Pedersen AG. Tumor markers in patients with lung cancer. *Chest* 1986;89(Suppl 4):219S–224S.
112. Glover DJ, Glick JH. Metabolic oncologic emergencies. *CA Cancer J Clin* 1987;37:302–320.
113. Hantman D, Rossier B, Zohlman R, Schrier R. Rapid correction of hyponatremia in the syndrome of inappropriate secretion of antidiuretic hormone. An alternative treatment to hypertonic saline. *Ann Intern Med* 1973;78:870–875.
114. Katzman R. Effect of electrolyte disturbance on the central nervous system. *Annu Rev Med* 1966;17:197–212.
115. Vassilopoulou-Sellin R, Newman BM, Taylor SH, Guinee VF. Incidence of hypercalcemia in patients with malignancy referred to a comprehensive cancer center. *Cancer* 1993;71:1309–1312.
116. Pruitt AA. Central nervous system infections in cancer patients. *Neurol Clin* 1991;9:867–888.
117. Haan J, Caekebeke JF, van der Meer FJ, Wintzen AR. Cerebral venous thrombosis as presenting sign of myeloproliferative disorders. *J Neurol Neurosurg Psychiatry* 1988;51:1219–1220.
118. Beal MF, O'Carroll CP, Kleinman GM, Grossman RI. Aspergillosis of the nervous system. *Neurology* 1982;32:473–479.
119. Walsh TJ, Hier DB, Caplan LR. Aspergillosis of the central nervous system: clinicopathological analysis of 17 patients. *Ann Neurol* 1985;18:574–582.
120. Bach MC, Davis KM. Listeria rhombencephalitis mimicking tuberculous meningitis. *Rev Infect Dis* 1987;9:130–133.
121. Fujita NK, Reynard M, Sapico FL, Guze LB, Edwards JE Jr. Cryptococcal intracerebral mass lesions: the role of computed tomography and nonsurgical management. *Ann Intern Med* 1981;94:382–388.
122. Viscoli C, Garaventa A, Ferrea G, Manno G, Taccone A, Terragna A. Listeria monocytogenes brain abscesses in a girl with acute lymphoblastic leukaemia after late central nervous system relapse. *Eur J Cancer* 1991;27:435–437.
123. Lukes SA, Posner JB, Nielsen S, Armstrong D. Bacterial infections of the CNS in neutropenic patients. *Neurology* 1984;34:269–275.
124. Nemunaitis J, Buckner CD, Dorsey KS, Willis D, Meyer W, Appelbaum F. Retrospective analysis of infectious disease in patients who received recombinant human granulocyte-macrophage colony-stimulating factor versus patients not receiving a cytokine who underwent autologous bone marrow transplantation for treatment of lymphoid cancer. *Am J Clin Oncol* 1998;21:341–346.
125. Yoshida Y, Nakahata T, Shibata A, Takahashi M, Moriyama Y, Kaku K, et al. Effects of long-term treatment with recombinant human granulocyte-macrophage colony-stimulating factor in patients with myelodysplastic syndrome. *Leuk Lymphoma* 1995;18:457–463.
126. Macdonald DR. Neurologic complications of chemotherapy. *Neurol Clin* 1991;9:955–967.

127. Chabner BA, Collins JM (eds.). *Cancer and Chemotherapy: Principles and Practice.* Philadelphia, PA: JB Lippincott, 1990.

128. Hurwitz RL, Mahoney DH Jr, Armstrong DL, Browder TM. Reversible encephalopathy and seizures as a result of conventional vincristine administration. *Med Pediatr Oncol* 1988;16:216–219.

129. DeFronzo RA, Thier SO. Pathophysiologic approach to hyponatremia. *Arch Intern Med* 1980;140:897–902.

130. Goldberg M. Hyponatremia. *Med Clin North Am* 1981;65:251–269.

131. Jaffe N, Takaue Y, Anzai T, Robertson R. Transient neurologic disturbances induced by high-dose methotrexate treatment. *Cancer* 1985;56:1356–1360.

132. Packer RJ, Grossman RI, Belasco JB. High dose systemic methotrexate-associated acute neurologic dysfunction. *Med Pediatr Oncol* 1983;11:159–161.

133. Walker RW, Allen JC, Rosen G, Caparros B. Transient cerebral dysfunction secondary to high-dose methotrexate. *J Clin Oncol* 1986;4:1845–1850.

134. Martino RL, Benson AB, III, Merritt JA, Brown JJ, Lesser JR. Transient neurologic dysfunction following moderate-dose methotrexate for undifferentiated lymphoma. *Cancer* 1984;54:2003–2005.

135. Rubinstein LJ, Herman MM, Long TF, Wilbur JR. Disseminated necrotizing leukoencephalopathy: a complication of treated central nervous system leukemia and lymphoma. *Cancer* 1975;35:291–305.

136. Spencer MD. Leukoencephalopathy after CNS prophylaxis for acute lymphoblastic leukaemia. *Pediatr Rehabil* 1998;2:33–39.

137. Szeto HH, Inturrisi CE, Houde R, Saal S, Cheigh J, Reidenberg MM. Accumulation of normeperidine, an active metabolite of meperidine, in patients with renal failure of cancer. *Ann Intern Med* 1977;86:738–741.

138. Gregory RE, Grossman S, Sheidler VR. Grand mal seizures associated with high-dose intravenous morphine infusions: incidence and possible etiology. *Pain* 1992;51:255–258.

139. Wijdicks EF, Sharbrough FW. New-onset seizures in critically ill patients. *Neurology* 1993;43:1042–1044.

140. Heim ME, Fiene R, Schick E, Wolpert E, Queisser W. Central nervous side effects following ifosfamide monotherapy of advanced renal carcinoma. *J Cancer Res Clin Oncol* 1981;100:113–116.

141. Pratt CB, Green AA, Horowitz ME, et al. Central nervous system toxicity following the treatment of pediatric patients with ifosfamide/mesna. *J Clin Oncol* 1986;4:1253–1261.

142. Cattaneo MT, Filipazzi V, Piazza E, Damiani E, Mancarella G. Transient blindness and seizure associated with cisplatin therapy. *J Cancer Res Clin Oncol* 1988;114:528–530.

143. Hiesiger EM, Green SB, Shapiro WR, et al. Results of a randomized trial comparing intra-arterial cisplatin and intravenous PCNU for the treatment of primary brain tumors in adults: Brain Tumor Cooperative Group trial 8420A. *J Neurooncol* 1995;25:143–154.

144. Phillips GL, Fay JW, Herzig GP, et al. Intensive 1,3-bis(2-chloroethyl)-1-nitrosourea (BCNU), NSC #4366650 and cryopreserved autologous marrow transplantation for refractory cancer. A phase I-II study. *Cancer* 1983;52:1792–1802.

145. Madajewicz S, West CR, Park HC, et al. Phase II study—intra-arterial BCNU therapy for metastatic brain tumors. *Cancer* 1981;47:653–657.

146. Stein DA, Chamberlain MC. Evaluation and management of seizures in the patient with cancer. *Oncology* 1991;5:33–39.
147. De Reuck J, vander EH. The anatomy of the late radiation encephalopathy. *Eur Neurol* 1975;13:481–494.
148. Werner-Wasik M, Rudoler S, Preston PE, et al. Immediate side effects of stereotactic radiotherapy and radiosurgery. *Int J Radiat Oncol Biol Phys* 1999; 43:299–304.
149. Gelblum DY, Lee H, Bilsky M, Pinola C, Longford S, Wallner K. Radiographic findings and morbidity in patients treated with stereotactic radiosurgery. *Int J Radiat Oncol Biol Phys* 1998;42:391–395.
150. Bortin MM, Horowitz MM, Rimm AA. Increasing utilization of allogeneic bone marrow transplantation. Results of the 1988–1990 survey. *Ann Intern Med* 1992;116:505–512.
151. Chen RE, Ramsay DA, deVeber LL, Assis LJ, Levin SD. Immunosuppressive measles encephalitis. *Pediatr Neurol* 1994;10:325–327.
152. Mookerjee BP, Vogelsang G. Human herpes virus-6 encephalitis after bone marrow transplantation: successful treatment with ganciclovir. *Bone Marrow Transplant* 1997;20:905–906.
153. Antonini G, Ceschin V, Morino S, et al. Early neurologic complications following allogeneic bone marrow transplant for leukemia: a prospective study. *Neurology* 1998;50:1441–1445.
154. Graus F, Saiz A, Sierra J, Arbaiza D, et al. Neurologic complications of autologous and allogeneic bone marrow transplantation in patients with leukemia: a comparative study. *Neurology* 1996;46:1004–1009.
155. Madan B, Schey SA. Reversible cortical blindness and convulsions with cyclosporin A toxicity in a patient undergoing allogeneic peripheral stem cell transplantation. *Bone Marrow Transplant* 1997;20:793–795.
156. Gijtenbeek JM, van den Bent MJ, Vecht CJ. Cyclosporine neurotoxicity: a review. *J Neurol* 1999;246:339–346.
157. Dalmau J, Graus F. Paraneoplastic syndromes. In: Loeffler JS, Black PMcL (eds.), *Cancer of the Nervous System*. Boston, MA: Blackwell Science, 1996.
158. Dalmau J. Paraneoplastic syndromes of the nervous system: General pathogenic mechanisms and diagnostic approaches. In: Vinken PJ, Bruyn GW, editors: Handbook of Clinical Neurology, vol. 25. Amsterdam: Elsevier, 1997:319–328.
159. Dalmau J, Furneaux HM, Rosenblum MK, Graus F, Posner JB. Detection of the anti-Hu antibody in specific regions of the nervous system and tumor from patients with paraneoplastic encephalomyelitis/sensory neuronopathy. *Neurology* 1991; 41:1757–1764.
160. Graus F, Elkon KB, Cordon-Cardo C, Posner JB. Sensory neuronopathy and small cell lung cancer. Antineuronal antibody that also reacts with the tumor. *Am J Med* 1986;80:45–52.
161. Dalmau J, Furneaux HM, Gralla RJ, Kris MG, Posner JB. Detection of the anti-Hu antibody in the serum of patients with small cell lung cancer—a quantitative Western blot analysis. *Ann Neurol* 1990;27:544–552.
162. Furneaux HF, Reich L, Posner JB. Autoantibody synthesis in the central nervous system of patients with paraneoplastic syndromes. *Neurology* 1990;40:1085–1091.
163. Corsellis JA, Goldberg GJ, Norton AR. "Limbic encephalitis" and its association with carcinoma. *Brain* 1968;91:481–496.

164. Alamowitch S, Graus F, Uchuya M, Reñé R, Bescansa E, Delattre JY. Limbic encephalitis and small cell lung cancer—Clinical and immunological features. *Brain* 1997;120:923–928.

165. Lucchinetti CF, Kimmel DW, Lennon VA. Paraneoplastic and oncologic profiles of patients seropositive for type 1 antineuronal nuclear autoantibodies. *Neurology* 1998;50:652–657.

166. Dalmau J, Graus F, Rosenblum MK, Posner JB. Anti-Hu-associated paraneoplastic encephalomyelitis/sensory neuronopathy. A clinical study of 71 patients. *Medicine* 1992;71:59–72.

167. Gultekin SH, Voltz R, Gerstner E, et al. Characterization of a novel antineuronal antibody (anti-Ta) in the serum of 6 patients with testicular cancer and paraneoplastic limbic encephalopathy (PLE). *Neurology* 1998;50:A383.

168. Voltz R, Gultekin SH, Rosenfeld MR, et al. A serologic marker of paraneoplastic limbic and brain-stem encephalitis in patients with testicular cancer. *N Engl J Med* 1999;340:1788–1795.

169. Forman AD. Neurologic complications of cytokine therapy. *Oncology* 1994; 8:105–110.

170. Adams F, Fernandez F, Mavligit G. Interferon-induced organic mental disorders associated with unsuspected pre-existing neurologic abnormalities. *J Neurooncol* 1988;6:355–359.

171. Sherman ML, Spriggs DR, Arthur KA, Imamura K, Frei E, III, Kufe DW. Recombinant human tumor necrosis factor administered as a five-day continuous infusion in cancer patients: phase I toxicity and effects on lipid metabolism. *J Clin Oncol* 1988;6:344–350.

172. Steis RG, Urba WJ, VanderMolen LA, et al. Intraperitoneal lymphokine-activated killer-cell and interleukin-2 therapy for malignancies limited to the peritoneal cavity. *J Clin Oncol* 1990;8:1618–1629.

173. Moseley RP, Benjamin JC, Ashpole RD, et al. Carcinomatous meningitis: antibody-guided therapy with I-131 HMFG1. *J Neurol Neurosurg Psychiatry* 1991; 54:260–265.

14

Seizures Associated with Hypoxic–Ischemic Cardiopulmonary Disorders

Muredach Reilly, MB, MRCPI

Introduction

Seizures are associated with a broad range of cardiopulmonary disorders and may be encountered in a variety of pediatric and adult settings ranging from the emergency room to the intensive care unit (ICU) and the operating room **(Table 1).** It is important to recognize potential relationships between a specific cardiopulmonary presentation and possible seizure activity, including syncope, drug toxicity, and cardiopulmonary arrest. In clinical practice, it may be difficult to differentiate between a syncopal episode and true seizure activity or to recognize that seizures may represent a complication of a cardiopulmonary disorder such as myocardial infarction or stroke. Seizures may occur without tonic-clonic convulsive movements, and typical motor effects of seizures may be masked by the presence of muscle relaxants. This is of particular relevance given the large number of patients supported in the ICU following cardiac surgery and interventional cardiac procedures.

Cardiopulmonary disorders are associated with many factors that may lead to a lowering of the seizure threshold. These include hypoxia–ischemia (HI), electrolyte disturbance, medications, immunosuppression, diffuse atherosclerotic vascular disease, previous stroke, and hypertension. As in any systemically ill patient with seizures, it is important to exclude a primary neurological cause and to identify specific precipitating factors. Prompt treatment of the underlying cause is critical in certain cardiopulmonary settings, where recognition of an acute precipitant, such as cardiac arrhythmia or cardiopulmonary failure, is key to the successful management of such patients. Thus, it is essential that physicians, from the emergency room to the operating room, are able

From: *Seizures: Medical Causes and Management*
Edited by: N. Delanty © Humana Press, Inc., Totowa, NJ

Table 1
Potential Causes and Settings of Seizures in Cardiopulmonary Disorders

Potential Causes	Settings
Acute HI injury	
perinatal asphyxia	Neonatal
cardiopulmonary resuscitation	Emergency room/ICU
arrhythmia	Coronary/ICU
cardiovascular surgery	Operating room
Chronic HI injury	
chronic lung/heart failure	Outpatient/emergency room/inpatient
congenital heart disease	Pediatric patients
obstructive sleep apnea	Outpatient, nocturnal
Cerebral perfusion	
cardiogenic shock–hypotension	Emergency room/coronary/ICU
hypertensive encephalopathy	Emergency room/coronary/ICU
Cerebrovascular incidents	
embolic stroke	Emergency room/neurology
hemorrhagic stroke	Emergency room/neurosurgery
Electrolyte/medication/overdose	
hyponatremia/hypomagnesemia/heart failure	Coronary/ICU
cyclosporin/transplantation	Posttransplant/outpatient
chronic pulmonary disease/theophylline	Outpatient/pulmonary/inpatient
tuberculosis/isoniazid	Pulmonary
lidocaine/arrhythmia	Coronary/ICU
tricyclic antidepressant overdose/arrhythmia	Emergency room/psychiatry
anesthesia/cardiac surgery	Operating room/ICU
narcotic withdrawal	ICU/oncology
Alcohol/illicit drug abuse	
alcohol withdrawal/heart failure	Inpatient/psychiatry
cocaine/chest pain	Emergency room
Systemic inflammatory disease/infections	
sarcoidosis/pulmonary disease/heart block	Pulmonary/cardiology
systemic lupus erythematosus	Emergency room/rheumatology
bacterial endocarditis	Inpatient/cardiology

to recognize and manage the precipitants and manifestations of seizures in patients with cardiopulmonary disorders. The purpose of this chapter is to provide an overview of cardiopulmonary diseases that are associated with seizures and to elaborate on specific disorders relating to hypoxia and ischemia.

Pathophysiology of Seizures in Cardiopulmonary Disorders

Any event that disturbs the delicate balance between neuronal excitation and inhibition can cause a seizure *(1)*. Cardiopulmonary disorders can result in multiple pathophysiologic derangements that can markedly increase the likelihood of seizures. Hypoxia, resulting in seizures, can be caused by acute disorders such as cardiopulmonary arrest, or chronic cardiopulmonary failure seen in heart failure and sleep apnea. Alterations in excitatory neurotransmitters, such as glutamate, and inhibitory compounds such as γ-aminobutyric acid (GABA), formed during HI injury may increase neuronal excitability *(2,3)*. Changes in cerebral perfusion, ranging from acute circulatory collapse during cardiac arrhythmia to loss of autoregulation seen in hypertensive encephalopathy, have distinct effects on the cerebral metabolic environment. Changes in the permeability of the blood–brain barrier may permit the entry of drugs and toxins, which can alter neuronal excitability and lead to seizures. Patients with chronic cardiopulmonary disease who have electrolyte disorders and are taking medications such as theophylline or immunosuppressants, or receiving anesthetic agents, may be most at risk for neuronal excitotoxicity *(4)*. Disturbance of central electrolyte homeostasis, particularly that of potassium, may be important in the pathophysiology of seizures in critically ill patients *(5)*.

The effect of multiple, chronic cardiac risk factors, such as diabetes, hypertension, cigarette smoking, and oxidant stress may have subtle effects on cerebral endothelial function and the extracellular neuronal environment that predispose to seizures. Indeed, hyperglycemia and oxidant stress appear to have a role in the development of seizures in animal models *(6,7)*. Genetic factors may increase the risk of seizures during systemic illness, although the molecular mechanisms of this predisposition are presently unclear. The finding that a mutation in the *Drosophilia* human ether-a-go-go-related gene *(HERG)* gene, a gene for a K^+ channel implicated in hereditary long QT syndrome in humans, is responsible for seizure activity in *Drosophilia* offers an intriguing insight into genetic predisposition to both cardiac arrhythmia and seizures *(8)*.

Etiology

Cardiopulmonary diseases represent a major cause of secondary seizures and can occur in almost any setting. Specific disorders that can result in seizures are extensive and include cardiac arrhythmia, hypoxic–ischemic encephalopathy (HIE), hypertensive encephalopathy, acute and chronic cardiopulmonary failure, myocardial infarction, stroke, cardiovascular surgeries, cardiac transplantation, medication toxicity, sleep apnea, and cardiopulmonary infectious and inflammatory diseases **(Table 1)**. Many of these specific syndromes are discussed in detail in other chapters. In patients with syncope, a careful history and focused evaluation, including tilttable testing, can lead to the proper recognition of underlying cardiac arrhythmia or convulsive syncope and avoid the inappropriate diagnosis of epilepsy (chapter 14). Seizures attributable to electrolyte disturbance, medication toxicity, and medication withdrawal in patients with chronic cardiopulmonary disorders, particularly in the ICU, result in a significant clinical burden. Seizures may be the presenting feature of hypertensive encephalopathy (chapter 16) and are not uncommon following heart and lung transplantation (chapter 17). A number of specific cardiopulmonary disorders that are associated with symptomatic seizures attributable to hypoxia and ischemia are described below.

Hypoxic–Ischemic Encephalopathy

Seizures and myoclonus are common clinical manifestations of HIE and may be difficult to control *(9–12)*. In one series of consecutive adult patients who survived cardiopulmonary resuscitation (CPR), seizures occurred in 36%, myoclonus alone in an additional 8%, and myoclonic status epilepticus occurred in 32% *(9)*. Although seizure activity after CPR is not always associated with a worse prognosis *(9,13,14),* status epilepticus, particularly of the myoclonic form, is associated with markedly increased risk of death and poor neurological outcome *(9,11,12,14)*. The incremental prognostic value of seizure activity, when added to clinically based multivariate algorithms *(13–16),* is unclear. However, poor outcome in patients with sustained seizures could relate to the consequences of the increased metabolic demands and neuronal injury produced by seizures *(17)* in a brain already compromised by HI insult. Therefore, patients with HIE are monitored closely and treated aggressively for seizure activity in the hope of improving outcome. The routine use of anticonvulsant therapy (thiopental) in comatose survivors ($n = 262$) of cardiac arrest was examined in the Brain Resuscitation Clinical Trial I *(18)*. There was no difference in survival (23% vs 20%) or survival with neurological recovery (20% vs 15%) at 1-yr follow-up in thiopental-treated patients compared to controls.

The use of anticonvulsants or neuroprotective strategies in patients at high risk for seizures and poor outcome has not been examined prospectively. One potential approach involves the use of electrophysiological testing to identify patients at high risk for poor outcome. Indeed, sustained electroencephalographic abnormalities such as alpha coma pattern, burst suppression pattern, or isoelectric activity and absent or delayed somatosensory-evoked potentials (SSEPs) are highly predictive of a poor outcome in coma patients following CPR *(12,19–21)*. However, the utility of an early electroencephalogram (EEG) may be limited by the observation that cortical activity is commonly absent early after resuscitation in patients who subsequently show sequential and parallel recovery of both electrocortical activity and neurological functions. Jorgensen and Holm performed serial EEG and neurological exams over 1 yr in 231 patients following CPR and found that 125 had no detectable electrocortical activity in the immediate postresuscitation EEG *(22)*. Although the rate of recovery of consciousness was lower in this group compared to those with early EEG activity (30% vs 74%; $p < 0.001$), the time course of EEG and neurological improvement in patients who recovered was similar in both groups. In patients who regained consciousness, an ordered pattern of EEG recovery preceded awakening, but the time course of this recovery varied for individual patients. Abnormal recovery courses in individuals were identified by incomplete EEG recovery or by the appearance of spikes and sharp waves in the EEG. Early SSEP determination represents one of the most specific methods for determining poor outlook in HIE following CPR *(20,21)*. A multivariable approach, combining clinical, electrophysiological, and biochemical variables (e.g., serum neuron-specific enolase), may facilitate more reliable prediction of outcome in postanoxic coma patients without increasing falsely pessimistic outcomes *(12)*. Whether this approach will help to identify a group of patients with intermediate risk that might benefit most from novel therapies is not clear at present.

Between 2 and 4 per 1000 newborn infants suffer asphyxia at or shortly before birth, and related HIE is a major cause of neonatal seizures and subsequent severe neurological handicap *(23)*. Experimental evidence shows an increased susceptibility of the immature brain to the toxic and epileptogenic effects of hypoxia and ischemia *(24)*. A recent prospective, population-based study in Newfoundland found that clinical seizure activity occurred 6 times more frequently (11% vs 2%) in preterm infants than in term infants, was most often caused by HIE (40%), and was associated with a 9% neonatal death rate *(25)*. Clinical seizures and their time of onset, particularly if less than 4 h, predict poor prognosis in neonates with HIE *(26,27)*. Indeed, the time of onset of clinical seizures provides an earlier measure of severity of HIE than distinct clinical algorithms do. In neonatal seizures attributable to HIE, the EEG is abnormal in up to 80% of patients, with confirmatory epileptiform discharges in 60% *(28)*. A low-voltage or attenuated-voltage pattern, or the presence of burst-suppression pattern on early, continuous EEG, particularly in the first 12 h after birth, can also accurately predict outcome in neonates with birth asphyxia *(29,30)*. A small, randomized controlled trial of high-dose phenobarbital therapy in term newborn infants with severe perinatal HIE showed a 27% reduction in the incidence of seizures and a significant improvement in neurologic outcome at 3 yr of age *(31)*. However, results are not consistent in all clinical trials of short-acting barbiturates in perinatal asphyxia *(32)*. The early recognition of clinical seizures or abnormal EEG activity may permit the identification of newborns with birth asphyxia who may be the most suitable candidates for clinical trials of novel therapies aimed at reducing HI injury.

At the cellular level, cerebral HI sets in motion a cascade of biochemical events, including progressive cellular energy failure, acidosis, glutamate and nitric oxide generation, free radical formation, and calcium accumulation, which ultimately lead to neuronal death, neurologic injury, and related seizures *(2,23)*. However, there may be a therapeutic window, during which interventions might be efficacious in reducing the severity of the ultimate brain damage. This may be hours to days in adults but appears to be limited to a few hours in neonatal HIE *(23)*. Agents with promising neuroprotective effects in experimental HIE models that are being considered for clinical use include free radical scavengers, such as the 21-aminosteroids *(33)*, platelet-activating factor receptor antagonists *(34)*, N-methyl-D-aspartate (NMDA) glutamate receptor antagonists *(35)*, magnesium (physiologic glutamate receptor antagonist) *(36)*, nitric oxide (NO) synthase inhibitors *(37)*, and monosialogangliosides *(38)*.

Evidence from adult animal models and human observational studies suggest that hyperglycemia superimposed on cerebral HI injury *(23,39)* increases the likelihood of neuronal damage, seizures, and poor neurologic recovery. Despite improved neurologic outcome with hypoglycemia in some animal models *(23)*, patients resuscitated with glucose-free intravenous fluids during out-of-hospital cardiac arrest showed no improvement in survival or neurologic outcome compared to patients given fluids with glucose *(40)*. Furthermore, hyperglycemia during HI injury in perinatal animal models may be protective *(23)*. Thus, the benefit of hypoglycemia or hyperglycemia in human perinatal or adult HIE remains ill-defined, and it appears prudent to maintain glucose concentrations in the physiologic range following HIE in clinical practice. Hypothermia has been used for decades to preserve neurologic function during total circulatory arrest in adults and infants undergoing cardiac surgery. Mild hypothermia after cardiopulmonary arrest in mature animals *(41)* and selective head cooling following ischemia in fetal models *(42)* reduces seizures and improves neurologic outcomes. This has led to preliminary studies of hypothermia in adults with cardiac arrest *(43)* and selective head cooling in newborn infants after perinatal asphyxia *(44)*. Currently, there is no data from randomized controlled trials of hypothermia in either setting. However, there was no apparent benefit of hypothermia in a randomized clinical trial of 392 patients following acute brain injury *(45)*.

Cardiac Surgery

Cardiovascular surgeries involving bypass are a controlled form of HI brain injury. Neurological complications are a significant cause of mortality and morbidity following cardiac surgery (6–20%) *(46–48)*. The Multicenter Study of Perioperative Ischemia Research Group reported that seizure without focal injury occurred in 8 of 2000 patients (0.4%) following coronary artery bypass grafting (CABG) *(46)*. This accounted for 6.2% of all neurological complications. Seizure or deterioration in mental function was classified as a type II outcome ($n = 55$). Type II outcome was predicted by older age, systolic hypertension, pulmonary disease, and excessive consumption of alcohol and was associated with a 5-fold increased in-hospital mortality (10%), and a doubling in the length of hospital stay compared to patients without neurological complications. Stroke occurred in 3.0% of patients in this study and was associated with 21% in-hospital mortality. In a previous report by this group, seizures occurred in 1.1% of 273 high-risk patients (valve surgery and CABG), and stroke occurred in 8.4% *(49)*. Type II outcomes were predicted by proximal aortic atherosclerosis, preoperative arrhythmia, and a history of endocarditis, in addition to hypertension and alcohol abuse. However, nonconvulsive seizures were unlikely to have been detected given the study design. In addition, seizure data were not reported separately in either study, and it is not clear if the findings reflect the true predictors and outcomes of seizures. The incidence of seizures in patients undergoing complex aortic surgery, in which the risk of neurological complications is believed to be greatest *(47,50),* has not been examined in a large prospective series.

Up to 6% of children undergoing cardiac surgery may experience acute neurological complications such as seizures depending on the nature of the surgery and the age at operation *(51)*. Additionally, clinical and subclinical seizures are common (6% and 20%, respectively) following hypothermic circulatory arrest and appear to be associated with a poorer outcome *(52)*. The Boston Circulatory Arrest Study Group found that transient postoperative clinical and subclinical seizures following arterial switch operation were associated with worse neurodevelopmental outcomes at ages 1 and $2\frac{1}{2}$ yr, and neurological and magnetic resonance imagery (MRI) abnormalities at 1 yr of age *(53)*. Importantly, recent studies suggest that multimodality, neurophysiologic monitoring can be used to reduce acute neurological morbidity following pediatric cardiac surgery *(54)*.

Both children and adults undergoing complex cardiac and aortic surgeries with circulatory arrest have a significant risk of adverse neurological events *(46,51)*. Retrograde cerebral perfusion has been combined with deep hypothermia, with the intention of delivering oxygen to the brain during the period when the antegrade blood flow is interrupted. A number of centers have applied multimodality, neurophysiologic monitoring to assess the adequacy of retrograde cerebral perfusion during prolonged arrest periods *(54–58)*. These techniques include quantitative electroencephalography or SSEP-based monitoring of cerebrocortical function, cerebral blood flow velocity determination using transcranial Doppler (TCD) ultrasonography, and regional cerebral venous oxygen saturation as assessed by transcranial near-infrared spectroscopy. In general flat-line EEG is used to determine the adequacy of hypothermia, and TCD and cerebral oximetry are used to define the perfusion pressure required to achieve adequate retrograde cerebral perfusion and minimize cerebral desaturations. In small uncontrolled studies, retrograde cerebral perfusion guided by neurophysiological monitoring appears to be associated with a more rapid return of continuous EEG activity, an earlier return of consciousness, and reduced neurologic complications compared to hypothermic arrest alone *(54,56)*.

Most studies have shown that postoperative serum concentrations of bio-chemical markers, such as neuron-specific enolase and protein S-100B, are predictive of both early and late neurologic and neuropsychological outcome after cardiac surgery in adults *(59,60)*. Excitotoxicity is likely to be an important mechanism of seizure activity and brain injury after cardiopulmonary bypass, and there is evidence of the benefit of neuroprotective agents in animal models of cardiac surgery *(61)*. However, there is limited clinical data with neuroprotective strategies *(58)*, and the use of early postoperative biochemical and/or neurophysiological testing to identify patients at risk who might benefit from such therapies has not been studied to date.

Cerebrovascular Accidents

The incidence of stroke is increased in patients with cardiovascular disorders, including atherosclerosis, hypertension, heart failure, and atrial fibrillation *(62)*. In addition, cerebrovascular disease is an important and sometimes unrecognized cause of epilepsy, particularly in the elderly *(63–70)*. The Oxfordshire Community Stroke Project examined the risk of seizure in 675 patients with first-ever stroke *(67)*. The 5-year actuarial risk of any seizure in stroke survivors was 11.5% with a 5% risk of multiple seizures, representing a 35-fold increased risk in the first year poststroke compared to the matched general population. Risk was greatest in survivors of subarachnoid and intracerebral hemorrhage and those with large anterior circulation ischemic strokes but was not increased significantly in patients with lesser ischemic events. Although lacunar subcortical infarcts occasionally can be associated with the development of seizures, the risk of seizures in ischemic stroke has been linked to anterior circulation events and stroke severity *(65,67,68)*, and seizures appear to be more frequent following atheroembolic events *(71)*. Seizure in the early phase of stroke occurs in approx. 2–5% of patients, is associated with increased risk of subsequent seizures, and may be related to worse outcome, although this remains controversial. *(67,68,70,72)*. Predictive factors for early seizures in 1220 first-ever stroke patients in a single Spanish center included cortical involvement and acute confusional state, perhaps related to the extent of cortical injury *(68)*. In this hospital-based study, patients with seizures had a higher in-hospital mortality rate (37.9% vs 14.4%; $p < 0.0005$) compared to nonseizure patients. However, in the prospective community-based Copenhagen Stroke Study of 1197 patients with acute stroke, early seizures were not associated with increased mortality and actually appeared to predict a better outcome in stroke survivors *(72)*. These contradictory findings may relate to differences in design (hospital vs community based) and analysis (the confounding effect of stroke severity may have been adjusted for differently).

An increased risk of seizure preceding first stroke *(67,73)* suggests that sub-clinical cerebrovascular disease may be a significant cause of epilepsy in older populations. The prophylactic use of anticonvulsant drugs in the management of acute stroke cannot be recommended presently, although their use in high-risk patients, including those with hemorrhagic strokes, may prevent exacerbation of stroke sequelae because of delayed seizures *(74)*. Overall, it is worth noting that although seizure after stroke is relatively common, it is unusual for epilepsy to be a major problem among stroke survivors, with less than 2% going on to have frequent seizures *(67)*.

Obstructive Sleep Apnea

Sleep apnea and epilepsy are common disorders, and coincidental cases are probably not rare *(75)*. In fact, obstructive sleep apnea (OSA) was first brought to prominence by Henri Gastaut, a French epileptologist. Seizures often have circadian periodicity and may occur exclusively during sleep or on awakening in some patients *(76)*. Furthermore, sleep deprivation is one of the most common seizure precipitants *(77)*. OSA can disrupt normal sleep–wake cycles and result in sleep deprivation *(78),* in addition to medical consequences such as nocturnal hypoxemia, hypertension, and cardiac arrhythmias *(79)*. Therefore, OSA may exacerbate epilepsy by causing sleep deprivation, hypoxemia, and reduced cerebral blood flow *(80)*. The overlap between sleep and seizures has sometimes led to the misdiagnosis of sleep apnea as seizures *(81)* or epilepsy as sleep apnea *(82)*. Selected, nonpopulation-based reports suggest that OSA is not uncommon in epilepsy patients *(83,84)*. In a recent study of 50 patients suspected of having seizures and sleep disorder, epilepsy was found in half and OSA requiring therapy in over three-quarters of patients *(83)*. A pathogenic association between these disorders is supported by the existence of familial diseases characterized by sleep apnea and epilepsy *(85),* and the presence of both in children with neurodevelopmental disorders *(86)*.

Small studies in adult and pediatric epilepsy patients have shown that treatment of concomitant OSA with continuous positive airway pressure (CPAP), without changes in antiepileptic medications, can lead to dramatic improvements in seizure control *(80,82,86–89)*. Therefore, a careful sleep history should be obtained in epileptic patients, and a low threshold for diagnostic testing, including video–EEG polysomnography, may assist in the management of refractory or nocturnal seizures. The presence of daytime somnolence in epileptic patients should not be discounted as medication-related, particularly if other markers of OSA (obesity, habitual snoring) are present. Notably, apnea disorders in infancy can be the first sign of underlying epilepsy *(90),* and infants with apnea requiring resuscitation who subsequently develop seizures are at marked increased risk of sudden infant death *(91)*.

Diverse Associations

The range of clinical presentations of seizures in cardiopulmonary disorders is striking. Seizures may be associated with acute myocardial infarction independent of cardiac arrest, e.g., during thrombolysis *(92,93)*. Antiarrhythmic and local anesthetic doses of lidocaine have been implicated as a cause of seizures and may be related to alterations in GABA and glutamate signaling pathways *(94,95)*. In contrast, severe seizures in newborn infants have been treated successfully with intravenous lidocaine *(96)*. Associations of seizures with distinct antiarrhythmic drugs are rare but have been reported *(97)*. Chronic obstructive pulmonary disease (COPD) *per se* does not increase the risk of seizure. However, theophylline, which is used extensively in COPD patients, as well as in patients with asthma, may lead to seizures, particularly as a feature of insidious chronic toxicity *(98)*. Alcohol abuse is a significant cause of both heart failure *(99)* and seizures *(100)*. Typically, alcohol-related seizures occur 6–48 h after alcohol withdrawal *(100)* and may therefore be observed in heart failure patients following admission. Over the past two decades, cocaine has become the most frequently used illicit drug among patients presenting to hospital emergency departments *(101)*. Chest pain and myocardial ischemia are the most common cocaine-related medical problem *(101)*, but seizures are seen in up to 5% of all cocaine-related emergency room visits *(102)*. The majority of these patients have a history of epilepsy, but cocaine appears to be the only provocative factor in 25% of cases. Bacterial endocarditis can be associated with seizures secondary to embolism, metabolic disturbance, or antibiotic toxicity *(103)*. Seizures are often the initial central nervous system (CNS) manifestation of inflammatory diseases that commonly affect the cardiopulmonary system, such as sarcoidosis and systemic lupus erythematosus, and are usually associated with a worse prognosis *(104,105)*. Seizures in heart or lung transplant patients have multifactorial etiologies, with immunosuppressive therapy, metabolic derangement, cerebroembolic events, and HI brain injury being the most common precipitants *(106,107)*. Congenital diseases such as Down's syndrome may have an increased incidence of seizures because of neonatal HIE and chronic hypoxia related to congenital heart disease *(108)*.

Summary

Patients with cardiopulmonary diseases have multiple distinct mechanisms that increase their risk of seizures. On occasion, seizure activity may delay the diagnosis of an underlying life-threatening cardiopulmonary event. Furthermore, the prognosis of the underlying illness may be adversely affected by the development of seizures, as in the case of HIE, cardiac surgery, and possibly stroke. Seizure management in patients with cardiopulmonary disorders is similar to that in other medically ill patients but requires a high index of suspicion of acute precipitants such as arrhythmias, myocardial infarction, stroke, and drug toxicity. This is particularly the case during cardiac surgery, in cardiovascular interventions, and in the ICU setting. A careful review of all drugs being taken and the metabolic status is critical, particularly in the Emergency Room and ICU and in patients with chronic cardiopulmonary failure and following transplantation. In specific instances, neurophysiologic monitoring may be useful in detecting early neurological complications, including seizure activity, in patients undergoing extensive cardiovascular procedures or after CPR. Whether these techniques will result in improved outcome is not yet clear. In addition, the use of such an approach to identify patients who might benefit from novel therapeutic strategies has not been tested prospectively. Finally, a primary neurological event such as stroke or vasculitis is not uncommon in cardiopulmonary patients with seizures and should be ruled out once the patient is stable.

References

1. McNamara JO. Cellular and molecular basis of epilepsy. *J Neurosci* 1994; 14:3413–3425.
2. Meldrum BS. The role of glutamate in epilepsy and other CNS disorders. *Neurology* 1994;44(Suppl 8):S14–S23.
3. Olsen RW, Avoli M. GABA and epileptogenesis. *Epilepsia* 1997;38:399–407.
4. Delanty N, Vaughan CJ, French JA. Medical causes of seizures. *Lancet* 1998;352:383–390.
5. Reid KH, Guo SZ, Iyer VG. Agents which block potassium-chloride cotransport prevent sound-triggered seizures in post-ischemic audiogenic seizure-prone rats. *Brain Res* 2000;864:134–137.
6. Uchino H, Smith ML, Bengzon J, Lundgren J, Siesjo BK. Characteristics of postischemic seizures in hyperglycemic rats. *J Neurol Sci* 1996;139:21–27.
7. Tan S, Zhou F, Nielsen VG, Wang Z, Gladson CL, Parks DA. Sustained hypoxia-ischemia results in reactive nitrogen and oxygen species production and injury in the premature fetal rabbit brain. *J Neuropathol Exp Neurol* 1998;57:544–553.
8. Wang XJ, Reynolds ER, Deak P, Hall LM. The seizure locus encodes the Drosophila homolog of the human ether-a-go-go-related gene (HERG) potassium channel. *J Neurosci* 1997;17:882–890.
9. Krumholz A, Stern BJ, Weiss HD. Outcome from coma after cardiopulmonary resuscitation: relation to seizures and myoclonus. *Neurology* 1988;38:401–405.
10. Edgren E, Hedstrand U, Kelsey S, Sutton-Tyrrell K, Safar P. Assessment of neurological prognosis in comatose survivors of cardiac arrest. BRCT I Study Group. *Lancet* 1994;343:1055–1059.
11. Wijdicks EF, Parisi JE, Sharbrough FW. Prognostic value of myoclonus status in comatose survivors of cardiac arrest. *Ann Neurol* 1994;35:239–243.
12. Bassetti C, Bomio F, Mathis J, Hess CW. Early prognosis in coma after cardiac arrest: a prospective clinical, electrophysiological, and biochemical study of 60 patients. *J Neurol Neurosurg Psychiatry* 1996;61:610–615.

13. Levy DE, Caronna JJ, Singer BH, Lapinski RH, Frydman H, Plum F. Predicting outcome from hypoxic-ischemic coma. *JAMA* 1985;253:1420–1426.

14. Snyder BD, Gumnit RJ, Leppik IE, Hauser WA, Loewenson RB, Ramirez-Lassepas M. Neurologic prognosis after cardiopulmonary arrest: IV. Brainstem reflexes. *Neurology* 1981;31:1092–1097.

15. Longstreth WT Jr, Diehr P, Inui TS. Prediction of awakening after out-of-hospital cardiac arrest. *N Engl J Med* 1983;308:1378–1382.

16. Berek K, Schinnerl A, Traweger C, Lechleitner P, Baubin M, Aichner F. The prognostic significance of coma-rating, duration of anoxia and cardiopulmonary resuscitation in out-of-hospital cardiac arrest. *J Neurol* 1997;244:556–561.

17. Meldrum BS. First Alfred Meyer Memorial Lecture. Epileptic brain damage: a consequence and a cause of seizures. *Neuropathol Appl Neurobiol* 1997;23:185–201

18. Randomized clinical study of thiopental loading in comatose survivors of cardiac arrest. Brain Resuscitation Clinical Trial I Study Group. *N Engl J Med* 1986; 314:397–403.

19. Moller M, Holm B, Sindrup E, Nielsen BL. Electroencephalographic prediction of anoxic brain damage after resuscitation from cardiac arrest in patients with acute myocardial infarction. *Acta Med Scand* 1978;203:31–37.

20. Madl C, Grimm G, Kramer L, Yeganehfar W, Sterz F, Schneider B, Kranz A, Schneeweiss B, Lenz K. Early prediction of individual outcome after cardiopulmonary resuscitation. *Lancet* 1993;341:855–858.

21. Zandbergen EG, de Haan RJ, Stoutenbeek CP, Koelman JH, Hijdra A. Systematic review of early prediction of poor outcome in anoxic-ischaemic coma. *Lancet* 1998;352:1808–1812.

22. Jorgensen EO, Holm S. The natural course of neurological recovery following cardiopulmonary resuscitation. *Resuscitation* 1998;36:111–122.

23. Vannucci RC, Perlman JM. Interventions for perinatal hypoxic-ischemic encephalopathy. *Pediatrics* 1997;100:1004–1014.

24. Vannucci RC, Palmer, C. Hypoxic-Ischemic encephalopathy: pathogenesis and neuropathology. In: Fanaroff AA, Nartin RJ (eds.), *Neonatal-Perinatal Medicine.* Philadelphia, PA: Mosby Yearbook, 1997, pp 856–877.

25. Ronen GM, Penney S, Andrews W. The epidemiology of clinical neonatal seizures in Newfoundland: a population-based study. *J Pediatr* 1999;134:71–75.

26. Ekert P, Perlman M, Steinlin M, Hao Y. Predicting the outcome of postasphyxial hypoxic-ischemic encephalopathy within 4 hours of birth. *J Pediatr* 1997; 131:613–617.

27. Ellenberg JH, Nelson KB. Cluster of perinatal events identifying infants at high risk for death or disability. *J Pediatr* 1988;113:546–552.

28. Sheth RD. Electroencephalogram confirmatory rate in neonatal seizures. *Pediatr Neurol* 1999;20:27–30.

29. Hellstrom-Westas L, Rosen I, Svenningsen NW. Predictive value of early continuous amplitude integrated EEG recordings on outcome after severe birth asphyxia in full term infants. *Arch Dis Child Fetal Neonatal Ed* 1995;72:F34–F38.

30. Sinclair DB, Campbell M, Byrne P, Prasertsom W, Robertson CM. EEG and long-term outcome of term infants with neonatal hypoxic-ischemic encephalopathy. *Clin Neurophysiol* 1999;110:655–659.

31. Hall RT, Hall FK, Daily DK. High-dose phenobarbital therapy in term newborn infants with severe perinatal asphyxia: a randomized, prospective study with three-year follow-up. *J Pediatr* 1998;132:345–348.

32. Goldberg RN, Moscoso P, Bauer CR, Bloom FL, Curless RG, Burke B, Bancalari E. Use of barbiturate therapy in severe perinatal asphyxia: a randomized controlled trial. *J Pediatr* 1986;109:851–856.
33. Lee SH, Kondoh T, Camarata PJ, Heros RC. Therapeutic time window for the 21-aminosteroid, U-74389G, in global cerebral ischemia. *Neurosurgery* 1996; 38:517–521.
34. Liu XH, Eun BL, Silverstein FS, Barks JD. The platelet-activating factor antagonist BN 52021 attenuates hypoxic-ischemic brain injury in the immature rat. *Pediatr Res* 1996;40:797–803.
35. Hattori H, Morin AM, Schwartz PH, Fujikawa DG, Wasterlain CG. Posthypoxic treatment with MK-801 reduces hypoxic-ischemic damage in the neonatal rat. *Neurology* 1989;39:713–718.
36. Levene M, Blennow M, Whitelaw A, Hanko E, Fellman V, Hartley R. Acute effects of two different doses of magnesium sulphate in infants with birth asphyxia. *Arch Dis Child Fetal Neonatal Ed* 1995;73:F174–F177.
37. Tsuji M, Higuchi Y, Shiraishi K, Kume T, Akaike A, Hattori H. Protective effect of aminoguanidine on hypoxic-ischemic brain damage and temporal profile of brain nitric oxide in neonatal rat. *Pediatr Res* 2000;47:79–83.
38. Tan WK, Williams CE, Mallard CE, Gluckman PD. Monosialoganglioside GM1 treatment after a hypoxic-ischemic episode reduces the vulnerability of the fetal sheep brain to subsequent injuries. *Am J Obstet Gynecol* 1994;170:663–669.
39. Mullner M, Sterz F, Binder M, Schreiber W, Deimel A, Laggner AN. Blood glucose concentration after cardiopulmonary resuscitation influences functional neurological recovery in human cardiac arrest survivors. *J Cereb Blood Flow Metab* 1997;17:430–436.
40. Longstreth WT Jr, Copass MK, Dennis LK, Rauch-Matthews ME, Stark MS, Cobb LA. Intravenous glucose after out-of-hospital cardiopulmonary arrest: a community-based randomized trial. *Neurology* 1993;43:2534–2541.
41. Safar P, Xiao F, Radovsky A, Tanigawa K, Ebmeyer U, Bircher N, Alexander H, Stezoski SW. Improved cerebral resuscitation from cardiac arrest in dogs with mild hypothermia plus blood flow promotion. *Stroke* 1996;27:105–113.
42. Gunn AJ, Gunn TR, de Haan HH, Williams CE, Gluckman PD. Dramatic neuronal rescue with prolonged selective head cooling after ischemia in fetal lambs. *J Clin Invest* 1997;99:248–256.
43. Zeiner A, Holzer M, Sterz F, Behringer W, Schorkhuber W, Mullner M, Frass M, Siostrzonek P, Ratheiser K, Kaff A, Laggner AN. Mild resuscitative hypothermia to improve neurological outcome after cardiac arrest. A clinical feasibility trial. Hypothermia After Cardiac Arrest (HACA) Study Group. *Stroke* 2000;31:86–94.
44. Gunn AJ, Gluckman PD, Gunn TR. Selective head cooling in newborn infants after perinatal asphyxia: a safety study. *Pediatrics* 1998;102:885–892.
45. Clifton GL, Miller ER, Choi SC, et al. Lack of effect of induction of hypothermia after acute brain injury. *N Engl J Med* 2001;344:556–563.
46. Roach GW, Kanchuger M, Mangano CM, Newman M, Nussmeier N, Wolman R, Aggarwal A, Marschall K, Graham SH, Ley C, Ozanne G, Mangano DT. Adverse cerebral outcomes after coronary bypass surgery. Multicenter Study of Perioperative Ischemia Research Group and the Ischemia Research and Education Foundation Investigators. *N Engl J Med* 1996;335:1857–1863.

47. Carrascal Y, Guerrero AL, Maroto LC, Forteza AP, Rodriguez-Hernandez JE, Rufi-lanchas JJ. Neurological complications of aortic artery surgery. *Rev Neurol* 1998;27:854–861.

48. Wimmer-Greinecker G, Matheis G, Brieden M, Dietrich M, Oremek G, Westphal K, Winkelmann BR, Moritz A. Neuropsychological changes after cardiopulmonary bypass for coronary artery bypass grafting. *Thorac Cardiovasc Surg* 1998; 46:207–212.

49. Wolman RL, Nussmeier NA, Aggarwal A, Kanchuger MS, Roach GW, Newman MF, Mangano CM, Marschall KE, Lcy C, Boisvert DM, Ozanne GM, Herskowitz A, Graham SH, Mangano DT. Cerebral injury after cardiac surgery: identification of a group at extraordinary risk. Multicenter Study of Perioperative Ischemia Research Group (McSPI) and the Ischemia Research Education Foundation (IREF) Investigators. *Stroke* 1999;30:514–522.

50. Welz A, Pogarell O, Tatsch K, Schwarz J, Cryssagis K, Reichart B. Surgery of the thoracic aorta using deep hypothermic total circulatory arrest. Are there neurological consequences other than frank cerebral defects? *Eur J Cardiothorac Surg* 1997;11:650–656.

51. Kirkham FJ. Recognition and prevention of neurological complications in pediatric cardiac surgery. *Pediatr Cardiol* 1998;19:331–345.

52. Bellinger DC, Jonas RA, Rappaport LA, Wypij D, Wernovsky G, Kuban KC, Barnes PD, Holmes GL, Hickey PR, Strand RD, et al. Developmental and neurologic status of children after heart surgery with hypothermic circulatory arrest or low-flow cardiopulmonary bypass. *N Engl J Med* 1995;332:549–555.

53. Rappaport LA, Wypij D, Bellinger DC, Helmers SL, Holmes GL, Barnes PD, Wernovsky G, Kuban KC, Jonas RA, Newburger JW. Relation of seizures after cardiac surgery in early infancy to neurodevelopmental outcome. Boston Circulatory Arrest Study Group. *Circulation* 1998;97:773–779.

54. Austin EH 3rd, Edmonds HL Jr, Auden SM, Seremet V, Niznik G, Sehic A, Sowell MK, Cheppo CD, Corlett KM. Benefit of neurophysiologic monitoring for pediatric cardiac surgery. *J Thorac Cardiovasc Surg* 1997;114:707–715.

55. Ganzel BL, Edmonds HL Jr, Pank JR, Goldsmith LJ. Neurophysiologic monitoring to assure delivery of retrograde cerebral perfusion. *J Thorac Cardiovasc Surg* 1997;113:748–755.

56. Cheung AT, Bavaria JE, Pochettino A, Weiss SJ, Barclay DK, Stecker MM. Oxygen delivery during retrograde cerebral perfusion in humans. *Anesthesiol Analg* 1999;88:8–15.

57. Stecker MM, Cheung AT, Patterson T, Savino JS, Weiss SJ, Richards RM, Bavaria JE, Gardner TJ. Detection of stroke during cardiac operations with somatosensory evoked responses. *J Thoracic Cardiovasc Surg* 1996;112:962–972.

58. Grieco G, d'Hollosy M, Culliford AT, Jonas S. Evaluating neuroprotective agents for clinical anti-ischemic benefit using neurological and neuropsychological changes after cardiac surgery under cardiopulmonary bypass. Methodological strategies and results of a double-blind, placebo-controlled trial of GM1 ganglioside. *Stroke* 1996;27:858–874.

59. Georgiadis D, Berger A, Kowatschev E, Lautenschlager C, Borner A, Lindner A, Schulte-Mattler W, Zerkowski HR, Zierz S, Deufel T. Predictive value of S-100beta and neuron-specific enolase serum levels for adverse neurologic outcome after cardiac surgery. *J Thoracic Cardiovasc Surg* 2000;119:138–147.

60. Herrmann M, Ebert AD, Galazky I, Wunderlich MT, Kunz WS, Huth C. Neurobehavioral outcome prediction after cardiac surgery: role of neurobiochemical markers of damage to neuronal and glial brain tissue. *Stroke* 2000;31:645–650.

61. Aoki M, Nomura F, Stromski ME, Tsuji MK, Fackler JC, Hickey PR, Holtzman D, Jonas RA. Effects of MK-801 and NBQX on acute recovery of piglet cerebral metabolism after hypothermic circulatory arrest. *J Cereb Blood Flow Metab* 1994; 14:156–165.

62. Wolf PA, D'Agostino RB, Belanger AJ, Kannel WB. Probability of stroke: a risk profile from the Framingham Study. *Stroke* 1991;22:312–318.

63. Olsen TS, Hogenhaven H, Thage O. Epilepsy after stroke. *Neurology* 1987; 37:1209–1211.

64. Viitanen M, Eriksson S, Asplund K. Risk of recurrent stroke, myocardial infarction and epilepsy during long-term follow-up after stroke. *Eur Neurol* 1988; 28:227–231.

65. Kilpatrick CJ, Davis SM, Tress BM, Rossiter SC, Hopper JL, Vandendriesen ML. Epileptic seizures in acute stroke. *Arch Neurol* 1990;47:157–160.

66. So EL, Annegers JF, Hauser WA, O'Brien PC, Whisnant JP. Population-based study of seizure disorders after cerebral infarction. *Neurology* 1996;46:350–355.

67. Burn J, Dennis M, Bamford J, Sandercock P, Wade D, Warlow C. Epileptic seizures after a first stroke: the Oxfordshire Community Stroke Project. *Br Med J* 1997;315:1582–1587.

68. Arboix A, Garcia-Eroles L, Massons JB, Oliveres M, Comes E. Predictive factors of early seizures after acute cerebrovascular disease. *Stroke* 1997;28:1590–1594.

69. Thomas SV, Pradeep KS, Rajmohan SJ. First ever seizures in the elderly: a seven-year follow-up study. *Seizure* 1997;6:107–110.

70. Arboix A, Comes E, Massons J, Garcia L, Oliveres M. Relevance of early seizures for in-hospital mortality in acute cerebrovascular disease. *Neurology* 1996; 47:1429–1435.

71. Kraus JA, Berlit P. Cerebral embolism and epileptic seizures—the role of the embolic source. *Acta Neurol Scand* 1998;97:154–159.

72. Reith J, Jorgensen HS, Nakayama H, Raaschou HO, Olsen TS. Seizures in acute stroke: predictors and prognostic significance. The Copenhagen Stroke Study. *Stroke* 1997;28:1585–1589.

73. Shinton RA, Gill JS, Zezulka AV, Beevers DG. The frequency of epilepsy preceding stroke. Case-control study in 230 patients. *Lancet* 1987;1:11–13.

74. Bogousslavsky J, Martin R, Regli F, Despland PA, Bolyn S. Persistent worsening of stroke sequelae after delayed seizures. *Arch Neurol* 1992;49:385–388.

75. Vgontzas AN, Kales A. Sleep and its disorders. *Annu Rev Med* 1999;50:387–400.

76. Janz D. The grand mal epilepsies and the sleeping-waking cycle. *Epilepsia* 1962;3:69–109.

77. Gunderson CH, Dunne PB, Feyer TL. Sleep deprivation seizures. *Neurology* 1973;23:678–686.

78. Guilleminault C. Clinical features and evaluation of obstructive sleep apnea. In: Kryer M, Roth T, Dement W (eds.), *Principles and Practice of Sleep Medicine.* Philadelphia, PA: WB Saunders, 1989, pp 552–558.

79. Shepard JW. Cardiorespiratory changes in obstructive sleep apnea. In: Kryer M, Roth T, Dement W (eds.), *Principles and Practice of Sleep Medicine.* Philadelphia, PA: WB Saunders, 1989, pp 537–551.

80. Devinsky O, Ehrenberg B, Barthlen GM, Abramson HS, Luciano D. Epilepsy and sleep apnea syndrome. *Neurology* 1994;44:2060–2064.
81. Malow BA, Fromes GA, Selwa LM. Sleep attacks mimicking epileptic seizures and pseudoseizures. *J Epilepsy* 1997;10:232–235.
82. Oldani A, Zucconi M, Castronovo C, Ferini-Strambi L. Nocturnal frontal lobe epilepsy misdiagnosed as sleep apnea syndrome. *Acta Neurol Scand* 1998; 98:67–71.
83. Beran RG, Plunkett MJ, Holland GJ. Interface of epilepsy and sleep disorders. *Seizure* 1999;8:97–102.
84. Malow BA, Fromes GA, Aldrich MS. Usefulness of polysomnography in epilepsy patients. *Neurology* 1997;48:1389–1394.
85. Manon-Espaillat R, Gothe B, Adams N, Newman C, Ruff R. Familial 'sleep apnea plus' syndrome: report of a family. *Neurology* 1988;38:190–193.
86. Koh S, Ward SL, Lin M, Chen LS. Sleep apnea treatment improves seizure control in children with neurodevelopmental disorders. *Pediatr Neurol* 2000;22:36–39.
87. Tirosh E, Tal Y, Jaffe M. CPAP treatment of obstructive sleep apnoea and neurodevelopmental deficits. *Acta Paediatr* 1995;84:791–794.
88. Vaughn BV, D'Cruz OF, Beach R, Messenheimer JA. Improvement of epileptic seizure control with treatment of obstructive sleep apnoea. *Seizure* 1996;5:73–78.
89. Beran RG, Holland GJ, Yan KY. The use of CPAP in patients with refractory epilepsy. *Seizure* 1997;6:323–325.
90. Tirosh E, Jaffe M. Apnea of infancy, seizures, and gastroesophageal reflux: an important but infrequent association. *J Child Neurol* 1996;11:98–100.
91. Oren J, Kelly D, Shannon DC. Identification of a high-risk group for sudden infant death syndrome among infants who were resuscitated for sleep apnea. *Pediatrics* 1986;77:495–499.
92. Caramelli P, Mutarelli EG, Caramelli B, Tranchesi B Jr, Pileggi F, Scaff M. Neurological complications after thrombolytic treatment for acute myocardial infarction: emphasis on unprecedented manifestations. *Acta Neurol Scand* 1992;85:331–333.
93. Effects of stroke on medical resource use and costs in acute myocardial infarction. GUSTO I Investigators. Tung CY; Granger CB; Sloan MA; Topol EJ; Knight JD; Weaver WD; Mahaffey KW; White H; Clapp-Channing N; Simoons ML; Gore JM; Califf RM; Mark DB. *Circulation* 1999;99:370–376.
94. Barat SA, Abdel-Rahman MS. Decreased cocaine- and lidocaine-induced seizure response by dextromethorphan and DNQX in rat. *Brain Res* 1997;756:179–183.
95. Ye JH, Ren J, Krnjevic K, Liu PL, McArdle JJ. Cocaine and lidocaine have additive inhibitory effects on the GABAA current of acutely dissociated hippocampal pyramidal neurons. *Brain Res* 1999;821:26–32.
96. Hellstrom-Westas L, Svenningsen NW, Westgren U, Rosen I, Lagerstrom PO. Lidocaine for treatment of severe seizures in newborn infants. II. Blood concentrations of lidocaine and metabolites during intravenous infusion. *Acta Paediatr* 1992;81:35–39.
97. Kerns W 2nd, English B, Ford M. Propafenone overdose. *Ann Emerg Med* 1994;24:98–103.
98. Cooling DS. Theophylline toxicity. *J Emerg Med* 1993;11:415–425.
99. McKenna CJ, Codd MB, McCann HA, Sugrue DD. Alcohol consumption and idiopathic dilated cardiomyopathy: a case control study. *Am Heart J* 1989; 135:833–837.

100. Earnest MP, Yarnell PR. Seizure admissions to a city hospital: the role of alcohol. *Epilepsia* 1976;17:387–393.
101. Hollander JE. The management of cocaine-associated myocardial ischemia. *N Eng J Med* 1995;333:1267–1272.
102. Koppel BS, Samkoff L, Daras M. Relation of cocaine use to seizures and epilepsy. *Epilepsia* 1996;37:875–878.
103. Lerner PI. Neurologic complications of infective endocarditis. *Med Clin North Am* 1985;69:385–398.
104. Krumholz A, Stern BJ, Stern EG. Clinical implications of seizures in neurosarcoidosis. *Arch Neurol* 1991;48:842–844.
105. Moore PM. Neuropsychiatric systemic lupus erythematosus. Stress, stroke, and seizures. *Ann N Y Acad Sci* 1997;823:1–17.
106. Grigg MM, Costanzo-Nordin MR, Celesia GG, Kelly MA, Silver MA, Sobotka PA, Robinson JA. The etiology of seizures after cardiac transplantation. *Transplant Proc* 1988;20(Suppl 3):937–944.
107. Sila CA. Spectrum of neurologic events following cardiac transplantation. *Stroke* 1989;20:1586–1589.
108. Stafstrom CE, Patxot OF, Gilmore HE, Wisniewski KE. Seizures in children with Down syndrome: etiology, characteristics and outcome. *Dev Med Child Neurol* 1991;33:191–200.

15

Seizures, Hypertension, and Posterior Leukoencephalopathy

Norman Delanty, MB, FRCPI, and Carl J. Vaughan, MD, MRCPI

Introduction

Seizures may be associated with hypertension in two ways. First, chronic hypertension is a risk factor for vascular disease, thus predisposing to both obvious and subclinical cerebrovascular disease. Such disease is a strong risk factor for late-onset seizures and epilepsy in the elderly (1). The second peak of epilepsy incidence that occurs in the elderly is appreciated more now than previously, and this is likely to become a greater problem as more people live to old age. Second, hypertension may also be complicated by hypertensive encephalopathy, a hypertensive emergency (2). This may or may not occur in the setting of preexisting known hypertension. Acute symptomatic seizures are a common clinical feature of hypertensive encephalopathy. A clinicoradiological syndrome, known as reversible posterior leukoencephalopathy is recognized in this setting, although this also can occur apparently unrelated to acute hypertension. In addition, reversible posterior leukoencephalopathy may have a number of overlapping and interacting causes.

Epidemiology of Hypertension

Blood pressure tends to increase with age in most societies, and hypertension is slightly more prevalent in men compared to women, especially in younger and middle age (3). About 20–30% adults in industrialized countries have hypertension. The incidence and prevalence of hypertension is about 1.5–2 times greater in African Americans in the United States compared to the Caucasian population (4). In general, definite hypertension has been defined as a blood pressure of greater than 160/100 in Britain, and 140/90 in North America on two or more clinic readings. Most guidelines for the treatment of

From: *Seizures: Medical Causes and Management*
Edited by: N. Delanty © Humana Press, Inc., Totowa, NJ

hypertension discuss the issue in relation to reduction of chronic end-organ damage and do not specifically address the prevention of acute hypertensive complications. However, it seems reasonable to presume that improved treatment of chronic hypertension would also lead to a reduction in the incidence of hypertensive emergencies. This is supported by data from a 1988 study of 100 patients with severe hypertension (two-thirds of whom had evidence of end-organ damage) admitted to a large urban hospital *(5)*. In this series, 93% of patients had been diagnosed previously with chronic hypertension, thus suggesting that improved management of preexisting known hypertension could reduce the incidence of hypertensive emergencies.

Seizures and Chronic Hypertension

In a case control study from Rochester, Minnesota, 145 patients, aged 55 or older with a first unprovoked seizure (without a clinically apparent stroke), were compared with 290 controls matched for age, gender, and duration of medical follow-up *(6)*. In this study, hypertension did not increase the risk of seizure occurrence significantly overall. However, patients with echocardiographically proved left ventricular hypertrophy, a marker of long-standing severe hypertension, had an 11-fold increased risk of new-onset unprovoked seizures, a risk that was abolished by diuretic treatment. The absence of risk without preexisting left ventricular hypertrophy is supported by two earlier studies *(7,8)*. Left ventricular hypertrophy has also been associated with a great degree of leukoaraiosis, or diffuse white matter changes, on magnetic resonance imaging (MRI) *(9)*, suggesting a link between leukoaraiosis and risk of seizures.

Seizures and Hypertensive Encephalopathy
Pathophysiology

The endothelium has a central role in blood pressure homeostasis by secreting substances such as nitric oxide (NO) and prostacyclin (PGI_2), which modulate vascular tone through vasodilation *(10)*. NO is released under the influence of certain endothelial agonists such as acetylcholine, norepinephrine, and substance P. It may also be released by the endothelium in response to mechanical forces such as shear stress *(11)*. The pathophysiology of hypertensive emergencies is not completely understood, but an initial abrupt rise in vascular resistance appears to be a necessary initiating step. Enhanced vasoreactivity may be precipitated by release of vasoconstricting substances such as angiotensin II or noradrenaline, or may occur as a result of relative hypovolemia. Activation of the renin/angiotensin/aldosterone system may be particularly important in the pathophysiology of severe hypertension. Transgenic animal models have highlighted the importance of the renin–angiotensin system in the pathogenesis of hypertension. Rats expressing the mouse renin gene, *Ren-2,* develop severe hypertension in comparison with nontransgenic controls *(12).* Moreover, rats that are doubly transgenic for the human renin and human angiotensinogen genes not only develop moderately severe hypertension but also develop an inflammatory vasculopathy similar to that seen in severe human hypertension *(13).* There is a growing body of data suggesting that angiotensin II has direct cytotoxic effects on the vessel wall *(14,15).* Some of these effects appear to be mediated through the activation of proinflammatory cytokine gene expression (such as interleukin-6) and activation of the transcription factor NF-κB by angiotensin II *(14,15).* Much of the vascular sequelae and target organ dysfunction seen in hypertensive emergencies may be attributable to the injurious effects of angiotensin II on the blood vessel wall. Moreover, inhibition of angiotensin-converting enzyme (ACE) activity has been shown to prevent the development of malignant hypertension in transgenic rats expressing the murine renin gene *(16).*

During an initial rise in blood pressure, the endothelium attempts to compensate for the change in vascular resistance through enhanced autocrine/paracrine release of vasodilator molecules such as NO. When hypertension is sustained or severe, these compensatory endothelial vasodilator responses may be overwhelmed, leading to endothelial decompensation, which promotes further elevation of blood pressure and endothelial damage. In turn, this initiates homeostatic failure, with progressive increases in vascular resistance and further endothelial dysfunction. Although the exact cellular mechanisms leading to loss of endothelial function in hypertensive syndromes are poorly understood, putative mechanisms include mechanical stretch-induced proinflammatory responses such as secretion of cytokines *(17),* monocyte chemotactic protein-1 (MCP-1) *(18),* increase in endothelial cell cytosolic Ca^{2+} *(19),* release of the vasoconstrictor endothelin-1 *(20),* and upregulation of endothelial adhesion molecule expression *(21).* Enhanced expression of vascular cell adhesion molecules, such as P-selectin, E-selectin, or intracellular adhesion molecule-1, by endothelial cells promotes local inflammation, which leads to additional loss of endothelial function. Ultimately, these molecular events may trigger increases in endothelial permeability, inhibit local endothelial fibrinolytic activity, and activate the coagulation cascade. Platelet aggregation and degranulation on damaged endothelium may promote further inflammation, thrombosis, and vasoconstriction. In the brain, local small vessel cortical infarction may then act as a focus for initiation of seizure activity.

Cerebral Autoregulation and Hypertensive Encephalopathy

Cerebral blood flow is autoregulated within specific limits. In normotensive subjects cerebral blood flow remains unchanged between a mean arterial pressure of 60–120 mmHg. As mean arterial pressure increases, compensatory cerebral vasoconstriction limits cerebral hyperperfusion. At a mean arterial pressure of approx. 180 mmHg, this autoregulation is overwhelmed and cerebral vasodilation ensues, which is accompanied by the development of cerebral edema. Previously normotensive subjects may develop signs of encephalopathy at blood pressures as low as 160/100 mmHg, whereas subjects with longstanding hypertension may not do so until a blood pressure of 220/110 mmHg or greater is attained. Hypertensive encephalopathy is defined as an acute organic brain syndrome (acute encephalopathy or delirium) that occurs as a result of failure of the upper limit of cerebral vascular autoregulation (autoregulation breakthrough). The pathogenesis of hypertensive encephalopathy appears to be related to hypertensive cerebrovascular endothelial dysfunction, disruption of the blood–brain barrier (BBB) with increased BBB permeability, cerebral edema, and microhemorrhage formation. There may be interindividual differences in the degree of hypertension that can give rise to autoregulatory dysfunction leading to encephalopathy, as well as differences in the same patient over time depending on comorbidfactors.

Clinical Features

Hypertensive encephalopathy is characterized by the acute or subacute onset of lethargy, confusion, headache, visual disturbance (including blindness and visual hallucinations), and seizures. Encephalopathy may occur with or without proteinuria and hypertensive retinopathy. Seizures may be the presenting manifestation (22,23); these may be focal or generalized, or focal with secondarily generalized tonic-clonic convulsions. If not adequately treated, hypertensive encephalopathy may progress to cerebral haemorrhage, coma, and death. It is associated with untreated or undertreated hypertension, as well as other known causes and associations of severe hypertension, such as renal disease, immunosuppressive therapy (24,25), erythropoietin use (26), and thrombotic thrombocytopenic purpura (TTP) (27); it may also occur in unique circumstances such as in pre-eclampsia/eclampsia (28). Eclampsia may present suddenly with seizures and may not always occur as a clinically obvious continuum from pre-eclampsia (29). Eclampsia may occur in the postpartum period and, again in this situation, may not be heralded by clinically obvious pre-eclampsia (30). In TTP, and in the syndrome of hemolysis, elevated liver enzymes, and low platelet count (HELLP) associated with pre-eclampsia/ eclampsia (31), thrombocytopenia may predispose to superimposed intracerebral hemorrhage.

Reversible Posterior
Leukoencephalopathy Syndrome

In hypertensive encephalopathy, MRI demonstrates a characteristic posterior leukoencephalopathy that predominantly (but not exclusively) affects the white matter of the parieto-occipital regions (Fig. 1) (32). These changes are

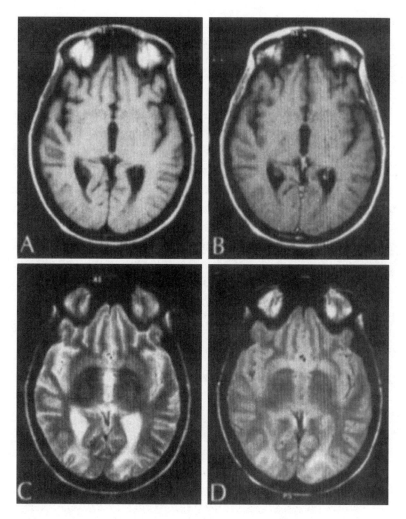

Fig. 1. Axial MR images of patient with erythropoietin-associated hypertensive encephalopathy showing unremarkable T1-weighted images before and after gadolinium **(A,B),** and occipital hyperintensity signal changes on T2-weighted **(C)** and proton-density **(D)** images, consistent with hypertensive posterior leukoencephalopathy.

best appreciated on T_2-weighted images, frequently involve other posterior structures such as the cerebellum and brainstem, may involve the cortex, and also sometimes may be seen more anteriorly in the temporal and frontal regions. Although the imaging changes are usually bilateral, they are often asymmetric. Posterior cerebral changes also may be seen on computerized tomography (CT) scanning in some patients. Recent studies using diffusion-weighted MRI indicate that the leukoencephalopathy is primarily a result of vasogenic rather than cytotoxic edema *(33,34)*. In one patient, magnetic resonance spectroscopy (MRS) has demonstrated a reduced ratio of occipital *N*-acetyl-aspartate (NAA) to creatine, thus indicating neuronal dysfunction

(35). The reason for the anatomical predilection to the parieto-occipital areas is not clear, although it may be the result of a relative paucity of vascular sympathetic (and thus protective) innervation of the vessels of the posterior circulation arising from the basilar artery *(36,37).* Hypertensive encephalopathy predominantly affecting the brainstem has also been reported *(38,39).* In parallel with the imaging findings, the electroencephalogram (EEG) may show loss of the posterior dominant alpha rhythm, generalized slowing, and posterior epileptiform discharges, which resolve following clinical improvement *(25,27,28).* Because hypertensive encephalopathy and its clinical and neuroimaging consequences are potentially fully reversible with timely and appropriate management, the recent popular label of hypertensive reversible posterior leukoencephalopathy syndrome (PLS) has ensued *(24,40,41).* This syndrome is a clinicoradiological diagnosis that is seen in both adults and children and has both hypertensive and nonhypertensive causes. PLS is not always fully reversible *(42),* emphasizing that awareness of the syndrome and institution of prompt management is vital in preventing permanent sequelae.

Nonhypertension-Associated Posterior Leukoencephalopathy

Nonhypertensive causes and associations of PLS include immunosuppressive and cytotoxic therapy (cyclosporine, tacrolimus [FK-506], cisplatin) *(24,25,43–46),* interferon-α *(24),* acquired immunodeficiency syndrome (AIDS) *(47),* TTP *(27),* postblood transfusion *(48),* and postcarotid endarterectomy hyperperfusion syndrome *(49,50).* However, some of the patients reported with these latter conditions also had acutely elevated blood pressure, e.g., patients treated with cyclosporine and tacrolimus *(24,25).* It is likely that in some patients, the etiology of PLS (and its underlying endothelial disturbance) is multifactorial, e.g., cyclosporine neurotoxicity and hypertension occurring following renal transplantation, and TTP, acute renal failure, and associated hypertension *(27).* Cyclosporine-associated PLS is usually associated with high drug levels, although levels may be within the therapeutic range *(51).* There is an associated hypocholesterolemia and/or hypomagnesemia in over half of the patients. Symptoms usually began on average after about 14 d of initiating therapy, and withdrawal or reduction of cyclosporine as well as management of associated hypertension leads to resolution of clinical symptoms and neuroimaging abnormalities within weeks. In a review of 50 patients with immunosuppressive-associated leukoencephalopathy, 31 occurred in liver, 8 in renal, 6 in lung, and 5 in heart transplant recipients, with median time to onset of 28 d *(52).* In this study, seizures occurred in 74% of patients, with altered mental status (50%) and visual disturbance (28%) being the other most common presenting symptoms. Resolution of the clinical features occurred at a median of 4 d, and imaging abnormalities at a median of 20 d on reduction or cessation of the offending drug.

Management

The management of hypertensive encephalopathy includes early recognition, withdrawal of exacerbating factors (e.g., erythropoietin), individualized antihypertensive drug treatment as for other hypertensive emergencies, and appropriate (and usually short-term) parenteral anticonvulsant treatment with either phenytoin or fosphenytoin, benzodiazepines, or barbiturates, or a combination of these drugs *(2,23)*. Although not evidence based, the use of anticonvulsant therapy in patients with hypertensive encephalopathy who are seizing is reasonable and will itself often help to lower blood pressure. In patients presenting with hypertensive encephalopathy, mean arterial pressure should be reduced by approx. 20% or to a diastolic blood pressure of 100 mmHg, whichever value is greater, within the first hour. Particular caution is necessary in the elderly or in those with preexisting hypertension in whom overaggressive reduction in blood pressure may be accompanied by worsening neurological status and even stroke. In these circumstances infusion of antihypertensive drugs should be discontinued or recommenced later at a lower dose.

Suitable agents in the management of hypertensive encephalopathy include sodium nitroprusside, labetalol, enalapril, and hydralazine. Clonidine should be avoided as it is a central nervous system depressant. Patients with elevated blood pressure and other risk factors for posterior leukoencephalopathy, such as immunosuppressive therapy or TTP, should be treated vigorously and carefully, as these patients may develop posterior autoregulatory failure at blood pressure levels lower than those classically associated with florid hypertensive encephalopathy.

In addition to delivery of the baby and placenta, parenteral magnesium is the treatment of choice to prevent the evolution of pre-eclampsia to eclampsia (seizures and worsening encephalopathy) *(53,54)*. There is also long-standing experience with a number of suitable antihypertensive drugs. The parenteral antihypertensive drugs used most commonly during pregnancy are hydralazine and labetalol. Hydralazine may lead to a reflex tachycardia that may require concomitant β-blockade. ACE inhibitors and angiotensin-receptor antagonists are contraindicated in pregnancy.

References

1. Hiyoshi T, Yagi K. Epilepsy in the elderly. *Epilepsia* 2000;41(Suppl 9):31–35.
2. Vaughan CJ, Delanty N. Hypertensive emergencies. *Lancet* 2000;356:411–417.
3. He J, Whelton PK. Epidemiology and prevention of hypertension. *Med Clin N Am* 1997;81:1077–1097.

4. Cooper R, Rotini C. Hypertension in blacks. *Am J Hypertens* 1997;7:804–812.

5. Bennett NM, Shea S. Hypertensive emergency: case criteria, sociodemographic profile, and previous care of 100 cases. *Am J Public Health* 1988;78:636–640.

6. Hesdorffer DC, Hauser WA, Annegers JF, Rocca WA. Severe, uncontrolled hypertension and adult-onset seizures: a case-control study in Rochester, Minnesota. *Epilepsia* 1996;37:736–741.

7. Ng SKC, Hauser WA, Brust JCM, Susser M. Hypertension and the risk of new onset unprovoked seizures. *Neurology* 1993;43:425–428.

8. Shapiro IM, Neufeld MY, Korczyn AD, Seizures of unknown origin after the age of 50: vascular risk factors. *Acta Neurol Scand* 1990;82:78–80.

9. Kawamoto A, Shimada K, Matsubayashi K, Nishinaga M, Kimura S, Ozawa T. Factors associated with silent multiple lacunar lesions on magnetic resonance imaging in asymptomatic elderly hypertensive patients. *Clin Exp Pharmacol Physiol* 1991; 18:605–610.

10. Furchgott RF, Zawadzky JV. The obligatory role of endothelial cells in the relaxation of arterial smooth muscle by acetylcholine. *Nature* 1980;288:373–376.

11. Kuchan MJ, Jo H, Frangos JA. Role of G proteins in shear stress-mediated nitric oxide production by endothelial cells. *Am J Physiol* 1994;267:C753–C758.

12. Mullins JJ, Peters J, Ganten D. Fulminant hypertension in transgenic rats harbouring the mouse Ren-2 gene. *Nature* 1990;344:541–544.

13. Ganten D, Wagner J, Zeh K, et al. Species specificity of renin kinetics in transgenic rats harboring the human renin and angiotensinogen genes. *Proc Natl Acad Sci* 1992;89:7806–7810.

14. Funakoshi Y, Ichiki T, Ito K, Takeshita A. Induction of interleukin-6 expression by angiotensin II in rat vascular smooth muscle cells. *Hypertension* 1999;34:118–125.

15. Muller DN, Dechend R, Mervaala EM, et al. NF-κB inhibition ameliorates angiotensin II-induced inflammatory damage in rats. *Hypertension* 2000; 35:193–201.

16. Montgomery HE, Kiernan LA, Whitworth CE, Fleming S, Unger T, Gohlke P, Mullins JJ, McEwan JR. Inhibition of tissue angiotensin converting enzyme activity prevents malignant hypertension in TGR (mREN2)27. *J Hypertens* 1998; 16:635–643.

17. Okada M, Matsumori A, Ono K, Furukawa Y, Shioi T, Iwasaki A, Matsushima K, Sasayama S. Cyclic stretch upregulates production of interleukin-8 and monocyte chemotactic and activating factor/monocyte chemoattractant protein-1 in human endothelial cells. *Arterioscler Thromb Vasc Biol* 1998;18:894–901.

18. Wung BS, Cheng JJ, Chao YJ, Lin J, Shyy YJ, Wang DL. Cyclic strain increases monocyte chemotactic protein-1 secretion in human endothelial cells. *Am J Physiol* 1996;270:H1462–H1468.

19. Naruse K, Sokabe M. Involvement of stretch-activated ion channels in Ca^{++} mobilization to mechanical stretch in endothelial cells. *Am J Physiol* 1993; 264:C1037–C1044.

20. MacArthur H, Warner TD, Wood EG, Corder R, Vane JR. Endothelin-1 release from endothelial cells in culture is elevated both acutely and chronically by short periods of mechanical stretch. *Biochem Biophys Res Commun* 1994;200:395–400.

21. Verhaar MC, Beutler JJ, Gaillard CA, Koomans HA, Fijnheer R, Rabelink TJ. Progressive vascular damage in hypertension is associated with increased levels of circulating P-selectin. *J Hypertens* 1998;16:45–50.

22. Bakshi R, Bates VE, Mechtler LL, Kinkel PR, Kinkel WR. Occipital lobe seizures as the major clinical manifestation of reversible posterior leukoencephalopathy syndrome: magnetic resonance imaging findings. *Epilepsia* 1998;39:295–299.

23. Delanty N, Vaughan CJ, French JA. Medical causes of seizures. *Lancet* 1998;352:383–390.

24. Hinchey J, Chaves C, Appignani B, et al. A reversible posterior leukoencephalopathy syndrome. *N Engl J Med* 1996;334:494–500.

25. Torocsik HV, Curless RG, Post J, Tzakis AG, Pearse L. FK506-induced leukoencephalopthy in children with organ transplants. *Neurology* 1999;52:1497–1500.

26. Delanty N, Vaughan C, Frucht S, Stubgen P. Erythropoietin-associated hypertensive posterior leukoencephalopathy. *Neurology* 1997;49:686–689.

27. Bakshi R, Shaikh ZA, Bates VE, Kinkel PR. Thrombotic thrombocytopenic purpura: brain CT and MRI findings in 12 patients. *Neurology* 1999;52:1285–1288.

28. Manfredi M, Beltramello A, Bongiovanni LG, Polo A, Pistoia L, Rizzuto N. Eclamptic encephalopathy: imaging and pathogenetic considerations. *Acta Neurol Scand* 1997;96:277–282.

29. Katz VL, Farmer R, Kuller JA. Preeclampsia into eclampsia: toward a new paradigm. *Am J Obstet Gynecol* 2000;182:1389–1396.

30. Veltkamp R, Kupsch A, Polasek J, Youry TA, Pfister HW. Late onset postpartum eclampsia without pre-eclamptic prodromi: clinical and neuroradiological presentation in two patients. *J Neurol Neurosurg Psychiatry* 2000;69:824–827.

31. Feske SK, Sperling RA, Schwartz RB. Extensive reversible brain magnetic resonance lesions in a patient with HELLP syndrome. *J Neuroimaging* 1997;7:247–250.

32. Schwartz RB, Jones KM, Kalina P, et al. Hypertensive encephalopathy: findings on CT, MR imaging and SPECT imaging in 14 cases. *AJR Am J Roentgenol* 1992;159:379–383.

33. Schaeffer PW, Buonanno FS, Gonzalez RJ, Schwamm LH. Diffusion weighted imaging discriminated between cytotoxic and vasogenic edema in a patient with eclampsia. *Stroke* 1997;28:1082–1085.

34. Schwartz RB, Mulkern RV, Gudbjartsson H, Jolesz F. Diffusion-weighted MR imaging in hypertensive encephalopathy: clues to pathogenesis. *AJNR Am J Neuroradiol* 1998;19:859–862.

35. Pavlakis SG, Frank Y, Kalina P, et al. Occipital-parietal encephalopathy: a new name for an old syndrome. *Pediatr Neurol* 1997;16:145–148.

36. Beausang-Linder M, Bill A. Cerebral circulation in acute arterial hypertension: protective effects of sympathetic nervous activity. *Acta Physiol Scand* 1981; 111:193–199.

37. Edvinson L, Owman C, Sjoberg N-O. Autonomic nerves, mast cells, and amine receptors in human brain vessels; histochemical and pharmacologic studies. *Brain Res* 1976;115:377–393.

38. Wang MC, Escott EJ, Breeze RE. Posterior fossa swelling and hydrocephalus resulting from hypertensive encephalopathy: case report and review of the literature. *Neurosurgery* 1999;44:1325–1327.

39. Chang GY, Keane JR. Hypertensive brainstem encephalopathy: three cases presenting with severe brainstem edema. *Neurology* 1999;53:652–654.

40. Hauser RA, Lacey DM, Knight MR. Hypertensive encephalopthy: magnetic resonance imaging demonstration of reversible cortical and white matter lesions. *Arch Neurol* 1988;45:1078–1083.

41. Pavlakis SG, Frank Y, Chusid R. Hypertensive encephalopathy, reversible occipitoparietal encephalopathy, or reversible posterior leukoencephalopathy: three names for an old syndrome. *J Child Neurol* 1999;14:277–281.
42. Antunes NL, Small TN, George D, Boulad F, Lis E. Posterior leukoencephalopathy syndrome may not be reversible. *Pediatr Neurol* 1999;20:241–243.
43. Gleeson JG, duPlessis AJ, Barnes PD, Rivello JJ Jr. Cyclosporin A acute encephalopathy and seizure syndrome in childhood: clinical features and risk of seizure recurrence. *J Child Neurol* 1998;13:336–344.
44. Ito Y, Arahata Y, Goto Y, et al. Cisplatin neurotoxicity presenting as reversible posterior leukoencephalopathy syndrome. *AJNR Am J Neuroradiol* 1998;19:415–417.
45. Schwartz RB, Bravo SM, Klufas RA, et al. Cyclosporine neurotoxicity and its relationship to hypertensive encephalopathy: CT and MR findings in 16 cases. *AJR Am J Roentgenol* 1995;165:627–631.
46. Small SL, Fukui MB, Bramblett GT, Eidelman BH. Immunosuppression induced leukoencephalopathy from tacrolimus (FK506). *Ann Neurol* 1996;40:575–580.
47. Frank Y, Pavlakis S, Black K, Bakshi S. Reversible occipital-parietal encephalopathy syndrome in an HIV-infected child. *Neurology* 1998;51;915–916.
48. Ito Y, Niwa H, Iida T, et al. Post-transfusion reversible posterior leukoencephalopathy syndrome with cerebral vasoconstriction. *Neurology* 1997;49:1174–1175.
49. Baptista MV, Maeder P, Dewarrat A, Bogousslavasky J. Conflicting images. *Lancet* 1998;351:414.
50. Dimakakos PB, Tsiligiris V, Gouliamos A, Kotsis TE, Katsaros G. Postcarotid endarectomy symptoms. Pre- and postoperative clinical and MRI findings. *Int Angiol* 1999;18:277–286.
51. Gijtenbeck JMM, van den Bent MJ, Vecht ChJ. Cyclosporine neurotoxicity: a review. *J Neurol* 1999;246:339–346.
52. Singh N, Bonham A, Fukui M. Immunosuppressive-associated leukoencephalopthy in organ transplant recipients. *Transplantation* 2000;69:467–472.
53. Lucas MJ, Leveno KJ, Cunningham FG. A comparison of magnesium sulfate with phenytoin for the prevention of eclampsia. *N Engl J Med* 1995;333:201–205.
54. Thomas SV. Neurological aspects of eclampsia. *J Neurol Sci* 1998;155:37–43.

16

Seizures Following Organ Transplantation

Jane Boggs, MD

Introduction

Seizures are common in transplant recipients but may also occur during the pretransplant screening and evaluation period because of underlying disease. Seizures are not considered a contraindication to transplantation but unfortunately are not routinely screened for, either by specific history or electroencephalogram (EEG). Knowledge that a patient has a lowered threshold for seizures before transplant could allow treatment to reduce the risk of seizures in the perioperative period. Care should be taken, however, to avoid further organ dysfunction while a patient waits for availability of a donor organ. This interval prior to transplantation may be the optimal time to reevaluate prior diagnosis of epilepsy by video–EEG monitoring or to consider revising antiepileptic drug (AED) therapy to reduce the likelihood of interactions with immunosuppressants and antibiotics following transplant. Epileptic donors are not excluded unless seizures are related to a disease that affects the viability of the donated organ.

Following transplantation, seizures result from toxic effects of immunosuppressant medication or infections secondary to immunosuppression. Transplant recipients are at significantly increased risk for central nervous system (CNS) and systemic infections or neoplasms, all of which can lower the threshold for seizures significantly. In new-onset seizures posttransplantation, a diligent search for localized neurologic infection or neoplasia must be conducted, especially if seizures have focal symptoms. A minimal diagnostic evaluation of such patients should include magnetic resonance imagery (MRI) using high-resolution sequences, usually pre- and postcontrast, as well as a carefully performed EEG with appropriately selected activation procedures.

Perioperative complications, as well as rejection, also can be a cause of

From: *Seizures: Medical Causes and Management*
Edited by: N. Delanty © Humana Press, Inc., Totowa, NJ

Table 1
Incidence of Seizures After Transplantation

Organ	Incidence of Seizures (%)	References
Kidney	1.5–67	*2,3*
Heart/heart–lung	15–40	*4–6*
Pancreas	13	*7*
Bone marrow	10	*8*
Liver	16–36	*9–11*

seizures. Overall, children are more susceptible to posttransplant seizures than are adults *(1)*. Some series have found that the incidence of seizures also varies by organ transplanted **(Table 1)**. As psychiatric complications of immunosuppression are common, consideration must also be given to the possibility of nonepileptic events. Distinguishing these events from true seizures is critical in the optimal management of transplant recipients to avoid complicating immunosuppressants therapy with interactions by AEDs.

This chapter will discuss the reported incidence, typical precipitants, and management of seizures in patients who have undergone liver, kidney, heart and lung, bone marrow, and pancreas transplants.

Liver Transplantation

Liver transplantation is considered in patients with irreversible and progressive liver dysfunction for which no alternative therapy is available. It is rarely performed over age 70 or with coexistent active alcohol or drug abuse. Allograft donors are matched for ABO blood compatibility and liver size, and should test negative for human immunodeficiency virus (HIV), and hepatitis B and C.

Following transplant, immunosuppression is usually accomplished by combinations of tacrolimus (FK-506) or cyclosporine (CsA), steroids, azathioprine, or OKT3 (monoclonal antithymocyte globulin). Posttransplantation complications include liver dysfunction from primary nonfunction, acute or chronic rejection, ischemia, hepatic artery thrombosis, and biliary obstruction or leak. Neurologic complications associated with seizures include cerebral hemorrhage and infarction, central pontine myelinolysis, basal ganglia demyelination, and encephalopathy. Bacterial, viral, fungal, and other opportunistic CNS and systemic infections may also occur, as well as renal disorders *(12)*. All of these disorders can result in altered mental status mimicking seizures, as well as seizures themselves. The possibility of psychiatric disorders, including nonepileptic events should be investigated by video–EEG monitoring.

Seizures have been found to occur in up to 16–36% of all liver transplant recipients *(9–11)*. Generalized tonic-clonic seizures are reported most commonly, and most patients have recurrent seizures within the first weeks after onset. Treatable metabolic causes may serve as precipitants of seizures posttransplantation and, once reversed, should not require chronic AED therapy. Hypoglycemia, hyponatremia, hypomagnesemia, hyperkalemia, and hypocalcemia are not uncommon. Nonketotic hyperosmolar hyperglycemia can occur through use of steroids or efforts to prevent hypoglycemia, and is more likely to occur with brief hepatic ischemia perioperatively *(13)*. As many of these electrolyte disturbances can result in altered levels of consciousness, an EEG can be useful in distinguishing encephalopathic behavior from subclinical seizures, as well as monitoring response to treatment *(14)*.

CsA has been strongly associated with a risk for seizures in liver and other transplant patients *(15)*. One series revealed that only 61% of liver transplant patients with seizures had elevated trough levels of CsA, but by decreasing the dose, neurotoxicity reversed even in patients with usually therapeutic levels. Substitution of CsA with FK-506 did not result in further seizures, suggesting this latter drug may have lower neurotoxicity in susceptible patients. A significant risk of seizure recurrence has been found in children with persistent EEG abnormalities after documented CsA encephalopathy *(3)*. Neoral, a newer formulation of oral CsA appears to have lower risk of seizures than older formulations do *(16)*. High-dose methylprednisolone appears to potentiate the risk of seizures in liver transplants receiving CsA *(17)*. Enzyme-inducing AEDs such as carbamazepine, phenytoin, and barbiturates will decrease CsA levels, resulting in impaired immunosuppression and a higher risk of rejection. Although valproic acid has minimal potential for interaction with CsA and therefore may be considered for use in transplant recipients in general, the high rate of hepatotoxicity in children under 2 yr is of concern, specifically in liver transplants. With an increasing selection of well-tolerated, nonenzyme-inducing AEDs (e.g., gabapentin, oxcarbazepine, levetiracetam), it is logical to consider newer AEDs if needed to control seizures in such patients. In cases of treatable metabolic derangements, short-term symptomatic use of benzodiazepines is appropriate.

Low serum cholesterol may be associated with a CsA syndrome of confusion, cortical blindness, and leukoencephalopathy on MRI *(18)*, which has been associated with a 25% risk of seizures. EEGs are typically abnormal with generalized or focal slowing but may not show epileptiform abnormalities unless actual seizures occur during the procedure.

There is a high risk of bacterial, viral, fungal, and opportunistic infections in all transplant patients. Although generalized seizures may be the result of any infection, focal onset seizures suggest localized CNS infection, especially when occurring between 1 and 6 mo after surgery. Evidence of partial seizure in a transplant patient should be evaluated promptly and carefully by high-resolution neuroimaging. Infection-related seizures have been noted most frequently in liver transplant patients with *Aspergillus* brain abscess and in *Listeria* meningoencephalitis *(19)*. Numerous opportunistic infections have been reported to cause seizures as well.

Kidney Transplantation

Renal transplantation is the treatment of choice for most patients with end-stage renal disease. It is usually contraindicated in active glumerulonephritis, infection, or malignancy, HIV, or hepatitis B, and relatively contraindicated in comorbid disease, in patients >70 yr, and in severe psychiatric disease.

Seizures attributable to cerebral infarction are less common following renal transplantation than after heart or liver transplantion *(20)*. CNS infection with *Listeria monocytogenes (21)*, fungi (especially *Aspergillus*) *(2)*, herpes simplex, and cytomegalovirus *(22)* are common causes of seizures. Cerebral neoplasia, typically lymphoma or sarcoma, may occur following renal transplantation but only occasionally present as either partial or generalized tonic-clonic seizures *(23)*. As in liver transplant patients, nonketotic hyperosmolar state and metabolic derangements can precipitate seizures. Use of high-dose steroids to treat acute rejection may alter glucose regulation and provoke such symptomatic seizures.

The incidence of seizures is higher before kidney transplantation but similar posttransplantation to other organ recipients. Seizures commonly occur pretransplantation as part of renal failure and dialysis, and on some occasions may be attributed incorrectly to symptoms of organ failure rather than epilepsy. Generalized tonic-clonic seizures have been reported in up to 86% and partial seizures in 57% of patients *(24)*. As nearly the entire latter group had abnormal EEGs, with half showing paroxysmal spike activity, it is especially important to evaluate all pretransplantation partial seizures by EEG and neuroimaging to identify the etiology and any ongoing risk of recurrence following transplantation. Posttransplantation series have documented a seizure incidence of 1.5% in adults *(25)* to 67% in children (2–16 yr) *(22)*. In infants with end-stage renal disease, however, over 80% of those who had seizures pretransplantation remained seizure-free 1 yr following renal transplantation without AEDs *(26)*.

A syndrome of rejection encephalopathy has been described in renal transplant recipients *(27)*. This syndrome consists of headache, focal neurologic signs, papilledema, altered mental status, and generalized tonic-clonic seizures occurring in about 6% of renal transplant patients. Other signs of acute organ rejection include fever, swelling, oliguria, hypertension, and graft tenderness. Metabolic parameters were similar to those of patients experiencing rejection without encephalopathy. EEGs usually were nonspecifically slow, but 25% had focal, potentially ictal, or interictal abnormalities. Although the generalized slow patterns improve with time, focal abnormalities often persist for months to years, raising controversy about discontinuing AEDs. Similar precaution should be used in selecting AEDs in all transplant patients treated with CsA. For patients in whom renal dysfunction persists or recurs with rejection, increased dosing interval and lower AED doses are appropriate, especially with medications exhibiting primarily renal elimination (e.g., gabapentin, oxcarbazepine, topiramate).

Rejection may be treated prophylactically or acutely with OKT3, a monoclonal CD3 antibody. A neurologic syndrome following this treatment includes seizures, lethargy, and altered mental status with patchy contrast-enhancing cerebral lesions seen on MRI *(28)*. Early use of OKT3 appears to be more likely to precipitate seizures, especially with uremia posttransplantation *(29)*. FK-506 has rarely been associated with seizures in renal transplant recipients *(4)*.

Heart and Heart–Lung Transplantation

Cardiac transplantation is indicated for progressive, terminal ischemic and idiopathic cardiomyopathies. Because patients with cardiac disease are at high risk for cerebral ischemia, perioperative risk for central neurologic sequelae is high. Immunosuppression also imposes similar neurologic risk to that of other transplanted organs, although lower doses of postoperative methylprednisolone are usually used in heart–lung recipients to expedite tracheal healing, with some reduction in seizure risk.

The incidence of seizures following cardiac transplantation is highest in the perioperative period and is typically the result of cerebral infarction. Seizures have been reported in up to 15% of adult cardiac transplants, with approximately half attributable to stroke *(5)*. In children, more than 40% of cyclosporine-treated cardiac transplant recipients had seizures, with half associated with rejection *(6)*. Cystic fibrosis and other primary lung failure patients may be treated by isolated lung transplantation, with a reported risk of seizures in 22% *(30)*. Isolated pediatric lung transplants have been associated with up to 27% risk of seizures *(31)*.

Although some investigators have suggested that long-term AED therapy may not be necessary in cardiac transplant patients with seizures, these recommendations were made largely with regard to the older, hepatic enzyme-inducing AEDs. Such medications decrease the blood levels of cyclosporine, making rejection more likely. Many of these medications also harbor significant risk for cardiac conduction abnormality and thus impose risk to the transplanted organ. Use of nonenzyme-inducing AEDs with a more favorable cardiac profile (e.g., valproic acid, gabapentin, etc.) may entail less risk of long-term complications to the patient than seizures would.

In addition to the direct risk of immunosuppressants, cardiac transplant recipients often later develop opportunistic infections that predispose to seizures. Focal necrotizing meningoencephalitis is caused most commonly by *Aspergillus,* which may be associated with hemorrhagic infarction and vascular thrombosis *(32).* This infection is usually the result of disseminated pulmonary infection and is suggested by increased signal intensity on both T1 and T2 MRI images, with evidence of rapid progression and hemorrhage. Confirmation by needle aspiration or biopsy should be performed urgently, as this infection is fatal if treatment is not instituted early. *Toxoplasma gondii* is the second most likely intracranial infection following cardiac transplantation and may be associated with chorioretinitis, myocarditis, and pneumonitis. As some patients may have reactivation of latent infection, comparison of sera with baseline values pretransplantation is imperative in avoiding misdiagnosis *(33).* Less commonly, cerebral abscesses are attributable to *Candida albicans, Nocardia asteroides, Klebsiella,* and phycomycoses including *Mucor.* Meningitides occur commonly with *Cryptococcus* and less frequently with *Coccidiodes immitis* and *Pseudoallescheria boydii (7).*

Altered mental status, including psychosis, may develop postoperatively and may be a subtle manifestation of subclinical seizures. An EEG recorded during symptoms is usually diagnostic but may require a prolonged or repeated study to evaluate cerebral rhythms as mentation waxes and wanes. In general, late psychosis is more suggestive of intracranial infection, whereas cognitive symptoms in the first 2 wk after transplant are often multifactorial. In either case, a thorough search for possible organic cause must be performed.

OKT3 has been described to cause aseptic meningitis with fever, headache, and seizures in 5% of cardiac transplant patients. These symptoms may occur during, or weeks after, exposure to this medication *(34).*

Bone Marrow Transplantation

Bone marrow transplantation is an important treatment for aplastic anemia, hematologic malignancies, and genetic immunologic deficiency diseases. It also allows treatment with otherwise fatal doses of chemotherapy in solid tumors and replacement of abnormal marrow in metabolic storage diseases. Conditioning regimens of myelotoxic irradiation and chemotherapy are administered prior to transplantation to reduce the risk of graft-versus-host disease (GVHD). GVHD manifests as rash, hepatic dysfunction, diarrhea, and abdominal pain and is the result of a donor lymphocytic reaction to non-HLA (human leukocyte antigen) host antigens. Bone marrow transplantation attempted with mismatched or unrelated donors has been found to have a higher risk of all neurologic complications, including seizures *(8).*

Seizures have been reported in 10% of bone marrow transplant recipients *(35).* The majority of seizures are associated with metabolic abnormalities and are most commonly generalized. Thrombocytopenia can precipitate cerebral hemorrhage and seizures and may be the result of either the underlying disease for which the transplantation was performed or of pretransplant conditioning regimens. Sinus venous thrombosis *(36)* or thromboembolic cardiogenic infarctions occur commonly and can also result in seizures *(37)*. Infections, as in other types of transplant, can also present with seizures.

Conditioning regimens that contain high-dose busulfan have been associated with isolated seizures within 96 h of initiation of dose *(38)*. As these patients did not have recurrent seizures, they were not maintained on AEDs. Cyclosporine neurotoxicity, with probable intracranial microhemorrhages coalescing into macrohemorrhages, has been reported as a cause of seizures in bone marrow recipients *(39)*.

In the selection of AEDs in patients who have undergone bone marrow transplantation, not only interactions with immunosuppressants but also risk for aplastic anemia must be taken into consideration. As many older generation AEDs have been associated with idiosyncratic aplastic anemia, it is reasonable to consider alternative newer medications. Because of its high risk of aplastic anemia, Felbamate should be avoided. As dose-related minimal thrombocytopenia is possible with the use of valproic acid, alternatives to this AED should be considered if platelet counts fall.

Pancreas Transplantation

Although pancreatic transplantation is an effective means of normalizing insulin secretion in refractory diabetics, the risks of surgery and long-term immunosuppression restricts this treatment to relatively few patients with multiple complications of diabetes mellitus. Renal, cardiac, and cerebrovascular disease is commonly encountered as part of end-stage diabetes prior to transplantation. Surprisingly, seizures have been reported in only 13% of transplant recipients *(40)*. Immunosuppression, infectious, and metabolic complications appear to occur in this transplant population in similar proportions to other organ recipients.

References

1. Gilmore RL. Seizures and antiepileptic drug use in transplant patients. *Neurol Clin* 1988;6:279–296.
2. Rifkind D, Marchioro TL, Schneck SA, Hill RB. Systemic fungal infectious complicating renal transplantation and immunosuppressive therapy. *Am J Med* 1967;43:28–38.
3. Gleeson JG, duPleiss AJ, Barnes PD, Riviello JJ. Cyclosporin A acute encephalopathy and seizure syndrome in childhood: clinical features and risk of seizure recurrence. *J Child Neurol* 1998;13:336–344.

4. Neu AM, Furth SL, Case BW, Wise B, Colombani PM, Fivush BA. Evaluation of neurotoxicity in pediatric renal transplant recipients treated with tacrolimus (FK506). *Clin Transplant* 1997;11:412–414.

5. Grigg MM, Costanzo-Nordin MR, Celesia GG, et al. The etiology of seizures after cardiac transplantation. *Transplant Proc* 1988;20(Suppl 3):937–944.

6. Fricker FJ, Bartley PG, Hardesty RL, et al. Experience with heart transplantation in children. *Pediatrics* 1987;79:138–146.

7. Hotson JR, Enzmann DR. Neurologic complications of cardiac transplantation. *Neurol Clin* 1988;6:349–365.

8. De Brabander C, Cornelissen J, Smitt PA, Vecht CJ, van den Bent MJ. Increased incidence of neurological complications in patients receiving allogenic bone marrow transplantation from alternative donors. *J Neurol Neurosurg Psychiatry* 2000; 68:36–80.

9. Adams HP, Ponsford S, Gunson B, et al. Neurological complications following liver transplantation. *Lancet* 1987;1:949–951.

10. Grant D, Wall W, Duff J, et al. Adverse effects of cyclosporine therapy following liver transplantation. *Transplant Proc* 1987;19:3463–3465.

11. Martinez AJ, Conrado E, Faris AA. Neurologic complications of liver transplantation. *Neurol Clin* 6:327–348.

12. Dienstag, JL. Liver transplantation In: *Harrison's Principle's of Internal Medicine,* 14th ed., Fauci AS, Braunwald E, Isselbacher KJ, et al. (eds.), New York: McGraw-Hill, 1998, Chapter 301.

13. Lampe EW Simmons RL, Najarian JS. Hyperglycemic nonketotic coma after liver transplantation. *Arch Surg* 1972;105:774–776.

14. Steg RE, Wszolek ZK. Electroencephalographic abnormalities in liver transplant recipients:practical considerations and review. *J Clin Neurophysiol* 1996;13:60–68.

15. Wijdicks EF, Wiesner RH, Krom RA. Neurotoxicity in liver transplant recipients with cyclosporine immunosuppression. *Neurology* 1995;45:1962–1964.

16. Wijdicks EF, Dahlke LJ, Wiesner RH, Oral cyclosporine decreases severity of neurotoxicity in liver transplant recipients. *Neurology* 1999;2:1708–1710.

17. Boogaerts MA, Zachee P, Verwilghen RL. Cyclosporine, methylprednisolone and convulsions. *Lancet* 1982;2:1216–1217.

18. De Groen PC, Aksamit AJ, Rakela J, Forbes GS, Krom RA. Central nervous system toxicity after liver transplantation: the role of cyclosporine and cholesterol. *N Engl J Med* 1987;317:861–866.

19. Hooper DC, Pruitt AA, Rubin RH. Central nervous system infection in the chronically immunosuppressed. *Medicine* 1982;61:166–188.

20. Adams HP, Dawson G, Coffman TJ, Corry RJ. Stroke in renal transplant recipients. *Arch Neurol* 1986;43:113–115.

21. Nicklasson PM, Hambraeus A, Lundgren G, Magnusson G, Sundelin P, Groth CG. Listeria encephalitis in five renal transplant recipients. *Acta Med Scand* 1978;203:181–185.

22. Kahan BD, Flechner SM, Lorber MI, Golden D, Conley S, Van Buren CT. Complications of cyclosporin-prednisone immunosuppression in 402 renal allograft recipients exclusively followed at a single center for from one to five years. *Transplantation* 1987;43:197–204.

23. Schneck SA, Penn I. Cerebral neoplasms associated with renal transplantation. *Arch Neurol* 1970;22:226–233.

24. O'Hare SA, Callaghan NM, Murnaghan DJ. Dialysis encephalopathy: medical, electroencephalographic and interventional aspects. *Medicine* 1983;62:129–141.

25. Nordal KP, Talseth T, Dahl E, Attramadal A, Albrechtsen D, Halse J, Brodwall EK, Flatmark A. Aluminum overload, a predisposing condition for epileptic seizures in renal transplant patients treated with cyclosporin? *Lancet* 1985;2:153, 154.

26. So SKS, Chang P, Najarian JS, Mauer SM, Simmons RL, Nevins TE. Growth and development in infants after renal transplantation. *J Pediatr* 1987;110:343–350.

27. Gross MLP, Sweny P, Pearson RM Kennedy J, Fernando ON, Moorhead JF. Rejection encephalopathy: an acute neurological syndrome complicating renal transplantation. *J Neurol Sci* 1982;56:23–34.

28. Parizel PM, Snoeck HW, van den Hauwe L, et al. Cerebral complications of murine monoclonal CD3 antibody (OKT3): CT and MRI findings. *AJNR* 1997; 18:1935–1938.

29. Seifeldin RA, Lawrence KR, Rahamtulla AF, Monaco AP. Generalized seizures associated with the use of muromonab-CD3 in two patients after kidney transplantation. *Ann Pharmacother* 1997;31:586–589.

30. Vaughn BV, Ali II, Olivier KN, Robertson KR, Messenheimer JA, Paradowski LJ, Egan TM. Seizures in lung transplant recipients *Epilepsia* 1996;37:1175–1179.

31. Wong M, Mallory GB, Goldstein J, Goyal M, Yamada KA. Neurologic complications of pediatric lung transplantation. *Neurology* 1999;53:1542–1549.

32. Britt RH, Enzmann DR, Remington JS. Intracranial infections in cardiac transplant recipients. *Ann Neurol* 1981;9:107–119.

33. Luft BJ, Naot Y, Araujo FG, Stinson EB, Remington JS. Primary and reactivated toxoplasma infection in patients with cardiac transplants. *Ann Int Med* 1983;99:27–31.

34. Adair JC, Woodley SL, O'Connell JB, Call GK, Baringer JR. Aseptic meningitis following cardiac transplantation: clinical characteristics and relationship to immunosuppressive regimen. *Neurology* 1991;41:249–252.

35. Patchell RA, Chite III CL, Clark AW, Beschomer WE, Santos GW. Neurologic complications of bone marrow transplantation. *Neurology* 1985;35:300–306.

36. Bertz H, Laubenberger J, Steinfurth G, Finke J. Sinus venous thrombosis: an unusual cause for neurologic symptoms after bone marrow transplantation under immunosuppression. *Transplantation* 1998;66:241–244.

37. Patchell RA, Chite CL III, Clark AW, Beschomer WE, Santos GW. Nonbacterial thrombotic endocarditis in bone marrow transplant patients. *Cancer* 1985; 55:631–635.

38. Marcus RE, Goldman JM. Convulsions due to high-dose busulfan. *Lancet* 1984;2:1463.

39. Shah AK. Cyclosporine A neurotoxicity among bone marrow transplant recipients. *Clin Neuropharmacol* 1999;22:67–73.

40. Kiok MC. Neurologic complications of pancreas transplants. *Neurol Clin* 1988;6:367–376.

17

Seizures and Syncope

Suneet Mittal, MD, and Bruce B. Lerman, MD

Introduction

Syncope, defined as an abrupt loss of consciousness and postural tone caused by cerebral hypoperfusion with spontaneous recovery, is a common clinical problem, accounting for 3% of emergency room visits and 6% of general hospital admissions in the United States *(1)*. A subset of these patients (up to 12%) have an associated convulsive reaction, which may be difficult to differentiate from epilepsy *(2)*. This entity has been designated convulsive syncope. It is estimated that as many as 20–30% of patients diagnosed with epilepsy may in fact suffer from convulsive syncope *(3,4)*. The intent of this chapter is to review the approach to the patient with syncope, with an emphasis toward differentiating syncope from seizures.

Syncope

Syncope can be caused by a variety of disorders. The differential diagnosis of syncope includes cardiac as well as noncardiac disorders. The cardiac causes of syncope can be classified into four general categories: (1) neurally mediated reflex syncope; (2) postural hypotension; (3) cardiac outflow obstruction, and (4) arrhythmic **(Fig. 1).** Each is associated with a transient reduction in cardiac output, resulting in cerebral hypoperfusion and syncope.

Neurally mediated syncope is the most common cause of fainting, particularly in the absence of structural heart disease *(1)*. Its subtypes include vasovagal syncope, carotid sinus syncope, as well as syncope attributable to reflex triggers (e.g., micturition, defecation, swallow, and tussive syncope). Of these subtypes, vasovagal syncope is the most common. A trigger for vasovagal

From: *Seizures: Medical Causes and Management*
Edited by: N. Delanty © Humana Press, Inc., Totowa, N

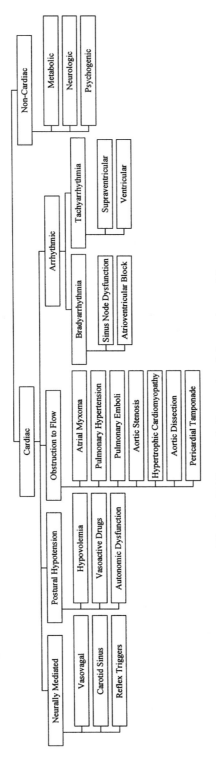

Fig. 1. Differential diagnosis of the patient with syncope.

272

syncope often is not readily identified, but psychological stress is a well-known precipitant *(5)*.

An episode of vasovagal syncope is usually marked by a premonitory period of symptomatic hypotension followed by bradycardia. The mechanism underlying the bradycardia and hypotension is not fully understood. One hypothesis is that a reduction in central blood volume and stroke volume in response to orthostatic stress results in vigorous contraction of a relatively empty left ventricle. This stimulus activates ventricular mechanoreceptors and results in an increase in nonmyelinated (C-fiber) vagal afferent activity and triggers the Bezold–Jarisch reflex. Stimulation of the reflex increases parasympathetic activity and inhibits sympathetic activity, producing brady-cardia, vasodilation, and hypotension *(6,7)*. Although some vasovagal episodes are attributable to bradycardia (cardioinhibitory response) or hypotension (vasodepressor response) alone, most episodes are associated with both bradycardia and hypotension (mixed response). The relative impor-tance of bradycardia and hypotension during a syncopal episode differs among patients and even varies within patients during different episodes *(8)*.

Syncope stemming from postural hypotension may be related to hypo-volemia, use of vasoactive drugs, or intrinsic autonomic dysfunction. The lat-ter may be idiopathic or secondary to a neuropathy caused by alcohol use, diabetes mellitus, or attributable to a central or spinal cord lesion. Disorders that cause either right- or left-sided obstruction to cardiac outflow can result in syncope. Such disorders include atrial myxoma, pulmonary hypertension and pulmonary emboli, aortic stenosis, hypertrophic obstructive cardiomy-opathy, aortic dissection, and pericardial tamponade.

Arrhythmias due to either bradycardia or tachycardia can be associated with syncope. Bradycardia may result from either sinus node dysfunction or atrioventricular (A-V) block. Sinus node dysfunction accounts for more than 50% of new pacemaker implants in the United States *(9)*. Patients with sinus node dysfunction may also manifest tachyarrhythmias, typically paroxysmal atrial fibrillation, flutter, or atrial tachycardia. Consequently, either bradycar-dia or tachycardia can account for symptoms of dizziness or syncope. Second- or third-degree A-V block is usually secondary to fibrosis of the conduction system. However, secondary causes of heart block, such as acute myocardial infarction, drug toxicity (e.g., digoxin), and an infectious etiology (e.g., Lyme disease) must be excluded.

Supraventricular arrhythmias, capable of causing hemodynamic collapse and syncope, include atrial fibrillation with a rapid ventricular response, atrial tachycardia (including atrial flutter) with 1:1 A-V conduction, A-V nodal reentrant tachycardia, and A-V reciprocating tachycardia utilizing an acces-sory pathway. Patients with an accessory pathway capable of anterograde con-duction (the Wolff–Parkinson–White syndrome) can develop syncope secondary to atrial fibrillation with rapid conduction to ventricles via the accessory pathway. Interestingly, syncope during supraventricular tachycardia is not always a reflection of the tachycardia rate; in some patients it may precipitate a vasovagal episode *(10)*. Consistent with this concept, patients with tachycardia-induced syncope have a greater decline in mean blood pressure when tilted upright during tachycardia as well a higher incidence of vasovagal syncope during tilt testing in sinus rhythm when compared to similar tachycardia patients who do not develop syncope *(10)*. Ventricular tachycardia is observed most commonly in patients with underlying structural heart disease, particularly in patients with ischemic heart disease. In addition, syncope (or seizures) caused by torsade de pointes ventricular tachycardia may be the initial manifestation in patients with the congenital or acquired forms of long QT interval syndrome *(11,12)*.

Important noncardiac causes of syncope include psychogenic disorders, metabolic disturbances (e.g., hypoglycemia), and neurologic disorders. Psychogenic disorders, most commonly panic disorders, may be responsible for presyncope or syncope in up to 25% of patients *(13)*. Compared with patients with nonpsychogenic syncope, patients with psychogenic syncope are younger, have more prodromal symptoms prior to syncope, have more frequent episodes of presyncope or syncope in the 6 mo prior to evaluation, and are more disabled because of their symptoms. Common prodromal symptoms include light-headedness, shortness of breath, dizziness, palpitations, chest pain, and tingling in the limbs. It is important to make the diagnosis, as relief of symptoms is possible in most patients with a combination of psychotherapy and pharmacotherapy *(13)*. Neurologic causes of syncope include vertebrobasilar insufficiency, migraine headaches, neuralgias (trigeminal and glossopharyngeal), and seizures.

Seizures

Syncope may be related to an underlying seizure disorder. In the ictal–bradycardia syndrome, for example, ictal episodes are accompanied by profound bradycardia, which results in syncope *(14,15)*. The diagnosis of this condition requires electroencephalographic documentation of a seizure followed by electrocardiographic documentation of bradycardia/asystole and resulting syncope. Therefore, simultaneous electroencephalogram (EEG) and electrocardiogram (EKG) recordings are necessary to make the appropriate diagnosis. In these patients, syncope mistakenly may be attributed only to the cerebral effects of the seizure or only to a cardiac disorder, without appreciation of an underlying neurologic condition. It should be noted that EEG documentation of the sequence of events is essential because it is possible for an episode of neurally mediated syncope to trigger an actual seizure, usually in patients with an underlying seizure disorder *(16,17)*.

The majority of patients with the ictal–bradycardia syndrome have temporal lobe epilepsy *(14,15,18)*. A 5:1 ratio of male to female patients has been reported *(14)*. Some investigators have reported lateralization to the left temporal lobe *(18)*. Of note, in patients who undergo temporal lobectomy, stimulation of the right insular area causes tachycardia, whereas stimulation of the left insular area causes bradycardia *(19)*. Recognition of the role of cortical activity in the genesis of cardiac arrhythmias is important to initiate proper therapy with anticonvulsant medications, usually in conjunction with a pacemaker.

Seizures vs Syncope

Initial Evaluation

A correct diagnosis is often made on the basis of the history and physical examination alone. However, the diagnosis may be elusive after just a single clinical episode. In one study, physicians were asked to differentiate between syncope and a seizure based on a patient's history. A final diagnosis was made in each patient after further evaluation; however, the physicians were given the results of the initial evaluation only. The overall initial agreement among physicians was only 31% *(20)*.

Although a variety of disorders can cause syncope, most are not typically associated with convulsions. In our experience, convulsive syncope is most commonly a manifestation of vasovagal syncope. Interestingly, patients with syncope and underlying structural heart disease rarely present with convulsions. The presence of a prodrome may not differentiate adequately between seizures and convulsive syncope. Features suggestive of the latter include the following: relationship to the upright position, absence of tonic-clonic movements or automatisms, rapid recovery, absence of postictal disorientation,and a normal interictal EEG *(15)*. In fact, postevent disorientation may be the most powerful discriminator in distinguishing convulsive syncope from sei-zures *(21)*.

EKG

An EKG should be obtained in all patients with syncope or suspected epilepsy. Abnormalities on the EKG that may suggest a specific cause for syncope include bundle branch block, A-V block, preexcitation (the hallmark of the Wolff–Parkinson–White syndrome), and prolonged QT interval. In addition, the presence of ventricular hypertrophy may suggest underlying cardiac pathology.

Often it is necessary to obtain a 24 to 48-h ambulatory EKG recording to correlate symptoms with a rhythm disturbance. Because symptoms may be sporadic in some patients, prolonged ambulatory EKG recordings may be required. An insertable loop recorder has been developed recently, which is capable of 14 mo of continuous EKG monitoring *(22)*. The recorder is a 61 $\times$ 19 $\times$ 8-mm recording device with a weight of 17 g and a volume of 8 cm^3. The device is inserted subcutaneously in the infraclavicular region, similar to

A

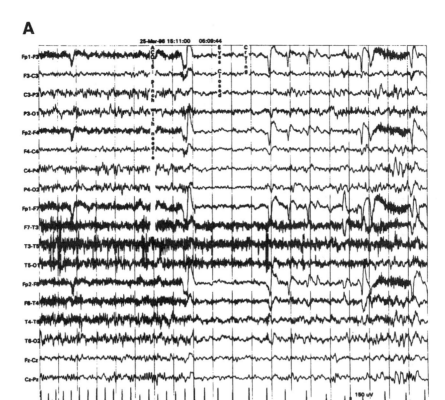

B

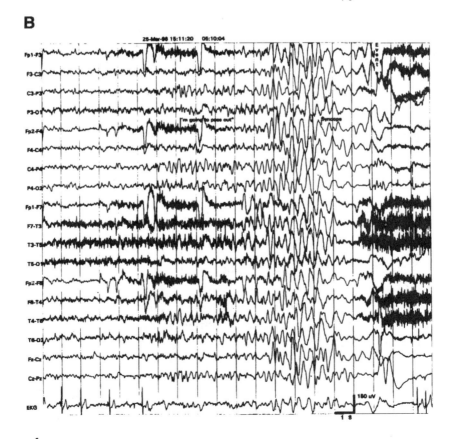

C

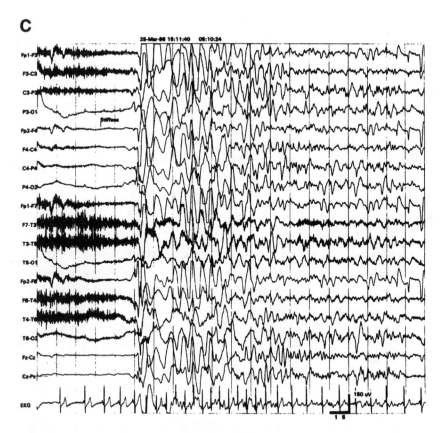

Fig. 2. One-minute epoch demonstrating a convulsive, syncopal episode in a 7-yr-old-girl following a venipuncture. (**A**) Venipuncture was performed at 15:11:05. (**B**) Patient feels as though she is going to pass out at 15:11:27. Syncope occurs at 15:11:34 following a burst of delta activity. (**C**) Patient stiffens at 15:11:44 after EEG has flattened. EEG then returns to baseline in reverse sequence. (Reproduced with permission from Ref. *24.*)

a pacemaker. The device has two sensing bipoles, which allow for the recording of a single-lead EKG. Patients trigger the device using a handheld activator during an episode of presyncope or syncope. The EKG during the episode can then be downloaded using a standard pacemaker programmer. Once a diagnosis is made, the recorder can be removed. Because documentation of bradycardia and syncope does not absolutely exclude a seizure, combined ambulatory EEG and EKG recordings may be necessary to determine the relationship between a cardiac arrhythmia and an EEG abnormality *(23)*.

EEG

The EEG can be used to distinguish syncopal events attributable to cerebral hypoperfusion from those that are epileptic in nature *(24)*. The EEG patterns during vasovagal syncope were first elucidated by Gastaut and Fischer-Williams (**Fig. 2**) *(25)*. Syncope was induced by ocular pressure. All patients underwent simultaneous EEG and EKG procedures. With an arrest lasting 3–6 s, there were no clinical or electrical abnormalities. With an arrest lasting 7–13 s, bilateral and synchronous slow waves appeared, usually accompanied by presyncope or syncope. With a longer period of arrest, one or two generalized clonic jerks appeared without affecting the EEG. This was followed by a generalized tonic contraction, which was accompanied by flattening of the EEG. Observation of an extensor tonic spasm and clonic jerks while the cortical EEG appears flat suggests that the observed convulsions are a brainstem release phenomenon (26). With recovery, the EEG normalizes in the reverse sequence.

More recent data suggest that no single EEG abnormality is pathognomonic in patients with syncope. Aminoff and colleagues reported EEG patterns in patients with an implantable cardioverter–defibrillator undergoing defibrillation threshold testing (27). Some patients had no EEG changes despite loss of consciousness. Sheldon et al. reported EEG results obtained in 18 patients with presyncope or syncope during tilt testing (28).

Abnormalities observed included theta wave slowing, delta wave slowing, and background suppression; however, each abnormality was not observed in every patient. An important observation was that there were abrupt changes in the EEG as patients progressed from presyncope to syncope. There was a sharp increase in the number of patients who developed delta slowing or background suppression. Importantly, epileptiform activity was not observed in any patient.

Tilt Table Testing

Over the past decade, tilt testing has become a widely accepted diagnostic tool for the evaluation of neurally mediated syncope (29–31). For a detailed review of tilt table testing the reader is referred to a recent American College of Cardiology expert consensus document on the subject (31).

Vasovagal episodes are associated with hypotension and bradycardia and may result in seizure-like activity (convulsive syncope) (2). Recently, it was proposed that tilt testing may assist in the differentiation of convulsive syncope and seizures (31,32). In one study, vasovagal syncope was diagnosed on the basis of a positive tilt test in 67% of patients with recurrent idiopathic seizures that were unresponsive to antiepileptic therapy (32). Concomitant with loss of consciousness, each patient developed a rigid flexed posture, followed by a rigid extended posture with upward eye rolling and head extension with nuchal rigidity. In some patients, these tonic spasms were followed by bilateral myoclonic rhythmic jerks as well as urinary incontinence. It is therefore not surprising that convulsive syncope can be mistaken for seizures or epilepsy.

A subset of these patients had an EEG during tilt testing. The EEG showed generalized brain wave slowing consistent with cerebral hypoxia. However, no epileptiform activity was noted. The EEG returned to normal when the patients were returned to the supine position. Of note, among patients with a positive tilt test, there was no significant difference in the degree of hypotension and bradycardia between patients with and without seizures. In addition, whereas all patients previously had failed therapy with anticonvulsant medications, therapy directed toward vasovagal syncope was successful in preventing further episodes of convulsive syncope in all patients.

A graded infusion of isoproterenol is often required to induce vasovagal syncope during tilt testing *(31–33)*. The rationale for isoproterenol provocation rests on the notion that variability in the magnitude of epinephrine/norepinephrine release may in part account for the unpredictable nature of spontaneous neurally mediated syncopal events and that the provision of exogenous catecholamines may facilitate induction of neurally mediated syncope in susceptible individuals *(31)*. Recently, we reported that bolus administration of adenosine facilitates induction of neurally mediated syncope *(34)*. Adenosine has a sympathoexcitatory effect, which is mediated via baroreflex and peripheral chemoreceptor activation *(35–37)*. The results with adenosine and isoproterenol tilt testing are often discordant, which may reflect differential patient sensitivities to the mechanisms of sympathetic activation by adenosine (chemoreceptor and baroreceptor activation) and isoproterenol (direct β-adrenergic stimulation and activation of baroreceptors) *(34)*. **Figure 3** illustrates an example of such a discordant response in a patient with a lifelong history of seizures unresponsive to anticonvulsant medications who was referred to our institution for tilt testing. The observed discordance suggests that adenosine and isoproterenol may have complementary roles during tilt testing; therefore, we currently use a tilt protocol that incorporates both agents *(34)*.

The tilt test can also distinguish between vasovagal and psychogenic syncope. Patients with psychogenic syncope faint during tilt testing without an alteration in their hemodynamics. These patients usually have an underlying psychiatric disorder, most commonly an anxiety disorder or major depression *(13)*.

Miscellaneous

Measurement of serum creatine kinase (CK) after an episode of transient loss of consciousness may also help differentiate syncope from a seizure. A CK level of ≥ 200 mU/mL on presentation or an increase in CK of >15 mU/mL over the first 24 h is highly suggestive of a seizure as opposed to an episode of vasovagal syncope *(38)*. Finally, the need for further diagnostic

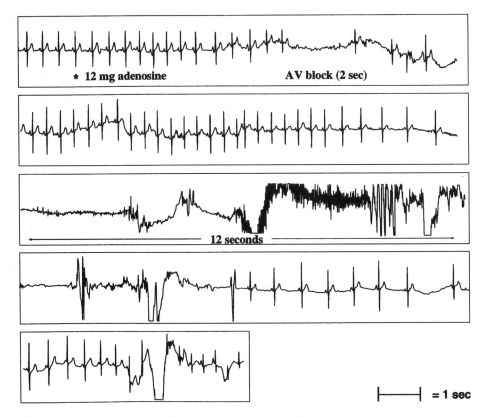

Fig. 3. Induction of neurally mediated syncope with adenosine. A continuous single-lead EKG recording (surface lead II) from a patient with a lifelong history of seizures precipitated by emotional distress and accompanied by nausea and light-headedness. The patient received 12 mg of adenosine while upright. Transient sinus tachycardia was followed by 2 s of A-V block, which was then followed by a reflex sinus tachycardia. Shortly thereafter, the patient experienced her typical preseizure prodrome followed by vasovagal syncope. This was characterized by a marked cardioinhibitory response, which reproduced her clinical seizures. A routine tilt test, with and without isoproterenol, was normal. (Reproduced with permission from Ref. *34.*)

testing, including echocardiography, exercise stress testing, cardiac catheterization, and/or invasive electrophysiologic testing, is typically determined by the suspicion of underlying structural heart disease.

Conclusions

Syncope and seizures are both common disorders. The clinician is often required to make a distinction based on the history of a single clinical episode. Convulsive syncope, which is most commonly a manifestation of vasovagal syncope, may easily be mistaken for epilepsy. Therefore, this entity should be considered in all patients with suspected epilepsy, especially when the history is atypical for epilepsy or when there is an inadequate response to anticonvulsant medication.

The tilt test is particularly useful in eliciting vasovagal syncope in patients with suspected convulsive syncope. Recent advances in tilt testing, such as the adenosine-based tilt test, may enhance the sensitivity of tilt testing and reproduce convulsive syncope in susceptible individuals. Proper recognition of convulsive syncope is important in preventing the emotional, physical, and financial consequences of inappropriately being diagnosed as having epilepsy.

References

1. Benditt DG, Remole S, Milstein S, Bailin S. Syncope: Causes, clinical evaluation, and current therapy. *Annu Rev Med* 1992;43:283–300.
2. Lin JT-Y, Ziegler DK, Lai C-W, Bayer W. Convulsive syncope in blood donors. *Ann Neurol* 1982;11:525–528.
3. Silbert PL, Graydon RH, Stewart-Wynne EG. Convulsive syncope and the diagnosis of a first epileptic seizure. *Med J Austral* 1992;157:72.
4. Zaidi A, Crampton S, Clough P, Scheepers B, Fitzpatrick AP. Misdiagnosis of epilepsy-Many seizure-like episodes have a cardiovascular cause. *PACE* 1999;22:457A.
5. Dohrmann ML, Cheitlin MD. Cardiogenic syncope: seizures versus syncope. *Neurol Clin* 1986;4:549–562.
6. Brooks R, Ruskin JN. Evaluation of the patient with unexplained syncope. In Zipes DP, Jalife J (eds.), *Cardiac Electrophysiology: From Cell to Bedside.* Philadelphia, PA: WB Saunders, 1995.
7. Mark AL. The Bezold-Jarisch reflex revisited: clinical implications of inhibitory reflexes originating in the heart. *J Am Coll Cardiol* 1983;1:90–102.
8. Benditt DG, Lurie KG, Fabian WH. Clinical approach to diagnosis of syncope. *Cardiol Clin* 1997;15:165–176.
9. Benditt DG, Sakaguchi S, Goldstein MA, Lurie KG, Gornick CC, Adler SW. Sinus node dysfunction: pathophysiology, clinical features, evaluation, and treatment. In Zipes DP, Jalife J (eds.), *Cardiac Electrophysiology: From Cell to Bedside.* Philadelphia, PA: WB Saunders, 1995.
10. Leitch JW, Klein GJ, Yee R, Leather RA, Kim YH. Syncope associated with supraventricular tachycardia: An expression of tachycardia rate or vasomotor response? *Circulation* 1992;85:1064–1071.
11. Sundaram MBM, McMeekin JD, Gulamhusein S. Cardiac tachyarrhythmias in hereditary long QT syndromes presenting as a seizure disorder. *Can J Neurol Sci* 1986;13:262–263.
12. Davis AM, Wilkinson JL. The long QT syndrome and seizures in childhood. *J Paediatr Child Health* 1998;34:410–411.
13. Linzer M, Varia I, Pontinen M, Divine GW, Grubb BP, Estes NAM III. Medically unexplained syncope: relationship to psychiatric illness. *Am J Med* 1992; 92:1A–18A.
14. Reeves AL, Nollet KE, Klass DW, Sharbrough FW, SO EL. The ictal bradycardia syndrome. *Epilepsia* 1996;137:983–987.
15. Constantin L, Martins JB, Fincham RW, Dagli RD. Bradycardia and syncope as manifestations of partial epilepsy. *J Am Coll Cardiol* 1990;15:900–905.

16. Bergey GK, Krumholz A, Fleming CP. Complex partial seizure provocation by vaso-vagal syncope: video-EEG and intracranial electrode documentation. *Epilepsia* 1997;38:118–121.

17. Tanaka T, Inoue H, Aizawa H, et al. Case of cough syncope with seizure. *Respiration* 1994;61:48–50.

18. Locatelli ER, Varghese JP, Shuaib A, Potolicchio SJ. Cardiac asystole and bradycardia as a manifestation of left temporal lobe complex partial seizure. *Ann Intern Med* 1999;130:581–583.

19. Oppenheimer SM, Gelb A, Girvin JP, Hachinski VC. Cardiovascular effects of human insular cortex stimulation. *Neurology* 1992;42:1727–1732.

20. Hoefnagels WAJ, Padberg GW, Overweg J, Roos RAC. Syncope or seizure? A matter of opinion. *Clin Neurol Neurosurg* 1992;94:153–156.

21. Hoefnagels WAJ, Padberg GW, Overweg J, van der Velde EA, Roos RAC. Transient loss of consciousness: the value of the history for distinguishing seizure from syncope. *J Neurol* 1991;238:39–43.

22. Krahn AD, Klein GJ, Yee R, Takle-Newhouse T, Norris C. Use of an extended monitoring strategy in patients with problematic syncope. *Circulation* 1999;99:406–410.

23. Beauregard LAM, Fabiszewski R, Black CH, et al. Combined ambulatory electroencephalographic and electrocardiographic recordings for evaluation of syncope. *Am J Cardiol* 1991;68:1067–1072.

24. Brenner RP. Electroencephalography in syncope. *J Clin Neurophysiol* 1997;14:197–209.

25. Gastaut H, Fischer-Williams M. Electro-encephalographic study of syncope: its differentiation from epilepsy. *Lancet* 1957;2:1018–1025.

26. Kempster PA, Balla JI. A clinical study of convulsive syncope. *Clin Exp Neurol* 1986;22:53–55.

27. Aminoff MJ, Scheinman MM, Griffin JC, Herre JM. Electrocerebral accompaniments of syncope associated with malignant ventricular arrhythmias. *Ann Internal Med* 1988;108:791–796.

28. Sheldon RS, Koshman ML, Murphy WF. Electroencephalographic findings during presyncope and syncope induced by tilt table testing. *Can J Cardiol* 1998;14:811–816.

29. Kenny RA, Bayliss J, Ingram A, Sutton, R. Head-up tilt: a useful test for investigating unexplained syncope. *Lancet* 1986;1:1352–1354.

30. Benditt DG, Remole S, Bailin S, Dunnigan A, Asso A, Milstein S. Tilt table testing for evaluation of neurally-mediated (cardioneurogenic) syncope: rationale and proposed protocols. *PACE* 1991;14:1528–1537.

31. Benditt DG, Ferguson DW, Grubb BP, et al. Tilt table testing for assessing syncope. *J Am Coll Cardiol* 1996;28:263–275.

32. Grubb BP, Gerard G, Roush K, Temesy-Armos P, Elliott L, Hahn H, Spann C. Differentiation of convulsive syncope and epilepsy with head-up tilt testing. *Ann Internal Med* 1991:115:871–876.

33. Almquist A, Goldenberg I, Milstein S, et al. Provocation of bradycardia and hypotension by isoproterenol and upright posture in patients with unexplained syncope. *N Engl J Med* 1989;320:346–351.

34. Mittal S, Stein KM, Markowitz SM, Slotwiner DJ, Rohatgi S, Lerman BB. Induction of neurally mediated syncope with adenosine. *Circulation* 1999;99:1318–1324.

35. Biaggioni I, Olafsson B, Robertson RM, Hollister AS, Robertson D. Cardiovascular and respiratory effects of adenosine in conscious man. Evidence for chemoreceptor activation. *Circ Res* 1987;61:779–786.
36. Biaggiono I, Killian TJ, Mosqueda-Garcia R, Robertson RM, Robertson D. Adenosine increases sympathetic nerve traffic in humans. *Circulation* 1991;83:1668–1675.
37. Engelstein ED, Lerman BB, Somers VK, Rea RF. Role of arterial chemoreceptors in mediating the effects of endogenous adenosine on sympathetic nerve activity. *Circulation* 1994;90:2919–2926.
38. Neufeld MY, Treves TA, Chistik V, Korczyn AD. Sequential serum creatine kinase determination differentiates vaso-vagal syncope from generalized tonic-clonic seizures. *Acta Neurol Scand* 1997:95:137–139.

18

Seizures in the Tropics

Nimal Senanayake, MD, PhD, DSc, FRCP, FRCPE

Introduction

Large parts of Asia, all of Africa, and most of Central and South America are located in the area between the tropics of Cancer and Capricorn, where more than one-third of the world's population lives. The two most populous countries, China and India, are largely and wholly in this region, respectively. Seizures are a major problem in tropical countries and are much more prevalent than in temperate countries *(1)*.

The prevalence of seizures, in terms of the prevalence of epilepsy, also is much higher in tropical countries than in temperate countries *(2,3)*. The age-adjusted prevalence for active epilepsy in tropical countries, in general, is between 10 and 15 per 1000 population, which is about twice the prevalence in temperate countries. This excess probably reflects the geographic and biologic disadvantages faced by these vast human populations in the tropics *(4)*.

The tropics have a relatively uniform climate with high temperature and humidity and mountains or plains that were formerly heavily forested. The rain forests and the heavy rainfall have attracted agriculture and massive deforestation, leading to soil erosion and the development of more swamps and free-flowing rivers, which favor the multiplication and spread of vectors of disease. The lack of winters further predisposes the region to vector-borne diseases such as malaria, dengue, trypanosomiasis, and schistosomiasis *(1)*. With agriculture and industry has come the use (often misuse) of pesticides and other toxic chemicals, many of which are known agents of seizures and epilepsy.

Poverty and illiteracy promote disease through undernutrition, poor sanitation, multiplication of insects and rodents, and inaccessibility of medical care. The despair brought about by these conditions leads to social diseases: drug

From: *Seizures: Medical Causes and Management*
Edited by: N. Delanty © Humana Press, Inc., Totowa, NJ

and substance abuse, violence, prostitution, and human immunodeficiency virus (HIV) infection. All of these factors, together with poor maternal and child health care, contribute to increased frequency of seizures and epilepsy in the tropics (1).

In most tropical diseases, epilepsy is either an acute or a remote symptomatic seizure disorder. The presence of other symptoms of brain involvement or the sudden onset of very frequent seizures may indicate an acute symptomatic disorder, whereas epilepsy *per se,* or seizures occurring with a long-standing neurologic deficit, is more suggestive of a remote symptomatic disorder (5).

This chapter reviews the tropical diseases that manifest with acute symptomatic seizures or lead to symptomatic epilepsy.

Parasitic Infections

Metazoan Infections

Neurocysticercosis

EPIDEMIOLOGY

Neurocysticercosis is the most frequent parasitosis of the central nervous system (CNS) in several countries in Latin America, Africa, and Asia (6). The disease is a scourge in Mexico, Brazil, Peru, and Ecuador (7), where, in some areas, the estimated prevalence, based on autopsies and biopsies in general hospitals, is over 3000 per 100,000 population (8). In Mexico, neurocysticercosis is responsible for 10% of all neurologic hospital admissions. There is a growing incidence of the disease in Africa, except in the Muslim countries along the Mediterranean, and in the center and south of the continent, because of the fact that the Koran prohibits consumption of pork (7). In Asia, the disease is widely distributed, particularly in China, and it is endemic in India and Thailand but uncommon in Pakistan, which is also a Muslim country (7). Because of migrating workers, neurocysticercosis is being recognized more frequently in North America, Europe (9), and Australia (10).

Seizures are the most common manifestation of neurocysticercosis (11,12) and in Mexico are the main cause of late-onset epilepsy, accounting for half the cases (6,13). In Ecuador, seizures account for nearly one-quarter of all new cases of epilepsy (14) and in Brazil, are the single most identifiable cause of epilepsy (15).

In Africa, neurocysticercosis is considered an important cause of epilepsy in Bantus and southern Rhodesians (16–19) but not in West Africans (20). However, a more recent survey in northern Togo of West Africa has attributed neurocysticercosis as the cause in about one-third of epilepsy patients over 15-yr-olds and two-thirds of those whose epilepsy began after the age of 50 (21,22).

In India, 2.5% of all intracranial space occupying lesions *(23)* and 2% of focal epilepsy *(24)* seen in patients in a hospital in New Delhi were attributable to neurocysticercosis. Neurocysticercosis also accounted for 5.1% of 253 patients aged 25 yr or more evaluated for recent onset epilepsy *(25)*. Neurocysticercosis has been suggested as the cause of many cases of epilepsy in southern India *(26)* as well, but the disease is more prevalent in the northern and northwestern regions of the country *(23,27)*.

Neurocysticercosis is the most common cause of epilepsy of late onset in Southeast Asia *(28)*. In Bali, 8% of the population in one village had epilepsy that was possibly related to neurocysticercosis *(29)*. It has also been identified as a frequent cause of accidental burns attributable to epilepsy among the Kapadoku people of Indonesia *(30)* and in New Guinea *(31)*. Among Nepalese adults (Gurkhas) based in Hong Kong who presented with adult-onset epilepsy, neurocysticercosis was the cause in seven of eight cases *(32)*.

PATHOGENESIS

Cysticercosis is caused by the larva of *Taenia solium,* the pork tapeworm. The adult worm is an intestinal parasite in man. Its eggs, expelled with feces, develop into larvae in pigs, and by eating poorly cooked pork, man contracts intestinal taeniasis. Cysticercosis results when man accidentally ingests the infective eggs of *T. solium,* usually via food such as vegetables or water that are contaminated with human feces. The eggs hatch in the duodenum, releasing hexacanth larvae. They penetrate the intestinal mucosa, enter the bloodstream, and disseminate by systemic embolization. The larvae show a marked preference for muscle and brain. There, they develop into cysticerci (*Cysticercus cellulosae* or *Cysticercus racemosae*) and evolve through vesicular, colloidal, granular–nodular, and calcified stages over a period of 2–5 yr *(9)*.

In the brain, the cysticerci are localized mainly subarachnoidally, in the cortex, in the ventricles, in the basal cistern, and also in the white matter of the cerebrum itself. Lesions may range from a solitary asymptomatic cysticercus, found at autopsy, to large, expansive lesions with allergic inflammatory reaction in the brain, vasculitis, and edema. The miliary form, with hundreds of parasites in the brain, represents a massive invasion of the bloodstream by the parasite. An inflammatory reaction in the cerebral spinal fluid (CSF) may occur with meningitis, reactive fibrosis, cranial nerve involvement, visual alteration, and obstructive hydrocephalus *(33)*.

CLINICAL FEATURES

Epilepsy and intracranial hypertension, with or without meningeal signs, followed by psychiatric syndromes, are the most common presentations of neurocysticercosis *(9)*. Epilepsy has been reported as the presenting symptom in 74% of patients with mixed-form (intra- and extraparenchymal) neurocysticercosis and in 92% of those with intraparenchymal form *(9)*. A high frequency of partial seizures, with or without secondary generalization, is characteristic *(6,9,34)*. A variety of seizure types, such as partial motor (Jacksonian) seizures alternating between right and left sides, or even more complex patterns related to multiple cortical cysts has been observed *(34)*.

Other manifestations vary from focal neurological signs to intermittent increases in intracranial pressure. Basal meningitis with involvement of cranial nerves, particularly the optic and the oculomotor nerves, and behavioral and mental alterations resembling those of tuberculous meningitis, may also occur *(33)*. Cases of acquired epileptic aphasia (Landau–Kleffner syndrome) have been attributed to cysticerci situated in the left Sylvian fissure *(35)*.

An acute encephalitic form of cysticercosis occurs predominantly in children and adolescents. Its rapid clinical course to death or resolution, as well as the observation that computerized tomography (CT) shows multiple areas of edema with ring enhancement, appears to indicate that initial invasion of the CNS by a cysticercus takes place with an immune-mediated parenchymal reaction *(9)*. The frequency of the encephalitic form varies from 10% *(9)* and 20% *(36,37)* to 65% *(38)*.

In India, attention has also been drawn to a rare form of disseminated cysticercosis in which literally thousands of cysticerci invade the body muscle mass, the brain, and even some other organs like the heart. Uncontrolled seizures, progressive dementia, behavior disorder, muscular pseudohypertrophy, and a relative paucity of localizing neurological signs or signs of raised intracranial pressure are the main features. CT of the brain shows numerous small discrete lesions with attenuation density values less than those of calcium, caused by the scolices within cysticerci *(39)*.

MANAGEMENT

In inactive cases, a simple skull X-ray film may show single or multiple calcifications in up to 10% of patients. CT or magnetic resonance imaging (MRI) allows precise localization of the viable cysticerci as well as the inactive calcified lesions. The presence of CSF lymphocytosis is evidence of active disease and arachnoiditis. More than half of the patients show pleocytosis of between 10 and 200 cells/µL, with a preponderant lymphocytic response. When the CSF has inflammatory cells, 50% of the cases show eosinophils in the spinal fluid. CSF glucose may be low, and there is occasional increase in protein and immunoglobulin G (IgG). Simultaneous use of complement fixation and ELISA tests on the CSF give positive results in up to 95% of cases *(40)*. Serum tests are unreliable in the diagnosis of neurocysticercosis because of the frequency of asymptomatic infection in the population in endemic areas, giving false-positive results *(33)*.

Praziquantel is often effective *(40–42)*. Corticosteroids may be required to treat the adverse reactions induced by the lysis of parasites. In cases with mass effect from a single cysticercus or with CSF obstruction, surgical treatment may be required. However, accidental rupture of the vesicles during surgical intervention may provoke a severe allergic reaction in the spinal fluid, causing fibrosis and angiitis. Shunting of CSF may also be needed. Albendazole also has been used with excellent result *(33,40)*.

Schistosomiasis

EPIDEMIOLOGY

Schistosomiasis (bilharziasis) is a major health problem in many parts of the tropics, with some 600 million people estimated to be at risk in 79 endemic countries *(43)*. Of the three major human schistosomes, *Schistosoma mansoni* is endemic in Africa and Latin America, *Schistosoma haematobium* in Africa, and *Schistosoma japonicum* in Southeast Asia. *S. japonicum* is responsible for the majority of reported cases of cerebral schistosomiasis *(44)*.

PATHOGENESIS

Schistosomes (blood flukes) are digenetic trematodes. They multiply in the intermediate snail host before entering the definitive mammalian host. The cercariae released from the snail may infect man by penetrating through the skin and entering subcutaneous tissue, venous blood vessels, and lymphatic tissue. The mature parasites mate in the portal system or liver and then migrate to the mesenteric or vesical veins to lay eggs. Eggs find their way into the lumen of ureters and urinary bladder, or intestine, and are carried to the outside world to complete the life cycle.

CLINICAL FEATURES

Acute schistosomiasis (Katayama fever) may occasionally produce an encephalopathy manifesting with impairment of consciousness, papilledema, partial and generalized seizures, and focal neurological signs *(45)*. A chronic form of cerebral schistosomiasis may be caused by schistosoma eggs embolizing to the brain. The most common manifestation of this is epileptic attacks, usually in the form of partial seizures. The chief pathologic changes are eosinophilic abscesses and tubercle formation, which may be disseminated to produce meningoencephalitis or conglomerated to form space-occupying granulomata *(46)*.

MANAGEMENT

Patients with epilepsy or suspected brain tumors in endemic areas should have repeated examinations of urine or stools for *Schistosoma* ova. Signs of schistosomiasis may be demonstrable by cystoscopy or sigmoidoscopy. Peripheral blood may show eosinophilia, and CSF may show a pleocytosis, occasionally with eosinophilia *(45)*. Radioimmunoassay and enzyme-linked immunosorbent assay on serum or CSF may indicate previous exposure to schistosomes. Demonstration of ova by biopsy is the final proof of CNS involvement, although therapeutic tests with schistosomicidal drugs (praziquantel, oxamniquine, metrifonate) may be advocated in specific cases *(9)*.

Paragonimiasis

EPIDEMIOLOGY

Paragonimiasis is another trematode infection caused by species of *Paragonimus*, with *Paragonimus westermani* (the oriental lung fluke) being the most common *(47)*. The disease is prevalent in the Far East, Southeast Asia, some parts of Africa, and South America *(48)*. The lung is the primary site of infection. Of the other organs, brain is involved with the highest frequency *(49)*. Cerebral paragonimiasis is one of the major neurological problems in endemic areas *(50)*. For instance, in Korea, it accounts for nearly one-fourth of cases of brain tumor *(51)*.

P. westermani requires a final host (man and other mammals), a first intermediate host (snails), and a second intermediate host (crustacea) for completion of its life cycle. The most common method of human infection is by eating raw or undercooked crabs or crayfish contaminated with metacercariae. The metacercariae exist in the small intestine, penetrate the intestinal wall, enter the peritoneal cavity, and travel through the diaphragm into the pleural cavity to enter the lung parenchyma *(52)*.

PATHOGENESIS

Cerebral lesions are thought to be caused by the entrance of semimature or mature worms into the brain through the foramina at the base of the skull *(53)*. Three distinct histopathological forms corresponding to the developmental stage of the disease have been identified, namely, a meningoencephalitic form, a granulomatous form, and an organization–calcification form *(52)*.

CLINICAL FEATURES

Seizures, usually focal motor, are the most common manifestation of cerebral paragonimiasis. Other common symptoms include headache, vomiting, visual disturbances, mental deterioration, hemiplegia, and hemihypesthesia. Pulmonary symptoms, usually cough with rusty sputum, are present in over half of the cases *(54)*.

MANAGEMENT

The criteria for the diagnosis of paragonimiasis include demonstration of *Paragonimus* ova in sputum, cytonodular-type lesions in the chest X-ray, and positive complement fixation test in the serum. For cerebral paragonimiasis, the criteria include demonstration of ova in the CSF, other CSF abnormalities, calcification in the skull X-ray, and focal electroencephalographic abnormalities. CT and MRI assays may also help. In the treatment of paragonimiasis, bithionol is the drug of choice *(52)*.

Sparganosis

Sparganosis is caused by the migrating larva (sparganum) of various pseudophyllidean cestodes, especially of the genera *Diphyllobothrium* and *Spirometra*. Human sparganosis is present worldwide and is most common in Asia (China, Japan, Korea, and Southeast Asia) *(55)*.

Adult worms reside in the intestine of cats, dogs, and racoons. Eggs hatch in fresh water and release coracidia that develop into procercoid larvae in *Cyclops* and then into spargana in fish, frog, or snake. Humans contract sparganosis by drinking water contaminated with *Cyclops* harboring procercoid larvae, by eating infected fish, frog, or snake, and by applying poultice of frog flesh to a wound or eye. When the sparganum penetrates the intestinal wall, it migrates to subcutaneous tissue, skeletal muscle, or viscera and rarely to the brain. Convulsions are a common symptom of cerebral sparganosis *(55)*.

Other Metazoan Diseases

Hydatid disease has been found to be associated with epileptic seizures in about one-third of cases *(56)*. Toxocariasis *(57)* and ascariasis *(58)* are also known to contribute to the etiology of symptomatic epilepsy.

Protozoan Infections

Toxoplasmosis

Toxoplasma gondii is an intracellular parasite found in domestic and wild animals, which is distributed worldwide. The sexual form develops in members of the cat family. Man is infected by ingestion of cysts from raw or undercooked meat, ingestion of sporulated oocysts from cat feces, or transplacental transmission *(57)*. Toxoplasmosis recently has assumed special status because of its frequency as an opportunistic infection in acquired immunodeficiency syndrome (AIDS) *(59)*. Seizures are a well-recognized consequence of toxoplasmosis and are seen in about 25% of affected individuals *(9)*. With the increasing incidence of AIDS in tropical countries, toxoplasmosis may become a more prevalent cause of epilepsy in the tropics.

Acquired toxoplasmosis is usually asymptomatic or only a mild illness in an otherwise healthy host. Encephalitis may occur as a rare complication *(60)*. However, in the case of those with decreased immunity, more than half the patients may develop encephalopathy, meningoencephalitis, or cerebral mass lesion(s) *(61)*. Cerebral toxoplasmosis is the most common cause of focal CNS disease complicating AIDS, affecting 10–15% of patients *(59)*.

Congenital toxoplasmosis manifests as chorioretinitis, hydrocephalus with aqueduct stenosis and cerebral calcification, mental retardation with seizures and cerebral palsy, or blindness *(62).* Some 40–60% of these patients have seizures *(63).* Toxoplasmosis also has been suggested as a possible cause of Landau–Kleffner syndrome *(64).*

Several serologic tests are available for the diagnosis of toxoplasmosis, with the Sabin–Feldman dye test being the most sensitive and specific. The CSF may show moderate elevation of protcin, a mononuclear pleocytosis, and normal or slightly reduced glucose. CT scan may show single or multiple lesions, mainly of subcortical structures with enhancing margins. MRI may be more sensitive in AIDS patients *(9).* Treatment consists of a combination of sulfadiazine, pyrimethamine, and folinic acid *(60).* Pregnant women are treated with spiramycin or clindamycin because of the teratogenic effects of pyrimethamine *(65).*

African Trypanosomiasis

African trypanosomiasis (sleeping sickness) caused by *Trypanosoma brucei* is widely distributed throughout sub-Saharan Africa, extending from the western to the eastern coasts and south to Zambia and Zimbabwe *(66).* About 40 million people are at risk of infection *(67).* The case fatality rate approximates 90%, making sleeping sickness one of the most lethal of diseases *(9).*

T. brucei is transmitted by the tsetse fly *Glossina* within which it undergoes important developmental changes. When the fly bites, the parasite present in the fly's saliva is injected into the victim's bloodstream. Within the vertebrate host, the parasite causes antigenic stimulation and production of large amounts of IgM. These effects probably underlie the pathological characteristics of the disease, including anemia, thrombocytopenia, glomerulonephritis, pancarditis, and a late-evolving diffuse meningoencephalitis with edema and arachnoiditis *(66,68).*

The trypanosome chancre is a local reaction at the site of the fly bite. Acute trypanosomiasis causes fever, anemia, lymphadenopathy, thrombocytopenia, and cardiac symptoms and signs. The acute stage is followed by a variable period of latent disease. The third stage is characterized by progressive neurological involvement, with mood changes, pyramidal, extrapyramidal, and cranial nerve signs, tremor, rigidity, choreoathetoid movements, muscle fasciculations, cerebellar ataxia, and generalized and partial seizures *(68,69).* Congenital cases may also occur and manifest as mental retardation and epilepsy *(70).*

Laboratory diagnosis, in the acute stage, is accomplished by demonstrating the parasite in thin and thick blood films stained with Giemsa or Field's stain. Trypanosomes may also be detected in chancre fluid, lymph node aspirates, bone marrow aspirates, serous effusions, and CSF. A variety of immunodiagnostic methods, including ELISA is also available. Examination of CSF shows a lymphocytosis and an increased IgM. Specific treatment in the acute stage is with suramin or pentamidine, and with melarsoprol in the late stage *(71)*.

American Trypanosomiasis

American trypanosomiasis (Chagas disease), a zoonotic disease caused by *Trypanosoma cruzi* is a public health problem in rural areas of Central and South America and is strongly linked with poor living conditions that allow proliferation of hematophagous insects (Reduvidae). The animal reservoirs are usually rodents, dogs, pigs, and marsupials *(33)*. Trypomasigotes are deposited by the *reduviid* insects when they defecate while biting the human host. The parasites enter the bloodstream through the skin and reach tissues. In late stages they continue to replicate intracellularly (as amastigotes) in muscle, cardiac tissue, and parasympathetic ganglion cells, causing immune-mediated tissue destruction, with cardiac and gastrointestinal dysfunction.

Clinically, the disease starts with a chagoma, a local reaction to the inoculation, followed by an acute stage with malaise, fever, headache, edema, skin rashes, lymphadenopathy, hepatosplenomegaly, myocarditis, and meningoencephalitis. It may lead to severe neurological impairment, including frequent seizures *(9,72)*. After a latent period, a chronic stage may develop, which is characterized by slowly progressive morphological and functional changes in the viscera, especially the heart, esophagus, and colon. Involvement of the CNS is secondary to cerebral embolization from the heart *(9)*. It may cause late-onset epilepsy, with a high frequency of partial seizures *(73)*.

The laboratory diagnosis is established by the demonstration of the parasite by direct or indirect methods, by histopathological examinations, and by serological demonstration of anti-*T. cruzi* antibodies. Specific treatment is with nifurtimox and benzonidazole *(74)*.

Malaria

EPIDEMIOLOGY

Malaria is endemic in tropical America, Africa, Asia, and subtropical areas of the eastern Mediterranean. One-fourth of humanity is exposed to the disease, which is held responsible for the death of at least 10% of African children under 3 yr of age *(9)*. Cerebral malaria is an acute encephalopathy that complicates exclusively the infection caused by *Plasmodium falciparum*. Cerebral involvement in malaria predominates in young adults, and children from 1 to 5 yr of age in hyperendemic areas. In adults, cerebral malaria occurs in nonimmunized subjects traveling from nonendemic areas, commonly when preventive treatment is interrupted. Pregnant women also are at risk because of decrease in immunity during pregnancy. AIDS may also predispose to cerebral malaria in the tropics *(33)*.

PATHOGENESIS

Cerebral malaria has been attributed to increased aggregability and sludging of the parasitized erythrocytes causing intravascular thrombosis. Erythrocytes parasitized with mature falciparum tropozoites and schizonts develop knob-like protrusions in the red cell membrane that cause adhesion to the vascular endothelium or cytoadherence. This may result in sequestration of parasitized erythrocytes in the brain *(75)* and occlusion of cerebral capillaries. Vasculitis, perhaps caused by circulating immune complexes, may also contribute *(76)*. Tumor necrosis factor has been shown to be crucial in producing brain lesions in experimental cerebral malaria *(77)*.

CLINICAL FEATURES

Cerebral malaria presents as an acute encephalitic illness, with fever, headache, delirium, and confusion progressing to coma. Generalized seizures occur in 40% of adult patients and in most children. Partial seizures may occur, and focal neurological signs are occasionally seen but tend to be transient. Despite appropriate treatment, cerebral malaria carries a mortality of 22% *(33)*.

Although reliable figures on the incidence of subsequent epilepsy in nonfatal cases following cerebral malaria are not available, epilepsy has long been recognized as a late complication of this illness. Generalized tonic-clonic seizures, as well as partial motor seizures, have been recorded *(78)*. Pathological examination of the brain in fatal cases, in late stages, have shown the malaric granuloma of Durck formed by an astroglial reaction *(76)*. It is conceivable that these lesions may act as epileptogenic foci in those who survive, giving rise to chronic epileptic seizures.

Even the benign forms of malaria have a role in the etiology of symptomatic seizures. Malaria is a common cause of febrile seizures in children in the tropics *(79,80)*. A study in the Congo showed that 9.6% of all children admitted to Brazzaville General Hospital between 1981 and 1983 presented with seizures *(81)*. Status epilepticus occurred in 13.6% of the patients, and 67% of the incidents were related to benign malaria. Febrile seizures occurred in 73.5% of all children, and 81% of these incidents were related to malaria, which was almost always benign (89%). Approximately 60% of all seizure disorders in children between 1 mo and 6 yr of age in a large general hospital were related to benign or malignant forms of malaria, and seizures were the reason for admission in 10% of all children in that age group.

Amebiasis

In addition to rare cases of involvement of the brain by the intestinal ameba *Entamoeba histolytica (82,83),* there is a growing number of cases of infection of the CNS with free-living amebae. These cases include *Naegleria* amebae, which is acquired by swimming in freshwater lakes *(84),* and

Acanthamoeba species *(85)*, which results from skin ulcers. These amebae produce a meningoencephalitis that clinically resembles either tuberculous meningitis, herpes encephalitis, or multiple brain abscesses. Granulomatous amebic encephalitis, presenting as a cerebral mass lesion, has also been reported *(85)*. Seizures are an important manifestation of cerebral amebiasis. Its role as an etiological factor in chronic epilepsy needs further evaluation.

Bacterial Infections

Tuberculous Meningitis

Tuberculous meningitis develops insidiously with nonspecific symptoms such as apathy, irritability, headache, low-grade fever, anorexia, and vomiting. Neck stiffness and Kernig's sign may be the only neurological sign at this stage. As the disease progresses, the patient becomes drowsy. Seizures and focal neurological deficits, such as cranial nerve palsies, hemiparesis, and involuntary movements, may occur. Intracranial hypertension, which is usually secondary to obstructive hydrocephalus, may develop, causing bulging fontanelles in young children and papilledema in adults. In late stages, the patient becomes deeply unconscious, often showing signs of brainstem dysfunction, such as decerebrate rigidity, fixed dilated pupils, and irregular pulse and respiration. Unless treated early and adequately, the patient may succumb or develop permanent neurological sequelae.

Epilepsy as a late sequel of tuberculous meningitis has been observed in 8 of 100 patients by Lorber *(86);* in 5 of them it was the only complication. In another series of 103 patients, 14 were found to have recurrent seizures; 9 of which had associated hemiplegia *(87)*. A form of tuberculous encephalopathy with or without meningitis has also been recognized *(88,89)*, affecting children and presenting with convulsions and coma.

Epilepsy is also a common manifestation of intracranial tuberculomas, which present as slow-growing, space-occupying lesions. In a recent series of 14 patients with intracranial tuberculoma in Saudi Arabia, 6 presented with epilepsy of late onset, including status epilepticus in 2 *(90)*. With the introduction of CT, small multiple tuberculomas are often found in patients with tuberculous meningitis. They can develop and enlarge at a time when tuberculous meningitis has been treated successfully *(91)*. They also may be discovered accidentally in asymptomatic individuals and in children with focal or generalized seizures *(92,93)*.

Ring or disk-enhancing lesions on CT in patients presenting with simple partial seizures recently have been described in India *(94)*. The lesions were more common in children and in those with a shorter duration of seizures (<6 mo). Of 39 patients with these abnormalities, 10 had evidence of tuberculosis elsewhere in the body, 3 had a past history of tuberculosis, and 4 had a history of close contact with a patient with tuberculosis. After 3 mo of antituberculosis treatment, 23 of 25 patients who were rescanned showed clearing of the lesion on CT. The two patients who did not were operated on, and the lesion was shown histologically to be a tuberculoma.

Pyogenic Meningitis

Pyogenic meningitis is common in the tropics. Epidemics of meningococcal meningitis occur in sub-Saharan Africa and Brazil. However, no reliable data are available on the long-term sequelae of pyogenic meningitis. In most cases, epilepsy that follows meningitis occurs within 5 yr of the acute illness, and the majority of patients have partial seizures *(95,96)*. Pathological studies have demonstrated that both large and small arteries and veins are involved in the inflammatory process of acute bacterial meningitis, often resulting in cerebral infarction *(97,98)*. This finding may explain the occurrence of focal neurological deficits and partial seizures in these patients. In a recent prospective study in the United States *(99)*, 185 infants and children were followed after bacterial meningitis for a mean duration of 8.9 yr (range, 0.1–15.5 yr). Of these children, 13 developed 1 or more afebrile seizures after the initial hospitalization. The majority of them had their first seizure within 2 yr of the acute illness. The seizures were of focal onset in all but one patient. Ten patients had recurrent seizures (epilepsy), with frequencies ranging from one to innumerable seizures a year. The association of recurrent seizures with persistent neurological signs was most striking and evident in 7 of the 10 patients with epilepsy. These findings add to the evidence that closely associates epilepsy with cerebral damage following intracranial infection.

Viral Infections

Viral encephalitis is a common neurological problem in the tropics, but information regarding its incidence, etiological agents, and sequelae are sparse, largely because of the lack of facilities for viral studies in many tropical countries, which are a prerequisite to accurate diagnosis. The disease may occur in epidemic form as with arbovirus infections, in sporadic form as with herpes simplex virus, mumps, and adenovirus infections, or in a subacute or chronic form as with subacute sclerosing panencephalitis. Japanese encephalitis (JE), perhaps, is the most important and the best documented viral encephalitis in the tropics.

Japanese Encephalitis

Since its first description in 1924, following a large epidemic in Japan, Japanese encephalitis (JE) has affected most countries of Asia. In China, as many as 10,000 cases are reported annually. It was subsiding in China, as well as in Japan and Korea, but increasing and spreading across parts of Bangladesh, Burma, India, Nepal, Thailand, and Vietnam *(100)*. It has also been found transiently as far east as the island of Guam *(92)*.

The disease is caused by an RNA Flavivirus whose main reservoirs are birds (herons and egrets) and mammals (pigs and cattle). The virus is transmitted to man by *Culex* mosquitoes, which breed prolifically in flooded rice fields. Children and nonimmune adults are particularly at risk of infection.

Following an incubation period of 6–16 d, the disease begins with a prodromal phase, which consists of malaise, fever, headache, and vomiting. In the encephalitic phase, the patient develops impairment of consciousness, seizures, signs of meningeal irritation, and focal neurological deficits. Peripheral blood smear usually shows a polymorphonuclear leukocytosis with lymphocytopenia. The CSF shows an increase in protein and pleocytosis, initially neutrophilic and later lymphocytic. The electroencephalogram (EEG) is grossly abnormal, showing marked slowing. Specific diagnosis of JE is made by demonstrating a fourfold rise in antibodies (hemagglutinin-inhibiting and complement-fixing) between acute and convalescent sera. The treatment is mainly symptomatic and supportive, including measures to reduce cerebral edema and to control seizures.

The mortality rates of JE vary from 5% to 50% *(101)*. Autopsies of brains show a diffuse meningoencephalitis, affecting both the gray and white matter of the cerebral hemispheres, basal ganglia, midbrain, brainstem, and cerebellum. Rather characteristic small punched-out necrotic areas are seen in the gray matter *(102)*.

Neurologic sequelae, including intellectual and emotional changes and motor impairment, occur in up to 80% of survivors, especially children *(103)*. The frequency of subsequent epilepsy is not well documented. In an outbreak affecting 128 patients in Bangalore, India, among 78 survivors, 1.3% developed epilepsy *(102)*. In a study of 59 children affected by JE in Chiang Mai, Thailand, 57% of the patients who survived had neurological sequelae, including epilepsy in 20% *(104)*.

Fungal Infections

Subacute or chronic meningitis resembling tuberculous meningitis is the usual presentation of certain fungal infections of the CNS, such as cryptococcosis, candidiasis, histoplasmosis, blastomycosis, coccidioidomycosis, and paracoccidioidomycosis. Some others, such as aspergillosis and dermatiomycosis, present as intracranial, space-occupying lesions. Acute symptomatic seizures are part of their symptomatology. No long-term studies on the incidence of chronic epilepsy following fungal infections are available.

Perinatal Factors

Poor antenatal and perinatal care in developing countries, which results in brain damage in the child, is often claimed to be a factor for the high prevalence of epilepsy in the tropics. In many developing countries, most deliveries in rural areas are conducted by traditional birth attendants. The families are large, and in certain areas the rate of twinning is high *(105)*. The incidence of preterm deliveries is at least twice as high as in developed countries *(106)*. Many of the mothers are multiparous, and it is not unusual to find women having babies well into their late 40s. It has been shown that the incidence of brain damage in the baby increases 5-fold in mothers aged over 30 *(106)*. The mothers may also be malnourished, anemic, and exposed to a variety of infections, which may affect the baby *in utero* or at the time of delivery. All of these factors may contribute to perinatal brain damage.

Neonatal bilirubinemic encephalopathy (NBE) is another disorder that may lead to epilepsy *(107)*. Although relatively uncommon in the West, it is a special problem in many developing countries. In Nigeria *(105)* it is the most common cause of cerebral palsy, accounting for 50% of cases. In Singapore, it is the most common cause of death in babies under the age of 1 wk *(108)*. Causative diseases, such as glucose 6-phosphate dehydrogenase (G6PD) deficiency (43% in the Singapore study *(108)*, and umbilical cord sepsis, probably explain the high incidence of NBE in the tropics.

Febrile Seizures

Febrile seizures are a common acute neurologic disturbance of childhood; the prevalence in the tropics varies from 0.64/1000 in a semiurban and rural area in southern India *(109)*, 2.4/1000 in the Parsi community in Bombay *(110)*, and 5.4/1000 in Ecuador *(111)*, to a high of 14% in the Mariana Islands *(112,113)*. In view of the high frequency of febrile illnesses caused by diseases such as malaria, a higher prevalence of febrile convulsions is expected in the tropics. A question worth appraising is whether the seizures accompanying fevers such as malaria in the tropics are febrile seizures, in the way the term is used in the West, or are the result of direct cerebral insult from infection. Unlike the situation in Caucasians, febrile convulsions in the African child are not a benign condition *(114)*. In one series, the mortality of febrile convulsions was 28% and the morbidity (hemiplegia, cortical blindness, iatrogenic burns with subsequent contractures, conjunctivitis, etc.) was high *(115)*. In survivors of febrile convulsions, 30% developed recurrent nonfebrile seizures within a period of 5 yr *(116)*. The toxic nature of some of the home remedies, such as cow's urine and herbal medicine used in the treatment of convulsions, may also contribute to brain damage *(105,117)*.

Head Injuries

Head injuries have been reported as an important cause of epilepsy in adults in certain communities, particularly in Africa *(118–120)*. These head injuries are attributed to fighting and jousting with heavy sticks and knobkerries, a pastime that serves both as a national sport and a means of settling grievances *(121)*. Cranial trauma related to personal attacks or to traffic accidents is a very common cause of epilepsy both in Brazil and in Uruguay *(122,123)*. In some tropical countries, people climb trees to make a living by plucking coconuts or tapping toddy from palmyra trees, and accidental falls often result in head injuries. Traffic accidents in countries with poor regulation of motor vehicle transit and lack of seat belts are a growing problem in developing nations.

Toxic Agents

Pesticides

Pesticide poisoning is a major public health problem in agricultural countries in the tropics. Self-poisoning with suicidal intent is responsible for over 90% of pesticide-related morbidity and mortality. The majority of patients are young males with a mean age of about 25 yr. Occupational exposure also occurs, for instance, during spraying, because of faulty equipment or techniques. Accidental ingestion of insecticides stored in households may also cause poisoning. Seizures are a common manifestation of both acute and chronic toxicity of most pesticides, especially organochlorine insecticides (OCIs).

OCIs (e.g., dichlorodiphenyltrichloroethane [DDT], benzene hexachloride [BHC], aldrin, dieldrin, endrin, chlordane, endosulfan) are absorbed through the gut, the lungs, and the skin in varying degrees. A significant part of the absorbed dose is stored in fat tissue as the unchanged parent compound. In the CNS, OCIs interfere with fluxes of cations across nerve cell membranes, increasing neuronal irritability. This effect manifests mainly as convulsions or myoclonic jerking. Hyperesthesia and paresthesia of the face and extremities, headache, dizziness, nausea, vomiting, incoordination, tremor, and mental confusion may precede convulsions. Coma and respiratory depression may follow convulsions, at times leading to death.

Epidemic epilepsy in the Lakhimpur Kheri district in India has been attributed to OCI toxicity. Farmers in this region were supplied with BHC for application on their sugar crop. Ignorantly, they used it as a food grain preservative and developed poisoning. Recurrent convulsive seizures often preceded by auditory and visual aura, headache, confusion and memory lapses, impaired vision, and staggering gait were common symptoms. Examination revealed abnormal mental state, pyramidal signs, myoclonic jerks, tremor, cerebellar ataxia, posterior column disorder, and eighth nerve palsies. The EEGs were grossly abnormal with diffuse epileptiform activity *(124)*. A similar epidemic occurred in Sitapur district of the same state in the same year *(125)*. These patients also presented with epilepsy, some in status epilepticus, but signs were few. Similar cases with slight variation in the clinical picture have been seen in various other states in India *(27)*.

There is no specific antidote for OCI poisoning. Morphine or its derivatives, and epinephrine or norepinephrine are contraindicated, because of their depressive effects on the respiratory center and because they may sensitize the myocardium and thus provoke serious cardiac arrhythmias, respectively. Fast-acting anticonvulsants, such as diazepam or clonazepam, are required for controlling convulsions. Benzodiazepines are relatively safe and carry a much smaller risk of sedation and respiratory depression than other sedatives such as barbiturates. Repeated intravenous administration may be required, because the central effects of both these drugs wane rapidly as a result of redistribution to other tissues. Lorazepam may also be used. Very high doses are tolerated without unwanted side effects. In endosulfan poisoning, we have used dexamethasone with a view to reducing cerebral edema, as well as magnesium sulfate on an empirical basis. The mortality seemed to improve, but controlled studies will be necessary before a firm recommendation can be made.

Heavy Metals

Lead poisoning is an important cause of seizures in children. Refining of jewelers' wastes to recover gold, and reconditioning and smelting of lead-containing batteries for recovery of scrap lead are sources of childhood plumbism in Sri Lanka *(126,127)*. Burning lead-containing batteries for cooking or to provide heat *(128)* have also caused lead poisoning in children in poor communities. Convulsions, vomiting, constipation, pica, abdominal colic, pallor, and mental retardation are common symptoms of childhood plumbism, but their nonspecificity makes the diagnosis difficult *(126,127)*.

Drugs

The antimalarial drugs chloroquine and mefloquine are known to be associated with seizures and mental abnormalities in some individuals *(129–131)*. A direct causal relationship has not been clearly established *(132)*. Quinine, the mainstay therapy for falciparum malaria, causes hypoglycemia and may lead indirectly to seizures. Isoniazid, used in the treatment of tuberculosis, has an effect on glutamate decarboxylase and can cause seizures. Often advertised in the Philippines as a "vitamin for the lungs," it is used commonly in high doses and frequently in suicide attempts. Surviving patients have intractable epilepsy *(1)*.

Alcohol

Seizures are a common withdrawal symptom in chronic alcoholics. Alcoholism is also an important cause of epilepsy. Data suggest that the prevalence of epilepsy among alcoholics is at least three times that in the general population and that alcoholism may be more prevalent among epileptic patients than in the general population *(133)*. Consumption of alcohol, illicit liquor in particular, is a growing problem in many tropical countries. Its contribution as an etiological agent of epilepsy in the tropics merits further evaluation.

Heredity

A number of diseases, which follow Mendelian patterns of inheritance, have seizures as part of their manifestation. Inbreeding is relatively common and customary in many developing countries in the tropics. In some communities, a patient with epilepsy, when looking for a marriage partner, may have no alternative but to find someone from a family afflicted by the same illness, because of the associated stigma *(134)*. These practices may increase the risk of seizure disorders in their offspring.

In isolated communities, specific diseases may manifest as seizure disorders. In the Grand Bassa county of Liberia, an environmental factor that possibly interacted with genes to determine host susceptibility was considered to be involved in etiology *(135)*. A hitherto unknown systemic disease of the CNS was thought to be responsible for the seizure disorder in the Wapogoro tribe in Tanzania *(136)*.

Conclusions

A large number of potential etiological factors of epilepsy exist in the tropics, and many diseases and disorders manifest with seizures. Many of these factors are preventable. Most of the infections, parasitic diseases in particular, can be eradicated if proper preventive measures are adopted. Where simple hygienic measures fail, the answer may lie in a vaccine, e.g., the control of epidemic meningococcal meningitis by vaccination. Epilepsy and other long-term sequelae of intracranial infections can be minimized by early detection and prompt, adequate treatment. The physician should, diagnose and treat meningitis by doing a lumbar puncture in every suspected case, especially in children *(137)*. Enforcement of strict traffic regulations, such as speed limits and motorcycle riders wearing helmets, as well as creating public awareness, is urgently needed in many tropical countries. This would slow the rapid increase of head injuries caused by road accidents and consequent posttraumatic epilepsy. Legislation and enforcement of regulations can minimize pesticide-related morbidity and mortality. Finally, some form of genetic counseling should be made available, at least in areas where a specific hereditary predisposition has been established as a cause of seizures or epilepsy *(138)*.

References

1. Bittencourt PRM, Adamolekum B, Bharucha N, Carpio A, Cossio OH, Danesi MA, Dumas M, Meinardi H, Ordinario A, Senanayake N, et al. ILAE Commission report. Epilepsy in the tropics: I. Epidemiology, socioeconomic risk factors, and etiology. *Epilepsia* 1996;37:1121–1127.
2. Senanayake N, Roman GC. Epidemiology of epilepsy in the tropics. *J Trop Geogr Neurol* 1992;2:10–19.
3. Senanayake N, Roman GC. Epilepsy in developing countries. *Bull WHO* 1993;71:247–258.
4. Commission on Tropical Diseases of the International League Against Epilepsy. Relationship between epilepsy and tropical diseases. *Epilepsia* 1994:35:89–93.
5. de Bittencourt PRM, Adamolekum B, Bharucha N, et al. Epilepsy in the tropics: II. Clinical presentations, pathophysiology, immunologic diagnosis, economics, and therapy. *Epilepsia* 1996;37:1128–1137.
6. Medina MT, Rosas E, Rubio-Donnadieu F, Sotelo J. Neurocysticercosis as the main cause of late-onset epilepsy in Mexico. *Arch Intern Med* 1990;150:325–327.
7. Trelles JO, Trelles L. Cysticercosis of the nervous system. In: Vinken PJ, Bruyn GW (eds.), *Handbook of Clinical Neurology,* vol 35. Amsterdam: North-Holland, 1978, pp 291–320.
8. Schenone H, Ramirez R, Rojas A. Aspectos epidemiologicos de la neurocisticercosis en America Latina. *Bol Child Parasitol* 1973;28:61–72.
9. Bittencourt PRM, Gracia CM, Lorenzana P. Epilepsy and parasitosis of the central nervous system. In: Pedley TA, Meldrum BS (eds.), *Recent Advances in Epilepsy,* vol 4. Edinburgh: Churchill Livingstone, 1988, pp 123–159.
10. Crimmins D, Collignon PJ, Dwyer D, Danta G. Neurocysticercosis: an under-recognized cause of neurological problems. *Med J Aust* 1990;152:434–438.
11. Alarcon G, Olivares L. Cysticercosis cerebral. Manifestaciones en un medio de alta prevelencia. *Rev Invest Clin* 1975;27:209–215.
12. Wei GZ, Li CJ, Meng JM, Ding MC. Cysticercosis of the central nervous system. A clinical study of 1,400 cases. *Chin Med J* 1988;101:493–500.
13. Sotelo J, Guerrero V, Rubio F. Neurocysticercosis: a new classification based on active and inactive forms. *Arch Intern Med* 1985;145:442–445.
14. Shorvon SD, Farmer PJ. Epilepsy in developing countries: a review of epidemiological, sociocultural, and treatment aspects. *Epilepsia* 1988;29:S36–S54.
15. Sakamoto AC. 1985. Estudio clinico e prognostico das crises epilepticas que niciam na infancia numa populacao Brasileira. Tese de doutorado. Universidade de Sao Paulo, Ribeirao Preto.
16. Gelfand M. Epilepsy in the African. *Cent Afr J Med* 1957;3:11–12.
17. Bird AV, Heinz HJ, Klintworth G. Convulsive disorders in Bantu mine-workers. *Epilepsia* 1962;3:175–187.
18. Levy LF, Forbes JI, Parirenyatwa TS. Epilepsy in Africans. *Cent Afr J Med* 1964;10:241–245.

19. Powell SJ, Proctor EM, Wilmot AJ, MacLeod IN. Cysticercosis and epilepsy in Africans. *Ann Trop Med Parasitol* 1966;60:152–615.
20. Osuntokun BO. Epilepsy in the African continent. In: Penry JK (ed.), *Epilepsy, the Eighth International Symposium.* New York: Raven, 1977, pp 365–378.
21. Dumas M, Grunitzky E, Deniau M, et al. Epidemiological study of neuro-cysticercosis in northern Togo (West Africa). *Acta Leiden* 1989;57:191–196.
22. Dumas M, Grunitzky K, Belo M, et al. Cysticercosis and neurocysticercosis: epidemiological survey in North Togo. *Bull Soc Pathol Exot Filiales* 1990; 83:263–274.
23. Tandon PN. Cerebral cysticercosis. *Neurosurg Rev* 1983;6:119–127.
24. Wani MA, Banerjee AK, Tandon PN, Bhargava S. Neurocysticercosis—some uncommon presentations. *Neurol India* 1981;29:58–63.
25. Ahuja GK, Mohanta A. Late onset epilepsy. A prospective study. *Acta Neurol Scand* 1982;66:216–226.
26. Veliath AJ, Ratnakar C, Thakur LC. Cysticercosis in South India. *J Trop Med Hyg* 1985;88:25–29.
27. Wadia NH. Clinical neurology. In: *Neurosciences in India: Retrospect and Prospect.* Trivandrum: Neurological Society of India, 1989, pp 437–507.
28. Vejajiva A. Neurological disorders in Southeast Asia. In: Weatherall DJ, Ledingham JGG, Warrell DA (eds.), *Oxford Textbook of Medicine.* Oxford: Oxford University Press, 1987, pp 21.269–21.272.
29. Simanjuntak GM, Margono SS, Sachlan R, Harjono C, Rasidi R, Sutopo B. An investigation of taeniasis and cysticercosis in Bali. *Southeast Asian J Trop Med Public Health* 1977;8:494–497.
30. Subianto DB, Tumada LR, Margono SS. Burns and epileptic fits associated with cysticercosis in mountain people of Irian Jaya. *Trop Geogr Med* 1978;30: 275–278.
31. Gadjusek DC. Introduction of Taenia solium into West New Guinea with a note on an epidemic of burns from cysticercus epilepsy in the Ekari people of the Wissel Lake area. *Papua New Guinea Med J* 1978;21:329–342.
32. Heap BJ. Cerebral cysticercosis as a common cause of epilepsy in Gurkhas in Hong Kong. *J R Army Med Corps* 1990;136:146–149.
33. Roman GC. Neurology in Latin America. In: Bradley WG, Daroff RB, Fenichel GM, Marsden CD (eds.), *Neurology in Clinical Practice.* Boston, MA: Butterworth-Heinemann, 1991, pp 1888–1898.
34. Arseni C, Cristescu A. Epilepsy due to cerebral cysticercosis. *Epilepsia* 1972;13:253–258.
35. Otero E, Cordova S, Diaz F, Garcia-Teruel I, Del Brutto OH. Acquired epileptic aphasia (the Landau-Kleffner syndrome) due to neurocysticercosis. *Epilepsia* 1989;30:569–572.
36. Mazer S, Antoniuk A, Ditzel LFS, Araujo JC. The computed tomographic spectrum of cerebral cysticercosis. *Comput Radiol* 1983;7:373–378.
37. Minguetti G, Ferreira MVC. Computed tomography in neurocysticercosis. *J Neurol Neurosurg Psychiatry* 1983;46:936–942.
38. Rodriguez-Carbajal J, Salgado P, Gutierrez-Alvarado R, Escobar-Izquierdo A, Aruffo C, Palacios E. The acute encephalitic phase of neurocysticercosis: computed tomographic manifestations. *Am J Neuroradiol* 1983;4:51–55.

39. Wadia N, Desai S, Bhatt M. Disseminated cysticercosis. New observations, including CT scan findings and experience with treatment by praziquantel. *Brain* 1988;111:597–614.

40. Sotelo J. Neurocysticercosis. In: Kennedy PGE, Johnson RT (eds.), *Infections of the Nervous System.* London: Butterworths, 1987.

41. Spina-Franca A, Machado LR, Nobrega JPS. Praziquantel in the cerebrospinal fluid in neurocysticercosis. *Arq Neuropsiquiatr* 1985;43:243–259.

42. Spina-Franca A, Nobrega JP, Machado LR, Livramento JA. Neurocysticercosis and praziquantel: long-term development in 100 patients. *Arq Neuropsiquiatr* 1989;47:444–448.

43. Mahmoud AAF, Wahab MFA. Schistosomiasis. In: Warren KS, Mahmoud AAF (eds.), *Tropical and Geographical Medicine.* New York: McGraw-Hill, 1990, pp 458–473.

44. Bird AV. Schistosomiasis of the nervous system. In: Vinken PJ, Bruyn GW, (ed), *Handbook of Clinical Neurology,* vol 35. Amsterdam: North-Holland, 1978, pp 231–241.

45. Scrimgeour EM, Gadjusek DC. Involvement of the central nervous system in *Schistosoma mansoni* and *S. haematobium* infection. *Brain* 1985;108:1023–1038.

46. Chang YC, Chu CC, Fan WK. Cerebral schistosomiasis. *Chin Med J* 1957; 75:892–907.

47. Harinasuta T, Bunnag D. Liver, lung, and intestinal trematodiasis. In: Warren KS, Mahmoud AAF (eds.), *Tropical and Geographical Medicine.* New York: McGraw-Hill, 1990, pp 473–489.

48. Belding DL. *Textbook of Parasitology.* New York: Meredith, 1965.

49. Chang H, Wang C, Yu C, Hsu C, Fang J. Paragonimiasis: a clinical study of 200 adult cases. *Chin Med J* 1958;77:3–9.

50. Oh SJ. The rate of cerebral involvement in cerebral paragonimiasis—an epidemiological study. *Jpn J Parasitol* 1969;18:211–215.

51. Cho WJ, Kim HJ. Ocular symptoms of intracranial tumour (clinical survey of 93 Korean cases). *J Korean Ophthal Soc* 1964;5:35–41.

52. Oh SJ. Paragonimiasis in the central nervous system. In: Vinken PJ, Bruyn GW (eds.), *Handbook of Clinical Neurology,* vol 35. Amsterdam: North-Holland, 1978, pp 243–266.

53. Yokogawa S, Suyemori S. An experimental study of the intracranial parasitism of the human lung fluke *(Paragonimus westermani). Am J Hyg* 1921;1:63–78.

54. Oh SJ. Cerebral paragonimiasis. *J Neurol Sci* 1968;8:27–48.

55. Fan K-J, Pezeshkpour GH. Cerebral sparganosis. *Neurology* 1986;36:1249–1251.

56. Arseni C, Marinescu V. Epilepsy in cerebral hydatidosis. *Epilepsia* 1974;15:45–54.

57. Elliot DL, Tolle SW, Goldberg L, Miller JB. Pet-associated illness. *N Engl J Med* 1985;313:985–995.

58. Dada T. Parasites and epilepsy in Nigeria. *Trop Geogr Med* 1970;22:313–322.

59. Navia BA, Petito CK, Gold JWM, Cho ES, Jordan BD, Price RW. Cerebral toxoplasmosis complicating the acquired immune deficiency syndrome: clinical and neurological findings in 27 patients. *Ann Neurol* 1986;19:224–238.

60. Krich JA, Remington JS. Toxoplasmosis in adult: an overview. *N Engl J Med* 1978;298:550–553.

61. Ruskin J, Remington JS. Toxoplasmosis of the compromised host. *Ann Intern Med* 1976;84:193–199.

62. Stern H, Elek SD, Booth JC, Fleck DG. Microbial causes of mental retardation. The role of prenatal infections with cytomegalovirus, rubella virus and toxoplasma. *Lancet* 1969;2:443–448.

63. Feldman HA. Toxoplasmosis. *Pediatrics* 1958;22:559–574.

64. Michaowicz R, Jozwiak S, Ignatowicz R. Landau-Kleffner syndrome—epileptic aphasia in children—possible role of *Toxoplasma gondii* infection. *Acta Paediatr Hung* 1988;29:337–342.

65. Toro G, Roman G, Navarro de Roman L. Toxoplasmosis. In: Toro G, Roman G, Navarro de Roman L (eds.), *Neurologia Tropical: Aspectos Neuropatologicos de la Medicina Tropical.* Bogota: Editorial Printer Colombiana, 1983, pp 113–117.

66. Lumsden WHR. Trypanosomiasis. *Br Med Bull* 1972;28:34–38.

67. Dumas M, Breton JC, Alexandre MP, Girad PL, Giodarno C. Etat actuel de la therapeutique de la trypanosomiase humaine africaine. *Presse Med* 1985;14:253–256.

68. Neves J. Trypanosomiase africana. In: Neves J (ed.), *Diagnostico e tratamento das doencas infectuosas e parasitarias.* Rio de Janeiro: Guanabara-Koogan, 1983, pp 725–731.

69. Ferreira FSC, Rocha LAC. Tripanossomfase africana. In: Veronesi R (ed.), *Doencas infecciosas e parasitarias.* Rio de Janeiro: Guanbara-Koogan, 1982, pp 713–723.

70. Lingam S, Marshall WC, Wilson J, Gould JM, Reinhardt MC, Evans DA. Congenital trypanosomiasis in a child born in London. *Dev Med Child Neurol* 1985;27:670–674.

71. Hajduk SL, Englund PT, Smith DH. African trypanosomiasis. In: Warren KS, Mahmoud AAF (eds.), *Tropical and Geographical Medicine.* New York: McGraw-Hill, 1990, pp 268–281.

72. Dias JCP, Cancado JR, Chiari CA. Doenca de Chagas. In: Neves J (ed.), *Diagnostico e Tratamento das Doencas Infectuosa e Parasitarias.* Rio de Janeiro: Guanabara-Koogan, 1983, pp 694–725.

73. Jardim E, Takayanagui OM. Epilepsia e doenca de Chagas cronica. *Arq Neuropsiquiatr* 1981;39:32–41.

74. Nogueira N, Coura JR. American trypanosomiasis (Chagas' disease). In: Warren KS, Mahmoud AAF (eds.), *Tropical and Geographical Medicine.* New York: McGraw-Hill, 1990, pp 281–296.

75. MacPherson GG, Warrell MJ, White NJ, Looareesuwan S, Warrell DA. Human cerebral malaria: a quantitative ultrastructural analysis of parasitized erythrocyte sequestration. *Am J Pathol* 1985;119:385–401.

76. Toro G, Roman GC. Cerebral malaria: a disseminated vasculomyelinopathy. *Arch Neurol* 1978;35:271–275.

77. Grau GE, Fajardo LF, Piguet P-F, Allet B, Lambert P-H, Vassalli P. Tumour necrosis factor (Cachectin) as an essential mediator in murine cerebral malaria. *Science* 1987;237:1210–1212.

78. Vietze G. Malaria and other protozoal diseases. In: Vinken PJ, Bruyn GW (eds.), *Handbook of Clinical Neurology,* vol 35. Amsterdam: North-Holland, 1978, pp 143–160.

79. Espinal CA, Toro G. Malaria. In: Chalem F, Escandon JE, Campos J, Esguerra R (eds.), *Medicina Interna.* Bogota: Editorial Norma, 1986, pp 278–288.

80. Toro G, Roman G, Navarro de Roman L. Paludismo. In: Toro G, Roman G, Navarro de Roman L (eds.), *Neurologia Tropical: Aspectos Neuropatologicos de la Medicina Tropical.* Bogota: Editorial Printer Colombiana, 1983, pp 106–113.

81. Senga P, Mayanda HF, Nzingoula S. Profile of seizures in infants and young children in Brazzaville (Congo). *Ann Pediatr* 1985;32:477–480.

82. Lombardo L, Alonso P, Arroyo LS, Saenz L, Brandt H, Mateos JH. Cerebral amebiasis: report of 17 cases. *J Neurosurg* 1964;21:704–708.

83. Toro G, Roman G, Navarro de Roman L. Amebiasis cerebral. In: Toro G, Roman G, Navarro de Roman L (eds.), *Neurologia Tropical: Aspectos Neuropatologicos de la Medicina Tropical.* Bogota: Editorial Printer Colombiana, 1983, pp 120–122.

84. Duma RJ, Rosemblum WI, McGehee RF, Jones M, Nelson EC. Primary amoebic meningoencephalitis caused by naegleria: two new cases. Response to amphotericin B and a review. *Ann Intern Med* 1971;74:861–869.

85. Martinez AJ. Is *Acanthamoeba encephalitis* an opportunistic infection? *Neurology* 1980;30:567–574.

86. Lorber J. Long term follow-up of 100 children who recovered from tuberculous meningitis. *Pediatrics* 1961;28:778–782.

87. Donner M, Wasz-Hockert O. Late neurological sequelae of tuberculous meningitis. *Acta Pediatr* 1962;51(Suppl. 141):34–38.

88. Dastur DK, Udani PM. Pathology and pathogenesis of tuberculous encephalopathy. *Acta Neuropathol* 1966;5:311–326.

89. Udani PM, Dastur DK. Tuberculous encephalopathy with and without meningitis. Clinical features and pathological correlations. *J Neurol Sci* 1970;10:541–561.

90. Bahemuka M, Murungi H. Tuberculosis of the nervous system. A clinical, radiological and pathological study of 39 consecutive cases in Riyadh, Saudi Arabia. *J Neurol Sci* 1989;90:67–76.

91. Teoh R, Humphries MJ, O'Mahoney SG. Symptomatic intracranial tuberculoma developing during treatment of tuberculosis: a report of 10 patients and review of the literature. *Q J Med* 1987;63:449–460.

92. Bharucha NE, Bharucha EP. Neurology in India. In: Bradley WG, Daroff RB, Fenichel GM, Marsden CD (eds.), *Neurology in Clinical Practice.* Boston, MA: Butterworth-Heinemann, 1991, pp 1925–1941.

93. Vyravanathan S, Senanayake N. Tuberculosis presenting with hemiplegia. *J Trop Med Hyg* 1979;82:38–40.

94. Wadia RS, Makhale CN, Kelkar AV, Grant KB. Focal epilepsy in India with special reference to lesions showing ring or disc-like enhancement on contrast computed tomography. *J Neurol Neurosurg Psychiatry* 1987;50:1298–1301.

95. Annegers JF, Hauser WA, Beghi E, Nicolosi A, Kurland LT. The risk of unprovoked seizures after encephalitis and meningitis. *Neurology* 1988;38:1407–1410.

96. Bergamini L, Bergamasco B, Benna P, Gilli M. Acquired etiological factors in 1785 epileptic subjects: clinical-anamnestic research. *Epilepsia* 1977;18:437–444.

97. Dodge PR, Swartz MN. Bacterial meningitis—a review of selected aspects. II. Special neurologic problems, postmeningitic complications and clinicopathological correlations. *N Engl J Med* 1965;272:954–960.

98. Rorke LB, Pitts FW. Purulent meningitis: the pathological basis of clinical manifestations. *Clin Pediatr* 1963;2:64–71.

99. Pomeroy SL, Holmes SJ, Dodge PR, Feign RD. Seizures and other neurologic sequelae of bacterial meningitis in children. *N Engl J Med* 1990;323:1651–1657.

100. Umenai T, Krzysko R, Bektimirov TA, Assaad FA. Japanese encephalitis: current worldwide status. *Bull WHO* 1985;63:625–631.

101. Weaver OM, Pieper S, Kurland R. Sequelae of the arthropod-borne encephalitides: V. Japanese encephalitis. *Neurology* 1958;8:888–889.

102. Gourie-Devi M, Deshpande DH. Japanese encephaltis. In: Prasad LS, Kulczycki LL (eds.), *Paediatric Problems.* New Delhi: S Chand, 1982, pp 340–356.

103. Monath TP. Japanese encephalitis—a plague of the orient. *N Engl J Med* 1988; 319:641–643.

104. Poneprasert B. Japanese encephalitis in children in northern Thailand. *Southeast Asian J Trop Med Public Health* 1989;20:599–603.

105. Animashaun A. Aetiology of cerebral palsy in African children. *Afr J Med Sci* 1971;2:165–171.

106. Malamud N, Itabashi HH, Castor J, Messinger HB. An etiologic and diagnostic study of cerebral palsy. *J Pediatr* 1964;65:270–293.

107. Bergamasco B, Benna P, Ferrero P, et al. Perinatal pathology and epilepsy. *Prog Clin Biol Res* 1983;124:185–198.

108. Boon WH. A surveillance system to prevent kernicterus in Singapore infants. *J Singapore Paediatr Soc* 1975;17:1–9.

109. Gourie-Devi M, Rao VN, Prakashi R. Neuroepidemiological study in semiurban and rural areas in South India: pattern of neurological disorders including motor neurone disease. In: Gourie-Devi M (ed.), *Motor Neurone Disease.* New Delhi: Oxford and IBH Publishing, 1987, pp 11–21.

110. Bharucha NE, Bharucha EP, Dastur HD, Schoenberg BS. Pilot survey of the prevalence of neurologic disorders in the Parsi community of Bombay. *Am J Prev Med* 1987;3:293–299.

111. Cruz ME, Schoenberg BS, Ruales J, et al. Pilot study to detect neurologic disease in Ecuador among a population with a high prevalence of endemic goiter. *Neuroepidemiology* 1985;4:108–116.

112. Mathai KV, Dunn DP, Kurland LT, Reeder FA. Convulsive disorders in the Mariana islands. *Epilepsia* 1968;9:77–85.

113. Stanhope JM, Brody JA, Brink E. Convulsions among the Chamorro people of Guam, Mariana Islands, I. Seizure disorders. *Am J Epidemiol* 1972;95:292–298.

114. Osuntokun BO. Malaria and the nervous system. *Afr J Med Sci* 1983;12:165–172.

115. Osuntokun BO, Odeku EL, Sinnettee CH. Convulsive disorders in Nigerians: the febrile convulsions. *E Afr Med J* 1969;46:385–394.

116. Osuntokun BO. Treatment of epilepsy: with special reference to developing countries. *Prog Neuropsychopharmacol* 1979;3:81–94.

117. Asirifi Y. Aetiology of cerebral palsy in developing countries. *Dev Med Child Neurol* 1972;14:230–232.

118. Cosnett JE. Neurological disease in Natal. In: Spillaine JD (ed.), *Tropical Neurology.* London: Oxford University Press, 1973, pp 259–272.

119. Haddock DRW. An attempt to assess the prevalence of epilepsy in Accra. *Ghana Med J* 1967;6:140.

120. Tellang BV, Hettiaratchi ESG. Patterns of epilepsy in Kenya—a clinical analysis of 115 cases. *E Afr Med J* 1981;58:437–444.

121. Cosnett JE. Neurological disorders in the Zulu. *Neurology* 1964; 14:443–454.

122. Bittencourt PRM, Turner M. Epilepsy in the Third World: Latin American aspects. In: Dam M, Gram L (eds.), *Comprehensive Epileptology.* New York: Raven, 1991, pp 807–820.

123. de Pasquet EG, Pietra M, Bonnevaure S, Silva NP, Gomensoro JB, Tenza M. Estudio epidemiologico de 500 epilepticos adultos procedentes de una poblacion hospitalaria. *Acta Neurol Latinoam* 1976;22:50–65.

124. Khare SB, Rizvi AG, Shukla OP, Singh RRP, Prakash O, Misra VD. Epidemic outbreak of neuromuscular manifestations due to chronic BHC poisoning. *J Assoc Physicians India* 1977;25:215–222.
125. Nag D, Singh GC, Sanong S. Epilepsy epidemic due to benzahexachlorine. *Trop Geogr Med* 1977;29:229–232.
126. Mirando EH, Gomez M. Lead poisoning in childhood in Ceylon. *Arch Dis Child* 1967;42:579–582.
127. Mirando EH, Ranasinghe L. Lead encephalopathy in children: uncommon clinical aspects. *Med J Aust* 1970;2:966–968.
128. Greengard J, Rowley W, Elam H, Perlstein M. Lead encephalopathy in children: intravenous use of urea and its management. *N Engl J Med* 1961;264:1027–1030.
129. Torrey EF. Chloroquine seizures. Report of four cases. *JAMA* 1968;204:867–870.
130. Fish DR, Espir MLE. Convulsions associated with prophylactic antimalarial drugs: implications for people with epilepsy. *Br Med J* 1988;297:526–527.
131. Bem JL, Kerr L, Stuercheler D. Mefloquine prophylaxis: an overview of spontaneous reports of severe psychiatric reactions and convulsions. *J Trop Med Hyg* 1992;95:167–179.
132. Hellgren U, Rombo L. Malaria prophylaxis and epilepsy. *Br Med J* 1988;297:1267.
133. Chan AWK. Alcoholism and epilepsy. *Epilepsia* 1985;26:323–333.
134. Aall-Jilek LM. Epilepsy in the Wapogoro tribe in Tanganyika. *Acta Psychiatry Neurol Scand* 1965;41:57–86.
135. Goudsmit J, van der Waals FW, Gajdusek DC. Epilepsy in the Gbawein and Wroughbarh Clan of Grand Bassa County, Liberia: the endemic occurrence of 'See-ee' in the native population. *Neuroepidemiology* 1983;2:24–34.
136. Jilek-Aall L, Jilek W, Miller JR. Clinical and genetic aspects of seizure disorders prevalent in an isolated African population. *Epilepsia* 1979;20:613–622.
137. Chandra B. Epilepsy in developing countries, Part I. Epilepsy in Indonesia. In: Laidlaw J, Richens A, Oxley J (eds.), *A Textbook of Epilepsy.* Edinburgh: Churchill Livingstone, 1988, pp 511–518.
138. Senanayake N, Roman GC. Aetiological factors of epilepsy in the tropics. *J Trop Geogr Neurol* 1991;1:69–80.

19

Seizures in the ICU Patient

Michael M. Frucht, MD
and Thomas P. Bleck, MD, FACP, FCCM, FCCP

Introduction

For many physicians, seizures represent one of the most disconcerting disease manifestations encountered. For family members of the afflicted patient, seizures are one of the few potential emergencies that they can identify (or misidentify) easily. This uneasiness can be amplified further for the critical care physician. Sudden thrashing about by a critically ill patient could remove delicately placed catheters and is a cause for real concern. Seizures remain a common cause of admission to caretakers in intensive care units (ICUs) *(1)*. In this patient population, prompt action is required to protect the patient from further complications.

Seizures themselves, however, are only a symptom of an underlying disease process. The physician must determine whether this process is a preexisting epilepsy, a readily treatable provoking condition, or a sign of a new, life-threatening neurologic problem. Prompt recognition of the underlying etiology is required for effective treatment. Seizures represent an imbalance between normal excitation and inhibition in the brain, and most of the currently available antiseizure agents act to reestablish more normal neuronal inhibition *(2)*.

Classification

To facilitate communication, a common understanding of terminology should be used. In 1989, the International League Against Epilepsy published a classification of epilepsy and epileptic syndromes *(3)*. Further classification is possible but may not help the ICU physician in either diagnosing the

From: *Seizures: Medical Causes and Management*
Edited by: N. Delanty © Humana Press, Inc., Totowa, NJ

etiology or treating the seizure. Whenever possible, the treating physician should attempt to classify a patient with seizures according to his or her epilepsy syndrome. This can help in the identification of more specific etiologies and therapeutic interventions. Additionally, by understanding the epilepsy syndrome, a more selective strategy may be possible for identifying which radiologic and laboratory investigations would be most beneficial.

Etiology

Seizures are the second most common neurologic complication in critically ill patients (*1*). However, rather than attempting to investigate all of the possible causes of seizures in critically ill patients, the physician should consider what disorders afflicting the patient may be epileptogenic. Some of the more frequently diagnosed causes for new-onset seizures in critically ill patients are metabolic encephalopathies (e.g., nonketotic hyperglycemia), new cerbrovascular diseases (e.g., intracerebral hemorrhage in the setting of thrombocytopenia), infections (e.g., aspergillosis in the leukopenic patient), and previously undiagnosed neoplasms.

Table 1 demonstrates some common etiologies of seizures arising in critically ill patients (*1,4*). The two series presented differed substantially in design, especially in their exclusion criteria, but provide a general guideline for differential diagnosis. The original publications should be consulted for more detail.

Nonconvulsive status epilepticus (NCSE) is a problem of growing recognition and importance in critically ill patients (*5*). It may occur *de novo* or as a consequence of incompletely treated convulsive status epilepticus (SE) (*6–8*).

Discrete Seizures

Regardless of the etiology, seizures can be divided into two temporal categories: discrete events, in which the seizure is followed quickly by a return to normal level functioning, and SE, in which seizure activity is ongoing. When diagnosing discrete seizures, it is important to make sure that the patient has completely returned to baseline. Subtle signs of decreased mental status or twitching may be signs of ongoing seizure activity. Electroencephalographic monitoring should be considered in such patients, as these signs may represent nonconvulsive SE (*9*).

Recognition of seizures is usually not difficult. Clinicians usually can identify a tonic-clonic seizure and most myoclonic, absence, or simple motor seizures. However, in the ICU, where patients often already have diminished consciousness, identification of subtle signs may be more difficult. Discrete seizures may simply manifest themselves with repetitive movements or intermittent symptoms, such as decreased mental status, hallucinations, or aphasia.

Table 1
Etiology of Seizures in Critically Ill Patients

Etiology	Prospective Rush Series[a]	Retrospective Mayo Series[b]
Vascular	24	5
Infectious	11	
Metabolic	11	18
Intracranial mass lesion	4	
Hypoxia	4	
CNS lupus	3	
Hypertensive encephalopathy	3	
Arrhythmia	2	
Other or unknown	3	6
Drug toxicity	(excluded from study)	8
Drug withdrawal	(excluded from study)	18

[a]Sample of 61 of 1850 patients; some had more than one etiology (1).
[b]Sample of 55 of 27,723 patients (4).

Although these conditions can be associated with other neurologic and psychiatric disturbances, seizures should enter into the differential diagnosis. If no other cause for these symptoms is apparent, a neurological consultation should be obtained, and an electroencephalogram (EEG) should be performed.

Managing some patients with discrete seizures may allow the luxury of time, letting the physician begin a thorough investigation of the process, as well as starting medications to prevent further seizure occurrences. Assuming the patient is stable from a cardiovascular standpoint, often obtaining basic chemistries, a blood count, and a urinalysis is beneficial. A review of the medical record to determine if there has been an inadvertent discontinuation of medications is also important. Patients who have been on long-term benzodiazepine therapy may seize upon abrupt withdrawal of the drug. If the patient has been in the hospital only a short time, review of the prehospital medication list may reveal a chronic centrally acting medication that has been discontinued.

Furthermore, discussion with the patient's family often reveals that the patient is dependent on ethanol, which is manifested only when the patient has not been able to drink in the ICU. Although alcohol withdrawal is commonly thought to lead to generalized seizures, focal seizures may result in a substantial minority (10). It is often prudent to screen the patient's serum and urine for drugs of abuse. If a patient has a suspected seizure history, contacting the treating physician may eliminate the need for costly and/or invasive tests. This may also be helpful in determining a more definite treatment strategy.

Neuroimaging is almost always indicated with new onset of seizures, whether focal or generalized. By definition, a focal seizure is associated with an area of cerebral cortex that is more irritable than other areas. This can be the result of previous cerebral infarction, tumor, arteriovenous malformation (AVM), hemorrhage, or abscess. In other cases, such as when a metabolic disturbance, including hyperglycemia, is involved, a partial seizure may have no identifiable cortical lesion. However, seizures in critically ill patients are often secondarily generalized, with any partial component unobserved or misinterpreted. Thus, unless the cause of the seizure is certain, magnetic resonance imaging (MRI) should be considered. If the patient's condition contraindicates an MRI study, then a computed tomographic (CT) study should be obtained.

Because infection is a cause of discrete seizures, a lumbar puncture (LP) is often part of the workup. There is debate as to whether coagulation studies and platelet counts are required before this test is performed because of the risks of epidural hematoma and intracranial bleeding. A recent survey of neurology departments suggests that if there is no personal or family history of a bleeding disorder, the LP can be performed *(11)*. Another issue is whether all patients need imaging prior to a LP. In the presence of focal abnormalities or impaired consciousness, many physicians opt to perform a scan prior to the LP. The risk of herniation may be higher in these patients, as there may be an underlying mass lesion. If there is a question of infection, appropriate antibiotic treatment should begin immediately after blood cultures are obtained.

Management of Discrete Seizures

If a patient is at risk for further worsening of an underlying condition should another seizure occur (e.g., unstable angina), an aggressive approach to preventing seizure recurrence is warranted. In general, the physician must weigh the prognosis of the patient, combined with the severity of the seizures and possible complications. If a metabolic insult or mass lesion can be treated, long-term therapy may not be needed. If abrupt cessation of seizures is needed, the use of a benzodiazepine such as lorazepam should be entertained. Lorazepam is preferred over other benzodiazepines for this purpose because of its longer half-life. If a more chronic antiepileptic medication is needed, fosphenytoin (or phenytoin as dictated by local practice) at 20 mg/kg may be used. Intravenous loading doses of fosphenytoin or phenytoin may produce sedation and eye-movement abnormalities, adverse effects that are not seen when the drug is given orally. Other intravenous choices include phenobarbital (15–20 mg/kg loading dose if a rapid effect is required) and valproate (20–30 mg/kg loading dose) *(12)*. The latter drug is usually well tolerated *(13)*, although large intravenous doses may produce hypotension in rare cases *(14)*. Valproate is a particularly useful agent in patients whose advance directives prohibit intubation, as benzodiazepines and phenobarbital may impair ventilation. It is also useful in patients in whom the sedating effects of the other drugs may make the neurologic examination difficult to follow.

Whether patients remain on long-term anticonvulsant therapy is a decision best made after the patient has left the ICU. Patients often remain on medications for months or years after such medications have been started in the ICU, often without careful thought about the need to continue them. Although anticonvulsant medications are relatively safe, some risk exists from both the medications and their drug–drug interactions. Therefore, if it is thought that the patient has only a certain window that needs to be treated, the ICU and other hospital physicians should communicate directly with the patient's primary physician to prevent unnecessary long-term medication.

Status Epilepticus

A standard definition of SE is a single seizure that persists for more than 30 min, or several seizures without return to baseline level of consciousness in between. The 30-min duration was chosen arbitrarily, and if treatment is delayed because of this definition it may be harmful to the patient *(15)*. When seizures are videotaped and timed, the average length of seizure is 62 s *(16)*; in this study, no generalized tonic-clonic seizure lasted more than 2 min. There is also evidence that the benzodiazepine receptor has a decrease in activity as SE progresses *(17)*. This has been seen both at the receptor level and at the organism level. In the latter, SE in experimental animals was terminated more readily with diazepam given after the first seizure as opposed to treatment after the second seizure *(18)*. This suggests that SE is a dynamic process, and what may be effective treatment early may not be as effective later.

Management of SE should be thought of similarly to any other emergency in the ICU. **Table 2** suggests an approach to management.

A recent study involving veterans, comparing four initial treatments for SE, found that lorazepam was statistically significantly superior to phenytoin treatment *(19)*. There was a nonstatistically significant trend toward better control compared with phenobarbital or diazepam treatment followed by phenytoin. There is no evidence that doses higher than 8 mg are efficacious *(20)*. Approximately 65% of patients with SE in the VA study involving veterans responded to this treatment. The use of a second or third conventional medication only controlled 9% and 3% of patients, respectively.

If a patient does not respond rapidly to lorazepam, fosphenytoin is normally used as a second-line agent for SE patients with peripheral intravenous access and phenytoin for those with central access.

Any patient whose seizures do not stop after use of a second conventional agent should be considered to be in refractory SE. If the patient has not been intubated previously, intubation is begun electively at this point and either

Table 2
Suggested Management of SE[a]

Elapsed Time from Recognition of SE (min)	Decision Point	Intervention	Comments
0	Recognition of SE	Obtain help and begin management	
0	Airway and ventilatory control	Terminate SE as rapidly as possible (see below); if intubation using a neuromuscular junction agent is indicated, use a nondepolarizing drug (e.g., 1.5 mg/kg rapacuronium)	
0	Monitor blood pressure	Do not treat hypertension (blood pressure will usually fall as anticonvulsant agents are administered) Treat hypotension with fluids and vasopressors as indicated by clinical setting	
0	Exclude hypoglycemia		
5	Terminate SE	0.1 mg/kg lorazepam	In hypotensive patients, consider using ketamine at an earlier stage than listed below
15	If SE persists, proceed to	20–25 mg/kg phenytoin or fosphenytoin	
40	If SE persists, proceed to	0.2 mg/kg midazolam loading dose, followed by an infusion of 0.1–2.0 mg/kg per hour (1.5–300 µg/kg per minute)	If SE is apparently terminated (at any step), observe for improvement in level of consciousness; if patient does not begin to improve, rule out NCSE by EEG
(depends on previous stage)	If SE persists or recurs, proceed to	1–3 mg/kg propofol loading dose, followed by an infusion of 1–15 mg/kg per hour (15–250 µg/kg per minute)	Intubation, mechanical ventilation, and continuous EEG monitoring required by this point; many patients will require arterial and central venous (or pulmonaryarterial) catheterization and hemodynamic support
(depends on previous stage)	If SE persists or recurs proceed to	1–4.5 mg/kg ketamine loading dose, followed by an infusion of 10–50 µg/kg per minute	Consider 20–30 mg/kg valproate as an alternative
(depends on previous stage)	If SE persists or recurs proceed to	12 mg/kg pentobarbital loading dose, followed by an infusion of 0.25–2.0 mg/kg per hour	

[a]Items at same elapsed time should be undertaken concurrently.

midazolam or propofol is started *(21,22)*. Recent experience suggests that midazolam should be the first choice, followed by propofol if midazolam fails or tachyphylaxis supervenes *(23)*. Most patients treated as such will require systemic arterial and central venous or pulmonary arterial catheterization for hemodynamic management unless their SE is terminated rapidly. Continuous electroencephalographic monitoring is required at this point; intermittent electroencephalographic sampling is inadequate to ensure that seizures have been suppressed. The dose of the drug is titrated to produce seizure suppression without regard for EEG background activity. Although there are many conflicting viewpoints on this topic *(24),* a burst-suppression background appears to be neither necessary nor sufficient to ensure control of seizures. The dose should be tapered by 50% every 12 h, returning to the last effective dose if more than a few brief seizures emerge. High concentrations of conventional anticonvulsants (e.g., phenobarbital concentrations in excess of 100 μg/mL) may be necessary to allow successful tapering of the agent being used for control of refractory SE.

For the patient who remains refractory at this point, pentobarbital coma would be initiated *(25)*. Recommended loading doses for pentobarbital range between 5 and 12 mg/kg, with maintenance doses beginning at 1 mg/kg per hour. Adverse effects from pentobarbital include hypotension, diminished myocardial contractility, immune suppression, poikilothermia, and interference with clearance of pulmonary secretions, as well as loss of gastric motility. Additionally, H_2 blockade *(26)* and deep venous thrombosis (DVT) prophylaxis are used.

Ketamine is emerging as a useful agent for the control of refractory SE, and has the added advantage of an intrinsic sympathomimetic effect *(27)*.

The role of long-term anticonvulsant medications is somewhat different in patients with SE when compared to patients with discrete seizures. In almost all cases of SE, the patient should remain on one or more anticonvulsant medications for a period of time because of the serious complications that can occur with repeated seizures or SE. Exceptions to this would include conditions such as ethanol withdrawal and altered metabolic states such as hyper- or hypoglycemia. In most cases, the patients will remain on their antiepileptic medications throughout their stay in the ICU and often throughout hospitalization. The decision to discontinue should be made by the primary physician or primary neurologist at some later time.

There are several main complications of SE. Certainly, patients are at risk for hypoxic injury attributable to tonic-clonic SE if the airway is threatened. In patients with NCSE, there remains debate about whether neuronal damage occurs, but this should not deter the ICU physician from treating such patients aggressively. Rhabdomyolysis is a common complication, especially in tonic-clonic SE. This is usually best treated with resolution of the seizures, as well as adequate hydration of the patient to protect against renal damage. Finally, hyperthermia can often be a complicating factor. The use of external cooling blankets may be of benefit, but again, as the seizures are treated, this should correct itself rapidly.

Overview for the Critical Care Physician

Introduction

1. Seizures are a common neurologic disorder in the critically ill patient.
2. Seizures are a manifestation of an underlying disease, and the treatment of the patient cannot be confined to symptomatic seizure suppression.
3. By rapidly identifying patients with seizures, morbidity and mortality can be reduced.

Discrete Seizures

1. There are many causes of seizures in the intensive care unit (ICU) patient.
2. Diagnosis should be on clinical grounds, i.e., tonic-clonic or focal seizures. In patients who do not regain their prior level of consciousness, the possibility of non-convulsive status epilepticus (NCSE) should be entertained.
3. Recognition and treatment or elimination of the cause of a seizure is often both the best short- and long-term management. The decision on long-term antiepileptic medication use should reflect the cause, prognosis, and severity of the seizure(s).

Status Epilepticus

1. The classic definition of status epilepticus (SE) is that of 30 min of continuous seizing or failure to return to baseline between seizures lasting over 30 min. This may not reflect the clinical and experimental data suggesting that spontaneously breaking seizures have a much shorter duration and that different mechanisms seem to be active throughout SE.
2. The etiology of SE is different for different age groups
3. A suggested treatment protocol is presented.

Conclusions

1. Rapid identification and treatment of patients with seizures is needed.
2. Treatment of the symptomatic seizure necessitates treating the underlying disease.
3. The careful use of electroencephalographic monitoring can help to identify when treatment needs to be adjusted.

Summary

A patient with seizures in the ICU will always remain a challenge for the treating physician. The successful physician will always be the one who can quickly identify the underlying etiology causing this symptom. By using electroencephalography and appropriate imaging and laboratory tests, patients can be managed positively.

Management of seizures, particularly SE, requires an organized approach to treat both the symptom and the underlying etiology. In treatment of SE, the physician should have a treatment strategy that he or she is comfortable with prior to initiation of treatment. In most cases, the use of lorazepam, followed by fosphenytoin or phenytoin, will be the first step. Patients in the ICU in refractory SE require excellent multidisciplinary critical care to treat the short- and long-term complications of this problem.

References

1. Bleck TP, Smith MC, Pierre-Louis JC, et al. Neurologic complications of critical medical illnesses. *Crit Care Med* 1993;21:98–103.
2. Fountain NB, Lothman EW. Pathophysiology of status epilepticus. *J Clin Neurophysiol* 1995;12:326–342.
3. Commission on Classification and Terminology of the International League Against Epilepsy: proposal for revised classification of epilepsies and epileptic syndromes. *Epilepsia* 1989;30:389–399.
4. Wijdicks EF, Sharbrough FW. New-onset seizures in critically ill patients. *Neurology* 1993;43:1042–1044.
5. Young GB, Jordan KG, Doig GS. An assessment of nonconvulsive seizures in the intensive care unit using continuous EEG monitoring: an investigation of variables associated with mortality. *Neurology* 1996;47:83–89.
6. Litt B, Wityk RJ, Hertz SH, et al. Nonconvulsive status epilepticus in the critically ill elderly. *Epilepsia* 1998;39:1194–1202.
7. Fagan KJ, Lee SI. Prolonged confusion following convulsions due to generalized nonconvulsive status epilepticus. *Neurology* 1990;40:1689–1694.
8. DeLorenzo RJ, Waterhouse EJ, Towne AR, Boggs JG, Ko D, DeLorenzo GA, Brown A, Garnett L. Persistent nonconvulsive status epilepticus after the control of convulsive status epilepticus. *Epilepsia* 1998;39:833–840.
9. Delanty N, Vaughan CJ, French JA: Medical causes of seizures. *Lancet* 1998;352:383–390.
10. Alldredge BK, Lowenstein DH. Status epilepticus related to alcohol abuse. *Epilepsia* 1993;34:1033–1037.
11. Waldman W, Laureno R. Precautions for lumbar puncture: a survey of neurologic educators. *Neurology* 1999;52:1296.
12. Venkataraman V, Wheless JW. Safety of rapid intravenous infusion of valproate loading doses in epilepsy patients. *Epilepsy Res* 1999;35:147–153.
13. Sinha S, Naritoku DK. Intravenous valproate is well tolerated in unstable patients with status epilepticus. *Neurology* 2000;55:722–724.
14. White JR, Santos CS. Intravenous valproate associated with significant hypotension in the treatment of status epilepticus. *J Child Neurol* 1999;14:822–823.
15. Lowenstein DH, Bleck T, Macdonald RL. It's time to revise the definition of status epilepticus. *Epilepsia* 1999;40:120–122.
16. Theodore WH, Porter RJ, Albert P, et al. The secondarily generalized tonic-clonic seizure: a videotape analysis. *Neurology* 1994;44:1403–1407.
17. Kapur J, Macdonald RL. Rapid seizure-induced reduction of benzodiazepine and Zn2+ sensitivity of hippocampal dentate granule cell $GABA_A$ receptors. *J Neurosci* 1997;17:7532–7540.
18. Walton NY, Treiman DM. Response of status epilepticus induced by lithium and pilocarpine to treatment with diazepam. *Exp Neurol* 1988;101:267–275.

19. Treiman DM, Meyers PD, Walton NY, et al. A comparison of four treatments for generalized convulsive status epilepticus. Veterans Affairs Status Epilepticus Cooperative Study Group. *N Engl J Med* 1998;339:792–798.
20. Leppik IE, Derivan AT, Homan RW, Walker J, Ramsay RE, Patrick B. Double-blind study of lorazepam and diazepam in status epilepticus. *JAMA* 1983;249:1452–1454.
21. Kumar A, Bleck TP. Intravenous midazolam for the treatment of refractory status epilepticus. *Crit Care Med* 1992;20:483–488.
22. Parent JM, Lowenstein DH. Treatment of refractory generalized status epilepticus with continuous infusion of midazolam. *Neurology* 1994;44:1837–1840.
23. Prasad A, Worrall BB, Bertram EB, Bleck TP. Propofol and midazolam in the treatment of refractory status epilepticus. *Epilepsia* 2001;42:308–386.
24. Krishnamurthy KB, Drislane FW. Depth of EEG suppression and outcome in barbiturate anesthetic treatment for refractory status epilepticus. *Epilepsia* 1999; 40:759–762.
25. Yaffe K, Lowenstein DH. Prognostic factors of pentobarbital therapy for refractory generalized status epilepticus. *Neurology* 1993;43:895–900.
26. Cook D, Guyatt G, Marshall J, et al. A comparison of sucralfate and ranitidine for the prevention of upper gastrointestinal bleeding in patients requiring mechanical ventilation. Canadian Critical Care Trials Group. *N Engl J Med* 1998;338:791–797.
27. Sheth RD, Gidal BE. Refractory status epilepticus: response to ketamine. *Neurology* 1998;51:1765–1766.

20

Status Epilepticus in the Critically Ill

Michael C. Smith, MD and Michele Del Signore, DO

Introduction

Status epilepticus (SE) and its subsequent sequelae have been described and documented since the seventh century, B.C. Despite this, it remains a significant medical and public health problem. According to a prospective, population-based study in Richmond, Virginia, a projected 126,000–195,000 cases of SE will occur in the United States each year with 22,000–42,000 resulting in death *(1)*. A retrospective, population-based study in Rochester, Minnesota, showed an age-adjusted incidence of 18.3/100,000, with the greatest incidence in children under 1 yr of age and adults over 60 yr of age *(2)*. The studies mentioned above report that a majority of patients (54%) presenting with SE had no prior history of epilepsy *(1,2)*, and only 18% of unprovoked SE occurred in patients with known epilepsy. There has been an increase in the incidence of SE in patients between 1975 and 1984 (22.4/1000 population) compared to 1965 and 1974 (13.9/1000) *(1,2)*. The majority of this increase is attributable to an increasing incidence in the elderly suffering SE secondary to anoxic encephalopathy, neurologic complications of medical illness, and other severe neurologic insults. Management of these patients poses unique challenges, and we can expect to treat an increasing number of these patients as the population ages and medical technology for the failing organ systems improves. Treatments, whether medical or surgical, carry multiple complication profiles. Other chapters in this book have dealt with specific medical illnesses and their propensity to precipitate seizures.

From: *Seizures: Medical Causes and Management*
Edited by: N. Delanty © Humana Press, Inc., Totowa, NJ

Definition of SE

This chapter is devoted to the medically ill patient found to be in SE. SE, as defined by the World Health Organization, is "a condition characterized by an epileptic seizure that is sufficiently prolonged or repeated at sufficiently brief intervals so as to produce an unvarying and enduring epileptic condition" *(3)*. The International League Against Epilepsy defined SE as a seizure that "persists for a sufficient length of time or is repeated frequently enough that recovery between attacks does not occur" *(4)*. However, these definitions lack a specific duration. The International Classification of Epileptic Seizures defined SE as "any seizure lasting ≥30 min or intermittent seizures lasting for >30 min from which the patient did not regain consciousness" *(5)*.

There is a growing consensus that the time period of continuous seizure or seizures without return to normal consciousness should be shortened. This impetus is driven by animal data showing excitotoxic damage occurring well before 30 min and clinical data suggesting that simple generalized tonic-clonic seizures rarely last longer than 5 min. Bleck proposed that a continuous seizure or repeated seizure lasting longer than 20 min be defined as SE *(6)*. Treiman et al. defined SE as a seizure or repeated seizure lasting 10 min or more as the inclusion criteria for the completed Veterans Affairs (VA) Cooperative Trial *(7)*.

Lowenstein et al. provided both a mechanistic and operational definition of SE. Mechanistically, SE occurs when there is failure of the seizure-terminating system or persistence of seizure-inducing factors. Operationally, they defined generalized convulsive SE in adults and children as continuous seizures lasting longer than 5 min or two or more discrete seizures over a brief period of time without regaining consciousness. In young children and infants, especially with fever, a longer time frame of 10–15 min was proposed *(8)*. Their proposal reflects the increased awareness that a prolonged seizure results in serious sequelae attributed to excitotoxic neuronal injury and that the successful treatment of seizures is related directly to duration of seizure. The earlier diagnosis of SE will prompt more aggressive and effective treatment.

Clinical Presentation

There is a continuum in clinical presentation of SE (plus elsewhere in text) from clinically obvious tonic-clonic seizure to only a change in mental status. This requires that the clinician be alert for subtle signs of muscle or eye movements in an intensive care unit (ICU) patient with new-onset convulsion and altered mental status. A low threshold for obtaining an immediate electroencephalogram (EEG) should be the rule rather than the exception.

Generalized convulsive status epilepticus (GCSE) is the most common presentation. This may represent either primary or secondary generalized seizure, depending on etiology. As the seizure continues, the clinically obvious tonic-clonic- or myoclonic movements give way to more subtle and intermittent muscle or eye movements in a patient with altered mental status. There is an increasing electrical–mechanical disassociation as the SE progresses. A common and troublesome clinical scenario is the patient who presents with an acute neurologic insult (stroke, hemorrhage, trauma), a generalized seizure, and coma. The clinical question is whether the abnormal mental status is attributable to the neurological insult or the potentially treatable ongoing subtle or nonconvulsive status epilepticus (NCSE). Continued electrographic seizures following treatment of GCSE occurred in over 14% of comatose patients studied prospectively at the Medical College of Virginia (2). NCSE carries a significant mortality and requires prompt diagnosis in the critically ill patient with mental status changes and coma.

Secondary neurological disorders in systemically ill patients constitute an underrecognized, but highly important, group (9). Epidemiologic studies cited above confirm that the majority of cases of SE in the ICU represent the elderly population with a new neurologic insult. This group suffers higher morbidity and mortality than medical ICU cohorts (10). Some of the higher morbidity and mortality is attributable to delay in recognition of potentially treatable neurological disorders such as NCSE (11). This condition must be considered and excluded in patients who have convulsed and are in coma, particularly of unknown etiology (11,12). Electroencephalographic monitoring is essential in making this diagnosis and monitoring success (13) of therapy. Although electroencephalographic monitoring is often difficult and sometimes impossible to obtain and interpret in the off hours in many ICUs, it is rapidly becoming the standard of care. In the near future, digital electroencephalogram (EEG) with off-site interpretation will improve this situation.

Pathophysiology

The pathophysiology of SE in the systemically ill patient may result from independent and coexisting abnormalities affecting the chemical milieu and structural integrity of the central nervous system (CNS). These abnormalities include glial cell dysfunction, alteration of the blood–brain barrier, extracellular ion concentration disturbance, altered neurotransmitter release and degradation, and opening of neuronal gap junctions—all leading to excessive neuronal excitation and synchronization (14). The balance between neuronal excitation and inhibition is regulated precisely, and once excessive glutamate excitation occurs, it sets off a cascade of events that increase excitation and synchronization in a positive feedback loop (14). Excessive glutamate activation occurs when the large metabolic pool of glutamate is intermixed with the small and tightly regulated synaptic pool. This occurs in hypoxic–ischemic encephalopathy, stroke, head trauma, seizure, and other neurological insults.

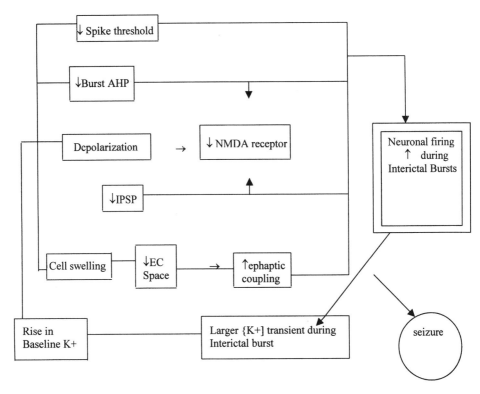

Fig. 1.

Once there is excessive accumulation of glutamate in the synaptic cleft, it activates N-methyl-D-aspartate (NMDA) and non-NMDA receptors, resulting in Na^+, Ca^{2+} and H_2O influx into the neuron **(Fig. 1)** *(14,15)*. This results in neuronal edema, shrinking the extracellular space, and creating a concomitant rise in extracellular K^+, a decrease in γ-aminobutyric acid (GABA) mediated after hyperpolarization, a depletion of GABA, and an opening of gap junctions leading to excessive neuronal depolarization, synchronization, and further seizures *(15)*. Glutamate is not solely responsible for the initiation and perpetuation of SE. GABA function is also critical in this process. GABA receptor desensitization and gross GABA depletion occur *(15)*, which further neuronal excitation.

Neuronal injury and death occur when there is excessive intracellular calcium accumulation that overwhelms calcium homeostatic mechanism *(15–17)*. This leads to activation of lipases, proteases, and free radical formation, producing permanent damage to the lipid bilayer or neuronal membrane. Once activated, this positive feedback activation leads to neuronal death. Those cortical areas most susceptible to excitotoxicity are those with the highest density of NMDA receptors *(18)*, producing deficits in memory and higher cortical function *(19)*. These deficits are often underrecognized without detailed neuropsychological testing. This underestimates the cognitive morbidity of SE, further complicating the data on prognosis and treatment success.

Acute Physiologic Changes

There are numerous physiologic effects and sequelae of an acute seizure, and the critically ill patient has little reserve to deal with these effects. They include dramatic changes in blood pressure and heart rate, acidosis, hypoxia, hyperthermia, respiratory compromise, leukocytosis, and renal dysfunction secondary to rhabdomyolysis *(20)*. In addition, SE further compromises CNS function by increasing intracranial pressure (ICP), pleocytosis, and disruption of the blood–brain barrier, increasing neurologic damage *(20)*.

In animal studies, SE increased systemic blood pressure and heart rate by 150% and returned to baseline within 60 min *(21)*. The cardiovascular changes are correlated with plasma epinephrine/norepinephrine levels. With prolonged SE, blood pressure drops below baseline, increasing the risk of cerebral hypoperfusion. Loss of cerebrovascular autoregulation furthers the risk of ischemic damage *(21)*. Marked acidosis, primarily metabolic because of lactic acidosis, with some respiratory component attributable to CO_2 accumulation, is commonly seen *(22)*.

Hypoxia is a common sequelae of SE primarily because of respiratory dysfunction related to pulmonary edema. SE produces a four- to sixfold increase in pulmonary capillary pressure, altering capillary permeability *(23)*. Hyperthermia occurs routinely with generalized tonic-clonic status epilepticus (GCSE). Although this is primarily attributable to muscle contraction, a paralyzed animal in SE also develops acidosis. Hyperthermia, with maximal core temperatures reaching 107°F, was recorded in 75 of 90 patients studied in SE *(22)*. The highest temperatures were seen in those with prolonged SE *(22)*. Leukocytosis that is attributable to demargination of white blood cells is common. Immature granulocyte bands are rarely elevated *(22)*. Rhabdomyolysis that is attributable to muscle damage associated with convulsive movements may lead to acute tubular neurosis because of myoglobinuria *(24)*.

The effects of SE on CNS physiology are significant. SE routinely increases ICP in a linear relationship to blood pressure *(25)*. The increase in ICP decreases the cerebral perfusion pressure, leading to ischemic damage. CSF pleocytosis occurs in approx. 20% of patients, but rarely over 30 cells *(22)*. Modest elevation of protein is also reported. Breakdown of the blood–brain barrier is common in SE, exposing the immunologic CNS to many larger proteins, including immunoglobulins that are not normally present. These combined systemic effects of SE are especially important to the compromised critically ill patient.

Table 1
Important Causes of SE in the Critically Ill

Cerebral infarction/intracranial hemorrhage
Meningitis/encephalitis
Severe head trauma
Hypoxic–ischemic encephalopathy
Hypertensive encephalopathy
Fulminant hepatic failure
Renal failure
Nonketotic hyperosmolar hyperglycemia
Medication-related (cyclosporine, theophylline, lidocaine, antibiotics)

Etiology, Diagnosis, and Initial Management

The etiology of the SE is critical in determining ultimate prognosis for the critically ill patient. Any cause of acute symptomatic seizure can also lead to acute symptomatic SE. SE that is attributable to an acute and devastating neurologic insult such as intracerebral hemorrhage, massive stroke, severe hypoxic–ischemic insult, multiorgan failure, and/or sepsis is difficult to treat and carries a high mortality, primarily because of the CNS insult and not the SE (*see* **Table 1**) *(26)*. The majority of the insults described above occur in the elderly population, increasing morbidity and mortality.

The initial management of these patients should consist of a detailed history and thorough physical and neurological evaluation *(26)*. The history should include a review of patient medications and other chemical exposures. Various blood tests should be performed, including drug/alcohol screens, liver function, coagulation studies, complete metabolic profiles, complete blood counts and differentials, erythrocyte sedimentation rate (ESR), arterial blood gas (ABG), creatinine phosphokinase (CPK), and blood cultures *(26)*. An emergent computerized tomography (CT) scan should be performed, to detect an acute neurologic insult such as hemorrhage, stroke, edema, tumor, or abscess. A lumbar puncture should be performed, if possible, to assess for infection, vasculitis, carcinomatosis, or hemorrhage. Magnetic resonance imagery (MRI), with and without gadolinium, may prove useful in assessing for structural lesions, as well as carcinomatosis and infectious etiologies. An EEG is necessary to make a diagnosis, guide treatment, and assure successful termination of SE. If the patient's mental status does not improve, after treatment of onset SE, electroencephalographic monitoring should be continued to rule out ongoing SE. EEG, clinical history, and response to therapy allow early prognostic information to be obtained *(26)*.

Management

Therapeutic options should begin with strategies of acute management of any medical emergency *(26)*. Airway management, ventilation, and circulatory issues must be addressed. A convulsing patient may be difficult to intubate; therefore, a short-acting paralytic agent, such as 0.1 mg/kg cevuronium may be used. When using paralytic agents, electroencephalographic monitoring is necessary to assess for therapeutic success and to rule out NCSE. A blood glucose assay should be performed, and thiamine, glucose and naloxone given. SE results in hyperthermia, which may worsen neurological outcome and should be treated with passive cooling. The presence of hyperthermia does not always indicate infection.

There are multiple treatment strategies for SE, and the protocol chosen depends on familiarity, type of SE, and an estimate of its severity. Short-acting agents such as midazolam or propofol may be preferable if the chances of successfully treating the SE rapidly are expected. A patient with known epilepsy that is noncompliant with treatment is one common example. A longer-acting agent (pentobarbital) would be preferable if a drug-induced coma in a patient is expected to last for days. A patient in prolonged SE or one with an acute insult, such as herpes simplex encephalitis, would be expected to require a longer drug-induced coma to be successful in abolishing SE.

In the patient with metabolic, drug, or other factors promoting the SE, removal of the offending agent or the correction of all metabolic abnormalities is paramount. Once that is accomplished, various SE treatment protocols could be offered.

Cessation of all clinical and electrical seizure activity is the ultimate goal. The ideal situation would be one where correcting the underlying etiology results in rapid resolution of SE. Unfortunately, many medical conditions resulting in SE are not treated easily and are intensely complicated.

The goal of therapeutic intervention is to achieve resolution within 5 min. Following the administration of thiamine, glucose, and naloxone, the physician should begin with a benzodiazepine. The VA Status Epilepticus Cooperative Study Group reported results of a double-blind study comparing four commonly used initial treatment regimens for GCSE *(7)*. Effective treatment of SE was defined as the cessation of all clinical and electrographic evidence of seizure activity in less than 20 min from the start of the infusion, with no recurrence of seizure activity in the next 40 min. This group found that lorazepam alone was more effective than phenytoin alone but that there was no significant difference in the effectiveness of lorazepam, phenobarbital, or diazepam followed by phenytoin. These first-line regimens were similar in incidence of side effects (including hypotension and respiratory depression), early recurrence of seizures, and long-term outcome. Lorazepam had a significantly shorter duration of infusion, giving it a distinct advantage over phenytoin. It is unclear if this superiority of lorazepam would persist if fosphenytoin administered at a faster rate were used. It is doubtful that these results will change the current practice of managing SE.

Fosphenytoin has become a popular alternative to for intravenous (IV) phenytoin in the acute treatment of seizures. An excellent review of the properties of fosphenytoin was provided by Browne (27). Fosphenytoin is metabolized rapidly to phenytoin, and therapeutic levels of phenytoin can be obtained within 10 min of rapid IV administration. The lower risk of cardiovascular side effects and a shorter infusion time as compared with that for phenytoin make fosphenytoin an excellent choice when managing critically ill patients with SE. However, because it takes approx. 1 hr to obtain therapeutic plasma concentrations when administered intramuscularly, this route is not recommended in SE, except when IV access is not possible. Postinfusion phenytoin levels should be obtained at least 2 hr after IV loading. The safety and efficacy of fosphenytoin have not been established for children less than 5 yr of age. Although fosphenytoin costs considerably more than IV phenytoin, the decreased risk of side effects and their associated costs may offset the initial price difference (28).

A barbiturate, commonly pentobarbital, is traditionally used in patients refractory to phenytoin and a benzodiazepine (26). The dose of barbiturate is tailored to maintain a burst-suppression pattern on EEG. A loading dose of 5 mg/kg with an infusion rate of 1–3 mg/kg per hour is the suggested initial dose. If phenobarbital is chosen, a loading dose of 20 mg/kg is used. The disadvantages of barbiturates are long half-life and respiratory depression. With prolonged treatment, depression of cardiovascular and immune function may occur.

IV valproate recently has been approved for patients on valproate who temporarily cannot take their medicine orally. There have been favorable reports of using IV valproate for acute seizures and SE in adults (29–31) and in children (32). In these reports, asymptomatic elevations of liver enzymes were sometimes found, but there were few other adverse reactions. Infusion rates up to 200 mg/min were well tolerated. More data on the safety of rapid infusions and the efficacy in acute treatment of convulsive seizures will be forthcoming with increased clinical use.

Midazolam may be used if cessation of seizures is not achieved with lorazepam or phenytoin or if the physician decides a midazolam infusion with its short half-life has clinical advantages (33–35). A dose of 0.2 mg/kg midazolam, in a slow IV bolus, followed by a maintenance dose of 0.1 mg/kg, is used. This dose may be doubled as needed every 15 min up to 2 mg/kg per hour, depending on clinical and EEG findings. Midazolam is beneficial because its short half-life will allow, theoretically, a rapid return of the patient to a desirable level of consciousness. However, tolerance to midazolam has been seen and once the SE is terminated with this drug, a slow wean off the infusion is at times necessary to prevent reoccurrence of SE. This negates somewhat the clinical advantages of midazolam.

Propofol (2,6-disopropylphenol) has become increasingly popular for the treatment of refractory SE *(36,37)*. Propofol may have unique mechanisms of action that are different from, and perhaps additive to, those of benzodiazepines and barbiturates. Cardiovascular side effects of propofol are less frequent when compared with those of high-dose barbiturates. Brown and Leven reported collective experience of propofol use in refractory SE in 28 patients *(38)*. Propofol infusion stopped clinical seizure activity and/or produced EEG burst suppression within seconds of a bolus. Propofol was compared with high-dose barbiturates in 16 critically ill adult patients with SE refractory to benzodiazepines and phenytoin *(38)*. Although both medications had similar efficacy in ultimately controlling SE, the mean time to seizure control was dramatically shorter with propofol (2.6 min) when compared with that for barbiturates (125 min). However, duration of mechanical ventilation and ICU stay, and the frequency of hypotension requiring intervention were not significantly different in the two groups. Propofol levels of 2.5 µg/mL were required in this study to control clinical and electrographic seizures. Of note, electrographic seizure activity resumed within 5 min of discontinuation of propofol in some patients, leading the investigators to recommend tapering propofol at a rate of 5% of the maintenance infusion rate per hour *(38)*. This would negate one of the principal advantages of propofol—the rapid clearing of consciousness and rapid extubation. The safe and efficacious use of propofol in pediatric patients was also reported recently. Propofol may be especially useful in patients developing tachyphylaxis to benzodiazepines (midazolam) or hemodynamic instability caused by high-dose barbiturates.

On one basis of the current literature, a protocol for managing generalized convulsive and complex partial SE is presented here (*see* **Table 2**). Fosphenytoin is used instead of phenytoin because of its faster rate of infusion and fewer side effects *(39)*. Also advocated for early use are midazolam or propofol in refractory SE because they both have a much faster onset and offset and appear to cause less hemodynamic instability when compared to high-dose barbiturates. Midazolam appears to produce even less hemodynamic effects than propofol *(35)*. Propofol may be useful in situations when tachyphylaxis to midazolam has developed *(35)*.

Outcome

The morbidity and mortality in SE remains significant despite advances in diagnosis and management. Literature review reveals a wide variability (5–50%) in acute mortality defined as death within 30 d *(40)*.

Table 2
Protocol for Treating SE

1. Give 100 mg thiamine, IV, and glucose, 50 mL of 50% solution, unless hypoglycemia excluded (for children, give 2 mL/kg of 25% glucose solution).
2. Consider contacting anesthesiology to be available for possible endotracheal intubation and EEG technologist to be available for possible prolonged EEG monitoring.
3. Give 0.1 mg/kg lorazepam, IV, at 2 mg/min up to total dose of 10 mg.[a]
4. If SE persists, give fosphenytoin, 20 mg phenytoin equivalents/kg IV at 150 mg phenytoin equivalents/min (3 mg phenytoin equivalents/kg per min for children). Give additional dose of fosphenytoin, 5 mg phenytoin equivalents/kg, if SE persists.
5. If SE persists, evaluate for endotracheal intubation and start EEG monitoring.
6. If SE persists, give either
   a. 0.2 mg/kg midazolam, slow IV bolus; then start maintenance infusion at 0.1 mg/kg per hour (1.7 µg/kg per min) and double dose as needed every 15 min up to 2 mg/kg per hour (33 µg/kg per min) based on clinical and electrographic evidence of seizures and/or burst-suppression EEG.
   b. 1 mg/kg propofol, IV bolus, over 2–5 min (rate based on blood pressure response). Repeat bolus if clinical or electrographic seizures persist. Start maintenance infusion at 2 mg/kg per hour (33 µg/kg per min) and increase as needed up to 15 mg/kg per hour (250 µg/kg per min).
7. Record EEG continuously for 1–2 h after seizures stop and then at least every 2 h for 30 min.
8. If SE persists after 1 h of midazolam or propofol, give 10 mg/kg pentobarbital, IV bolus, at maximum rate of 50 mg/min (0.4 mg/kg per min for children); then start maintenance infusion at 1 mg/kg per hour and increase as needed up to 10 mg/kg per hour to maintain burst-suppression EEG. Goal serum level is 10–20 µg/mL.
9. After SE has resolved for 12 h, attempt to taper midazolam and propofol over several hours. Attempt to taper pentobarbital over 12 h.

[a]If IV access not obtainable, consider rectal diazepam, buccal/sublingual midazolam, intramuscular (IM) midazolam, intranasal midazolam, or IM fosphenytoin.

More recent controlled studies report a 30-d mortality rate of 20.7% in the community-based Richmond study and 26% in patients with overt status in the VA multicenter study *(7,12)*. The predictors of mortality were the underlying etiology (acute CNS insult, infection), multiorgan failure, and type and duration of SE. In the VA study, subtle SE, occurring after overt SE, had a 65% mortality rate *(7)*.

The morbidity of SE is underestimated. This is primarily because of the unmeasured effects on memory and higher cognitive function. Those areas with the highest density of NMDA receptors (hippocampus, association neocortex) are those most at risk and difficult to evaluate clinically. Aicardi and Cheven reported in 1970 on 239 children with GCSE for over 1 hr. They reported a 11% acute morbidity rate but a 37% permanent neurologic morbidity rate, with a 20% morbidity rate attributable to the SE itself *(41)*. In adults, especially the elderly, there is a much higher morbidity, but this is primarily attributable to the underlying etiology. Although there are numerous case reports documenting the cognitive sequelae of SE, there is little prospective data. Dodril and Wilensky reported prospective neuropsychological data of 143 patients with epilepsy tested twice five years apart *(42)*. None of these patients had an episode of SE, either GCSE or complex partial SE. When compared to matched controls, the group with SE demonstrated only a slight drop in cognitive function as measured by their testing *(42)*. However, the group as a whole had lower base cognitive function, which supports the epidemiologic data that SE is more common in the neurologically impaired.

A major concern is the effect of SE causing permanent epilepsy. This literature is biased because of retrospective studies from tertiary epilepsy centers. In both adults and children who suffer an episode of SE, the risk of reoccurrence of both a seizure and SE is increased but not substantially *(39)*. This is concordant with the fact that continuous amygdala stimulation does not produce a kindling effect, whereas intermittent stimulation does. However, SE that produces neuronal injury and subsequent neuronal reorganization clearly may produce a chronic epileptic state *(39)*.

Animal studies have demonstrated that induced SE produces neuronal death through NMDA excitotoxic damage *(17,18)*. Mesial temporal sclerosis (MTS) first described by Falconer, is commonly associated with intractable complex partial seizures. In his surgical series, 47% of patients demonstrated MTS pathologically and 40% of these patients had had a prolonged episode of SE *(43)*.

Autopsy studies of five children who died after SE associated with a febrile illness revealed neuronal death in neocortex, basal ganglia, and cerebellum *(44)*. Neuronal injury and death occur with episodes of SE; however, the clinical sequelae are often difficult to demonstrate because of insensitive testing and underlying capacity of CNS to compensate for injury.

Conclusion

There has been significant improvement in the diagnosis and treatment of SE, especially in the critically ill patient, but there is a need for further progress. Morbidity, especially cognitive morbidity, remains unacceptably high. There have been important advances in the understanding of the pathophysiology of SE. The roles of glutamate excitotoxicity, intracellular calcium accumulation, free radical production, and neuronal membrane alteration in promoting SE and its neurologic sequelae are now well accepted and provide additional therapeutic targets to improve brain salvage and neurologic outcome. Many potential medications are currently in early clinical testing, and it is still too early to examine their benefits. However, the keys to successful treatment and reduction in the sequelae are early identification and aggressive management.

References

1. DeLorenzo RJ, Hauser WA, Towne AR, et al. A prospective, population-based epidemiologic study of status epilepticus in Richmond, Virginia. *Neurology* 1996;45:1029–1035.
2. Hesdorffer DC, Logroscino G, Cascino G, Annegers JF, Hauser WA. Incidence of status epilepticus in Rochester, Minnesota, 1965–1984. *Neurology* 1998; 50:735–741.
3. Gastaut H. Clinical and electroencephalographic classification of epileptic seizures. *Epilepsia* 1970;11:102–113.
4. Proposal for revised clinical and electroencephalographic classification of epileptic seizures from the Commission on Classification and Terminology of the International League against Epilepsy. *Epilepsia* 1981:22;489–501.
5. Gastaut H, Broughton R. *Epileptic Seizures: Clinical and Electrographic Features, Diagnosis and Treatment.* Springfield, IL: Charles C. Thomas, 1972, pp 25–90.
6. Bleck T. Convulsive disorders: status epilepticus. *Clin Neuropharmacol* 1991; 14:191–198.
7. Treiman DM, Meyers, PD, Walton NY, et al. A comparison of four treatments for generalized convulsive status epilepticus. *N Engl J Med* 1998;339:792–798.
8. Lowenstein DH, Bleck T, MacDonald RL. It's time to revise the definition of status epilepticus. *Epilepsia* 1999;40:120–122.
9. Bleck TP, Smith MC, Pierre-Louis SJ-C, Jares JJ, Murray J, Hansen CA. Neurologic complications of critical medical illnesses. *Crit Care Med* 1993;21:98–103.
10. Waterhouse EJ, Vaughan JK, Barnes TY, et al. Synergistic effect of status epilepticus and ischemic brain injury on mortality. *Epilepsy Res* 1998;29:175–183.
11. Litt B, Wityk RJ, Hertz SH, Mullen PD, Weiss H, Ryan DD, Henry TR. Nonconvulsive status epilepticus in the critically ill elderly. *Epilepsia* 1998;39:1194–1202.
12. DeLorenzo RJ, Waterhouse EJ, Towne AR, et al. Persistent nonconvulsive status epilepticus after the control of convulsive status epilepticus. *Epilepsia* 1998;39:833–840.
13. Jaitly R, Sgro JA, Towne AR, Ko D, DeLorenzo RJ. Prognostic value of EEG monitoring after status epilepticus: a prospective adult study. *Epilepsia* 1997; 14:326–334.
14. Dingledine R, McBain CJ, McNamara JD. Excitatory amino acid receptors in epilepsy. *Trends Pharmacol Sci* 1990;11:334–338.
15. Lothman E. Biological consequences of repeated seizures In: Engel J Jr, Pedley TA (eds.), *Epilepsy: A Comprehensive Textbook.* Philadelphia, PA: Lippincott-Raven, 1998, pp 481–497.
16. Kapur J, Stringer JL, Lothman EW. Evidence that repetitive seizures in the hippocampus cause a lasting reduction of Gabaergic inhibition. *J Neurophysiol* 1989;61;417–426.
17. Meldrum B. Excitotoxicity and epileptic brain damage. *Epilepsy Res* 1991; 10:55–61.
18. Meldrum BS. Excitoxicity and selective neuronal loss in epilepsy. *Brain Pathol* 1993;3:405–412.
19. Rice AC, DeLorenzo RJ. NMDA receptor activation during status epilepticus is required for the development of epilepsy. *Brain Res* 1998;782:240–247.
20. Meldrum BS. Metabolic factors during prolonged seizures and their relation to insure cell death. In: Delgado-Escueta AV, Wasterman CC, Treiman DM, Pater RJ (eds.), *Status Epilepticus: Mechanism of Brain Damage and Treatment.* New York: Raven, 1983, pp 261–275. Advances in Neurology, vol. 34.
21. Benowitz NL, Simon RP, Copeland JR. Status epilepticus: divergence of sympathetic activity and cardiovascular response. *Ann Neurol* 1986;19:197–199.

22. Aminoff MJ, Simon RP. Status epilepticus causes, clinical features and consequences in 98 patients. *Am J Med* 1980;69:657–666.
23. Bayne LL, Simon RP. Systemic and pulmonary vascular pressure during generalized seizures in sleep. *Ann Neurol* 1981;10:566–569.
24. Winocour PH, Waise A, Young G, Moriarity KJ. Severe self-limiting lactic acidosis and rhabdomyolysis accompanying convulsions. *Postgrad Med J* 1989;65:321–323.
25. Minns RA. Intracranial pressure changes associated with childhood seizures. *Dev Med Child Neurol* 1978;20:561–569.
26. Lukovits TG, Smith MC. Update on status epilepticus. *Curr Opin Crit Care* 1999; 5:107–111.
27. Browne T. Fosphenytoin. *Clin Neuropharmacol* 1997;20:1–12.
28. Ramsey RE, Wilder BJ. Parenteral fosphenytoin: efficacy and economic considerations. *Neurologist* 1998;4:S30–S34.
29. Koh HS, Hulihan JF. Intravenous valproic acid for acute inpatient seizure treatment. *Epilepsia* 1998;39(Suppl 6):S128 (abstract).
30. Mueed S, Naritoku DK. Intravenous loading and replinshment therapy with valproic acid (VPA). *Epilepsia* 1998;39(Suppl 6):S128 (abstract).
31. Lowe MR, DeToledo, JC, Vilavizza N, Ramsay RE. Efficacy, safety and tolearability of fast IV loading of valproate in patients with seizures and status epilepticus. *Epilepsia* 1998;39(Suppl 6):S235 (abstract).
32. Harrison AM, Lugo RA, Schunk JE. Treatment of convulsive status epilepticus with propofol case report. *Pediatr Emerg Care* 1997;13:420–422.
33. Kendall JL, Reynolds M, Goldberg R. Intranasal midzolam in patients with status epilepticus. *Ann Emerg Med* 1997;29:415–417.
34. Scott RC, Besag FM, Neville BG. Buccal midazolam or rectal diazepam for the acute treatment of seizures? *Epilepsia* 1998;39(Suppl 6):235.
35. Scott RC, Besad FMC, Boyd SG, Berry D, Neveille BGR. Buccal absorption of midazolam: pharmacokinetics and EEG pharmacodynamics. *Epilepsia* 1998; 39:290–294.
36. Stecker MM, Kramer TH, Rapps C, O'Meeghan R, Dulaney E, Skaar DJ. Treatment of refractory status epilepticus with propofol: clinical and pharmacokinetic findings. *Epilepsia* 1998;39:18–26.
37. Croutea D, Shevell M, Rosenblatt B, Dilenge M-E, Andermann F. Treatment of absence status in the Lennox-Gastaut syndrome with propofol. *Neurology* 1998;51:315–316.
38. Brown LA, Leven GM. Role of propofol in refractory status epilepticus. *Ann Pharmacother* 1998;32:1053–1059.
39. Hauser WA. Status epilepticus, frequency etiology and neurological sequelae. In: Delgado-Escueta AV, Wasterman CG, Treiman DM, et al. (eds.), *Status Epilepticus: Advances in Neurology,* New York: Raven, 1983, pp 3–14.
40. Simon R, Pellock JM, DeLorenzo RJ. Acute morbidity and mortality of status epilepticus. In: Engel J Jr, Pedley TA (eds.), *Epilepsy: A Comprehensive Textbook,* Philadelphia, PA: Lippincott-Raven, 1998, pp 741–753.
41. Aicardi J, Baraton J. A pneumoencephalographic demonstration of brain atrophy following status epilepticus. *Dev Med Child Neurol* 1971;15:77–81.
42. Dodrill CB, Wilensky AJ. Intellectual impairment as an outcome of status epilepticus. *Neurology* 1990;40(Suppl 2):23–27.
43. Falconer MA. Serafetinides EA, Corsellis JAN. Etiology and pathogenesis of temporal lobe epilepsy. *Arch Neurol* 1964;10:233–248.
44. Fowler M. Brain damage after febrile convulsion. *Arch Dis Child* 1957;32:67–76.

21

Anticonvulsants in Acute Medical Illness

Colin Roberts, MD and Jacqueline A. French, MD

Introduction

The choice of anticonvulsant agent for the medically ill patient with seizures will be influenced by a variety of factors. One important determinant will be the urgency with which seizure control is required. Both the severity of the patient's illness and the risk of additional seizures will be important to this decision.

A second, more confounding variable in antiepileptic drug (AED) selection and efficacy will be the spectrum of the patient's other medical conditions, both acute and chronic. The underlying health of primary organ systems, cardiac, hepatic, and renal, will have significant effects on drug absorption, protein binding, metabolism, and clearance. So too will the use of additional medications, including other anticonvulsants.

Some of the classically used anticonvulsants are highly plasma protein bound. Most are hepatically metabolized, via the cytochrome P450 enzyme system, and excreted renally. Many anticonvulsants have active secondary metabolites, which contribute substantially to drug toxicity and side effects. Most require maintenance of therapeutic serum concentrations, with monitoring of serum levels, and frequent oral dosing. The abundance of new anticonvulsants offers many alternatives to these characteristics. Although most are proposed for use as adjunctive therapy, some have proved quite effective when used alone. This has offered a significant improvement in seizure management to many patients, particularly those with more complex medical backgrounds.

In this chapter the spectrum of anticonvulsant choices as influenced by these issues will be discussed. The significant interactions with widely used medications will be reviewed briefly, as well as special considerations for AED initiation and monitoring in the setting of specific illnesses (see **Tables 1** and **2**).

From: *Seizures: Medical Causes and Management*
Edited by: N. Delanty © Humana Press, Inc., Totowa, NJ

Table 1
Anticonvulsants for Rapid Loading (1–3)

	Acute IV Load	Acute Oral Load	Maintenance	Considerations
Phenytoin	15–20 mg/kg In <5 mg/ml NSS Max rate, 50 mg/min	15–20 mg/kg[a] in 3 divided doses given q2 h	4–7 mg/kg (divided qd-bid)	EKG and BP monitoring with IV load Reduce rate if local or cardiovascular symptoms
Fosphenytoin (IV)	18–20 phenytoin equiv/kg Max rate, 150 mg PE/kg	(parenteral only)	4–7 mg PE/kg per day (divided bid)	EKG and BP monitoring with loading
Phenobarbital	10–20 mg/kg	10–20 mg/kg	1–3 mg/kg per day (divided qd-bid)	BP monitoring with loading. Sedation and respiratory depression with IV load
Valproic acid	10–15 mg/kg Max rate, 20 mg/min	5–10 mg/kg	15–50 mg/kg per day (divided bid-qid)	

[a]Use lower end for nonurgent treatment, higher for urgent.
NSS = normal saline solution.

334

Table 2
Anticonvulsant Information (1–3,4–6)

	Indication[a]	Dose Range (mg/d)	Ther. Range (mg/L)	$T_{1/2}$ (h)	Primary Excretion	Post-HD Supplementation	Hepatic Enzyme Induction
Phenytoin	P	5–7/kg	10–20	12–48[b]	hepatic (>95%)	no	++
Phenobarbital	P/G	1–3/kg	15–45	65–110	hepatic (75%) renal (25%)	++	++
Valproic Acid	P/G	15–30/kg	50–100	5–15	hepatic (>95%)	no	—
Carbamazepine	P	10–30/kg	4–12	5–20	hepatic (95%)	?	++
Oxcarbazepine[c]	P	600–2400	10–20	8–10	renal (45%) hepatic (45%)	?	+
Lamotrigine	P/G	200–500	2–15	20–30[d]	hepatic (85%)	+	—
Topiramate	P/G	200–800	2–15	18–24	renal (50–75%) hepatic (30–50%)	?	—
Gabapentin	P	30–40/kg	—	5–9	renal	++	—
Tiagabine	P	8–56	—	5–8	hepatic (90%)	?	—
Levetiracetam	P/G	1000–3000	—	6–8	renal/hydrolysis	+	—
Zonisamide	P/G	100–400	10–40	25–60	hepatic (>90%)	?	—

[a]Based on clinical data, but not necessarily indicating FDA approval. All listed drugs are effective in generalized tonic-clonic seizures. P = usefulness in partial or secondarily generalized convulsions. G = the drug may also be useful in other generalized seizure types, such as absence and myoclonus.
[b]Dose-dependent.
[c]Mono-hydroxy derivative.
[d]Monotherapy.
HD = hemodialysis.

335

Special Medical Considerations

The choice of anticonvulsant should be influenced by each patient's medical profile. Several anticonvulsants carry risks to patients with specific organ system dysfunction, including cardiac, hepatic, and renal disease. Many need dosage and administration adjustments when given to patients with altered renal or hepatic function. Additionally, several have side effect profiles, either idiosyncratic or via interactions with other common medications, which make them problematic in patients with certain medical conditions.

Patients with Cardiovascular Disease

Several anticonvulsants have potential cardiovascular side effects and should be used with caution in patients with known cardiac disease.

Phenytoin has the potential to cause hypotension and cardiac arrhythmias, primarily in the setting of rapid intravenous (IV) infusion. In patients with known heart disease, infusions of phenytoin should not exceed 25 mg/min, rather than the usual recommended maximum rate of 50 mg/min *(7)*. Symptoms of hypotension, bradyarrhythmias, and transient chest pain can be reversed by slowing or discontinuing the infusion. Some of the cardiovascular side effects are caused by the propylene glycol solvent used in IV phenytoin preparations. Use of the prodrug fosphenytoin has not been associated with any such reactions (it also does not contain propylene glycol) and, if available, should be the form of choice in patients with significant cardiac disease. IV infusions with phenytoin should be accompanied by continuous electrocardiogram (EKG) and blood pressure (BP) monitoring in all patients *(8–10)*.

Large overdoses of phenytoin have been associated with arrhythmias, usually in patients with preexisting cardiac dysfunction *(11)*. Given the drug's kinetic profile at the upper end of its therapeutic range, however, both phenytoin and fosphenytoin should probably be considered second-line agents for chronic use in patients with cardiac dysfunction.

Carbamazepine is a well-documented pro-arrhythmic agent and should be avoided in patients with cardiac disease. It has been shown to exacerbate known conduction abnormalities, as well as causing *de novo* arrhythmias in elderly patients *(12,13)*. Bradyarrhythmias, Stokes–Adams attacks, aggravation of sick sinus syndrome, or atrioventricular A-V block with resultant congestive heart failure have all been described *(14–16)*. Most cases arise after chronic carbamazepine therapy, although overdoses have significant acute arrhythmic effects *(13)*. Hypercholesterolemia may increase carbamazepine clearance, although the drug itself may alter high-density lipoprotein (HDL): total cholesterol ratio beneficially *(17,18)*.

Preliminary experience with oxcarbazepine suggests that it carries less risk of toxic conduction abnormalities, although long-term studies are not yet available *(19)*.

Phenobarbital carries a significant risk of hypotension with IV loading. Rapid dosing should be avoided in patients with limited cardiac reserve, as well as in any patient who cannot be monitored for hypotension *(20)*.

Recommendations

Although fosphenytoin may be used with caution when rapid loading is required, IV valproic acid carries less risk of arrhythmia or hypotension. In subacute circumstances, divided oral loading of phenobarbital will avoid its potential for hypotension. Oral loading with valproate is also safe, although more likely to cause nausea when initiated at full therapeutic doses.

When rapid loading is not required, current information indicates that newer agents such as topiramate or lamotrigine can be initiated safely in this population. Little data are available regarding cardiac side effects of zonisamide or levetiracetam.

Patients with Hepatic Disease

Hepatic disease will change the biotransformation and disposition of most of the commonly used anticonvulsants. Decreased hepatic blood flow and compromised hepatocyte function will alter drug metabolism. Alterations in serum protein levels will alter protein binding and levels of circulating free drug. The end effects on anticonvulsant activity can be variable.

Direct hepatotoxic effects of anticonvulsants are rare, although more common with valproic acid than any other. As with most drug-induced hepatic injury, most incidences are idiosyncratic, occurring in the setting of generalized hypersensitivity reactions.

Phenytoin protein binding correlates with serum albumin and total bilirubin levels, the latter presumably via competition for plasma protein binding sites *(21)*. Therefore, low albumin and bilirubin levels in combination with decreased biotransformation can result in high concentration of circulating drug, with a large unbound fraction. Careful monitoring of free phenytoin levels (target range, 1–2 mg/L) will help to avoid intoxication. Phenytoin-associated hepatic injury is rare and has occurred almost exclusively in the setting of hypersensitivity reactions. Patients are almost universally febrile, with a pruritic desquamating rash, lymphadenopathy, and peripheral eosinophilia *(22)*.

Valproic acid is generally contraindicated in the setting of hepatic failure because of direct hepatotoxicity and risks of fulminant hepatic failure. Protein binding is decreased, and clearance of free drug is decreased significantly with cirrhosis. Plasma half-life is also extended up to twice normal

(21). Accumulation of drug as a result of both of these factors may further enhance its hepatotoxic effect. Hyperammonemia may also be enhanced by valproate, particularly when it is used in combination with other anticonvulsants *(23)*.

Primary hepatic injury that is attributable to valproate therapy is uncommon, although well documented *(24,25)*. Although many patients who experience liver failure are subsequently found to have underlying metabolic disorders (urea cycle defects, ornithine transcarbamylase deficiency, etc.), the clinical presentation in these patients does not differ significantly from those without risk factors. Symptoms frequently begin with emesis, followed by icterus, encephalopathy, coagulopathy, and death.

Many patients on valproate therapy will have transient increases in hepatic enzymes. Although the majority return to normal, it may be impossible to identify those who will proceed to hepatic failure. The drug should be used with extreme caution in patients with compromised hepatic function and is best avoided, especially if other anticonvulsants may be used concurrently.

Phenobarbital is subject to fewer kinetic alterations with liver dysfunction than is phenytoin or valproate. Serum half-life, however, can be prolonged up to 130 ± 15 h. Serum levels should be followed to guide proper dosing intervals, which may be quite prolonged. Though protein binding may be decreased, there is no clinical value to monitoring free drug levels *(21)*.

Carbamazepine undergoes a significant reduction in protein binding with hepatic failure. This can accompany even mild hepatic dysfunction and does not appear to correlate with any measurable serum parameter. High free levels of carbamazepine and the 10–11-epoxide metabolite can increase toxic side effects significantly *(21)*. Both should be monitored closely to guide dosing.

Direct hepatotoxicity as a result of carbamazepine use is rare and occurs most commonly in the setting of hypersensitivity reactions *(26)*. Transient or persistent mild elevations of hepatic enzymes can occur with initiation of therapy and likely reflect enzyme autoinduction by the drug.

Oxcarbazepine has not been studied extensively in hepatic failure. Protein binding is decreased, although it may not lead to the same degree of toxicity as carbamazepine because of the absence of the epoxide metabolite. Levels should be followed closely.

Recommendations

Gabapentin and levetiracetam have profiles that uniquely suit them for use in this setting. Neither undergoes significant hepatic metabolism, neither is significantly protein-bound (gabapentin, 0%; levetiracetam, <10%), and both are excreted renally. Both would be useful when rapid loading is not required.

When acute therapeutic levels must be achieved, phenobarbital may be used, with careful monitoring of serum levels. Benzodiazepines may also be used acutely, although reduced protein binding and prolonged half-lives will also increase the risks of intoxication and respiratory depression. Oxazepam, a short-acting benzodiazepine, may have less potential problems because of its limited oxidative metabolism and may be preferred to diazepam, lorazepam, or clorazepate.

Patients with Renal Disease

Renal dysfunction will increase circulating levels of most anticonvulsants and their metabolites. In addition, uremia can significantly alter protein binding characteristics, with resultant increases in free drug fractions. Most patients can be maintained successfully on the traditional anticonvulsants with decreases in dosing and increased interdose intervals.

Both hemodialysis and peritoneal dialysis will clear fractions of unbound drug. Additionally, both have been shown to have effects on protein binding and kinetics in the period following completion of each cycle. Pre- and post-dialysis monitoring of drug levels with supplemental dosing is critical in maintaining therapeutic anticonvulsant concentrations.

Phenytoin has decreased protein binding in uremic patients. Free drug fractions can increase from 10% to 30% of total, without changes in total measured serum levels. These changes appear to correlate with the degree of renal failure as reflected by serum creatinine. The drug is 95% biotransformed, and accumulation of the glucuronimide metabolite is not associated with any toxicity. Free phenytoin levels should be followed (target, 1–2 mg/L), and total dosage adjusted accordingly. Serum half-life is decreased in uremia, and patients may require more frequent doses (every 8 h) of smaller amounts to maintain therapeutic levels *(21)*. The amount of drug removed by dialysis will increase as protein binding decreases.

Phenobarbital has significant accumulation in uremic patients, as elimination depends primarily on renal function. Increased levels and prolonged serum half-life can cause cardiovascular depression, potentially worsening renal function. Risks of intoxication are great. Dosages should be reduced and serum levels followed closely. As limited drug is protein-bound, free levels are of no use. Significant amounts of drug are removed by dialysis, and postdialysis levels should be followed to determine supplemental dosing *(21,27)*.

Carbamazepine does not appear to have altered protein binding in uremia. As less than 2% of the drug is excreted unchanged in the urine, accumulation of the drug or its toxic epoxide is unlikely. No studies are currently available on the effects of dialysis. Rare instances of carbamazepine-related renal injury have been reported. These have included idiosyncratic instances of protein-uria, hematuria, and oliguria, as well as rare cases of acute renal failure attributable to tubulo-interstitial nephritis or membranous glomerulonephropathy *(28,29)*. Oxcarbazepine has not been studied, although renal dysfunction has not been reported.

Valproic acid has decreased protein binding in uremic patients, correlating with the degree of renal dysfunction *(30)*. As it is primarily excreted by the liver, little is accumulated in renal failure. Various metabolites are renally excreted, but these are without established toxic potential. Patients should be followed clinically for evidence of toxicity. Free levels can be followed, with dosage reductions if free fractions exceed 10% of total *(21)*. Negligible amounts are removed by dialysis, though protein binding can be reduced postdialysis *(30)*. An increased incidence of valproate-induced pancreatitis has been described in patients with advanced renal failure *(31)*. As with all patients receiving this drug, serum amylase should be measured if abdominal pain or excessive nausea occurs.

Gabapentin is not metabolized, is not protein-bound, and is exclusively renally excreted. As such, serum concentrations and half-life can rise precipitously in correlation to dysfunction. The manufacturer has made dosing recommendations based on serum creatinine clearance (CrCl) *(1)*.

CrCl	Dosage
>60 ml/min	400 mg tid ($3\times$ a day)
30–60 ml/min	300 mg bid ($2\times$ a day)
15–30 ml/min	300 mg qd ($4\times$ a day)
<15 ml/min	300 mg qod

Significant amounts of drug are removed by dialysis, and it is recommended that an additional 200–300 mg be given after each 4 h of cycling *(32)*.

Although limited data are available about newer anticonvulsants, lamotrigine, topiramate, tiagabine, levetiracetam, and zonisamide are all completely or partially excreted renally. All may be expected to have accumulation and prolonged half-lives with renal failure. As tiagabine has the largest fraction of protein binding, it may have significant alterations in kinetics with uremia. Drugs with limited protein binding, such as topiramate, will likely require supplementation postdialysis.

Recommendations

Valproate, carbamazepine, and oxcarbazepine have the least potential for toxicity in renal failure. Uremia will alter protein binding, but most patients can be followed clinically for side effects. Patients on valproate should be monitored for pancreatitis via serum amylase. Free phenytoin levels should be monitored when used in uremic patients.

Gabapentin, levetiracetam, and phenobarbital carry risks of significant accumulation with renal dysfunction, and careful monitoring with dosage adjustments is warranted. Many drugs will require postdialysis dosage adjustments, as well as monitoring for postdialysis alterations in protein binding (Table 2).

Topiramate should be used with caution in patients with renal dysfunction. Its action as a weak carbonic anhydrase inhibitor increases the risk of renal calculi. Zonisamide has been associated with a similar risk of calculi, especially in patients with a history of prior stones.

Patients with Organ Transplantation

Seizures in this population are not infrequent in occurrence and may arise from a variety of sources. Although many seizures may be secondary to central nervous system (CNS) and systemic effects of the diseases that brought these patients to transplantation, equal numbers arise from the complications of surgery and therapy with immunologic modulators. Although some medications, such as cyclosporine A, busulfan, and cyclophosphamide, are potentially epileptogenic, others such as L-asparaginase can predispose to focal CNS injury, with seizures as a potential sequela *(33)*. Systemic and CNS infections can also cause seizures, both acute and chronic, in a population under chronic metabolic stress.

Anticonvulsant use in these complicated patients must follow careful investigation of the etiology of the seizure, with adjustments of concurrent medications and careful monitoring of metabolic parameters both pre- and post-AED initiation. Basic hepatic, renal, and cardiac function should be assessed to prevent AED-related toxicity. Finally, careful consideration of concurrent medications must be made, with an eye to potential interactions, both kinetic and dynamic (particularly of steroids, antibiotics, and antifungals).

Liver Transplantation

Although hepatic function may be normal following transplantation, it is prudent to avoid those medications associated with hepatotoxicity or significant alterations in hepatic enzymes. Phenobarbital may be used for generalized convulsions when rapid loading is required. Similarly, phenytoin or fosphenytoin may be used for rapid loading in treatment of partial seizures, and either is rarely associated with hepatotoxicity. As discussed below, some adjustment of immunosuppressive therapy may be required with phenytoin therapy.

Gabapentin, topiramate, and levetiracetam undergo minimal hepatic biotransformation and are excreted renally. They may be used when rapid loading is not required.

Valproate is a less ideal choice in this population, given the associated risks of hepatotoxicity. Most hepatically metabolized anticonvulsants will cause mild transaminasemias, and indices of hepatic function should be monitored so as not to confuse this effect with organ failure or rejection.

Renal and Cardiac Transplantation

Valproate therapy for both partial and generalized seizures is the best choice in either population given its limited renal excretion and absence of cardiac side effects. Fosphenytoin may be used with caution for IV loading, given its lower risk of arrhythmias relative to phenytoin, although the pro-arrhythmic risks of overdose are significant. Oxcarbazepine may also be used with caution, as preliminary experience does not suggest that it has the same pro-arrhythmic properties as carbamazepine.

In cardiac transplant patients without renal dysfunction, phenobarbital may be used with caution, given its potential for cardiovascular depression and hypotension. Topiramate, tiagabine, lamotrigine, gabapentin, levetiracetam, and zonisamide may also be used, although limited data are available regarding long-term side effects and potential interactions.

Bone Marrow Transplantation/Chemotherapy

Phenobarbital may be used during the 2- to 6-wk period of engraftment *(33)*. Hepatic enzyme induction by the drug may require increases in doses of cyclosporine and corticosteroids (generally by 25–30%).

Phenytoin and valproate should be avoided because of potential marrow suppression. Carbamazepine is relatively contraindicated because of potential hematopoetic side effects.

Special Considerations

Phenytoin has been associated with particular problems attributable to medication interactions in patients on antineoplastic therapies. Serum phenytoin levels are decreased with concurrent vinblastine, cisplatin, or bleomycin *(34)*. This is presumably caused by altered absorption, although it also may be exacerbated by concomitant use of steroids and antacids.

Phenytoin, carbamazepine, oxcarbazepine, phenobarbital, and primidone all induce microsomal enzyme systems involved with glucocorticoid and cyclosporine A metabolism. All can decrease the half-life, maximum concentration, and area under curve (AUC) of cyclosporine A. All will increase the clearance of both cyclosporine A and methylprednisolone. Monitoring of levels, with adjustments in dosages and dosing intervals, will help to prevent potential complications. Valproate and the newer anticonvulsants, with the exception of oxcarbazepine, are not hepatic enzyme inducers and, therefore, have no such interactions.

Hematologic Considerations

Hematologic side effects of anticonvulsant use range from mild alterations in circulating counts to marrow suppression and aplastic anemia. As with most classes of medication, these reactions are primarily seen in the setting of systemic hypersensitivity reactions, with antibody-mediated peripheral destruction of circulating platelets and white and red cells. Additional reactions can occur in the setting of drug-induced lupus-like syndromes. Others arise from direct toxic marrow inhibition. Instances of all three classes have been reported with all of the standard anticonvulsants. Several anticonvulsants can cause folate deficiency, with resulting megaloblastic anemia. Most reactions are idiosyncratic, and some are dose related. Review of specific hematologic profiles of the major anticonvulsants can help identify medication-related effects and avoid potential complications in patients at increased risk.

Carbamazepine has the widest range of anticonvulsant-related hematopoetic toxicity. Although aplastic anemia is rare (<1/50,000 patients), at least 10% of all patients exhibit a decline in neutrophil counts in the first months after initiation *(35)*. The vast majority rebound to normal, and drug withdrawal is not recommended unless counts decline below 2500 or absolute neutrophils count (ANC) < 750. Two percent of patients develop a persistent neutropenia, with the majority remaining asymptomatic *(36)*. Carbamazepine has additional suppressive effects on heme biosynthesis *(37)*. Inhibition of uroporphyrinogen-1-synthase has been linked to development of acute intermittent porphyria *(38)*. Oxcarbazepine has not been shown to have any of these hematologic side effects to date.

Valproate produces a dose-related decrease in circulating platelets *(39)*. This, in combination with negative effects on platelet adhesiveness *(40)*, can lead to an increase in ecchymoses (more common in children) but rarely symptomatic clotting dysfunction or spontaneous hemorrhage. Dosage should be reduced or withdrawn if purpura or petechiae appear. Valproate has also been associated with neutropenia, bone marrow suppression, pure red cell aplasia *(41)*, and fibrinogen depletion *(42)*.

Phenytoin has been associated with megaloblastic anemia after chronic use *(43)*. Although folate levels may be normal, supplementation reverses the condition. Thrombocytopenia and granulocytopenia are less common occurrences and resolve with dose reduction or drug withdrawal. Aplastic anemia is rare *(44)*.

Phenytoin can decrease circulating levels of immunoglobulin G (IgG) by 20–25% and, in some cases, IgA, without clinical changes in immune potency. This is an isolated B-cell loss, likely attributable to suppression of lymphocyte phytoagglutination transformation *(45)*.

Additionally, phenytoin has been implicated in an idiosyncratic pseudolymphoma syndrome *(46)*. Generalized lymph node hyperplasia is accompanied by fever, erythematous rash, and skin manifestations of mycoses fungoides. The drug has never been clearly implicated in induction or exacerbation of true lymphoma.

Phenobarbital has no significant systematic effects on hematologic indices. Patients in the Veterans Administration study were monitored over periods of 36 mo without statistically significant alterations in platelet or leukocyte counts or function. Rare aplastic anemia was reported *(47)*.

Levetiracetam has been associated with a statistically, but not clinically, significant reduction in red blood cell counts and total hemoglobin *(4)*.

Recommendations

Patients should be monitored both pre- and postinitiation for alterations in hematologic indices. Although most reactions are idiosyncratic, some respond to dose reduction or medication withdrawal. AEDs with a higher incidence of specific hematologic side effects (i.e., granulocytes with carbamazepine; platelets with valproate) should be avoided in patients with preexisting low levels or dysfunction of these cell lines, or in those for whom declining levels would pose acute risks because of infection, graft rejection, or hemorrhage.

Phenobarbital might be preferred over phenytoin and valproate for rapid IV loading in this population. No significant hematologic side effects have been reported with lamotrigine, or the other, newer agents, which should be chosen over carbamazepine.

Anticoagulation

Enzyme-inducing anticonvulsants such as carbamazepine (though not oxcarbazepine), phenytoin, and phenobarbital can increase the metabolism of warfarin and *bis*-hydroxycoumarin. Levels can be decreased by 25–50% by carbamazepine *(48)* and phenobarbital *(49)*. Phenytoin initially can inhibit metabolism, before inducing metabolism and clearance after 1–2 wk *(50)*. Careful monitoring of parameters in anticoagulated patients is highly recommended for 3–4 wk after initiation of therapy with these anticonvulsants.

Other Special Considerations

Autoimmune Disease/SLE

Various anticonvulsants have been found to precipitate the presentation or activity of autoimmune disorders, particularly systemic lupus erythematosis (SLE). Lupus-like syndromes have also been described as isolated drug reactions, with resolution of symptoms upon drug withdrawal. In drug-induced reactions, antibodies to double-stranded DNA normally are not induced, and clinical symptoms usually spare the skin, kidneys, and CNS *(51)*.

Without careful investigation, it may be difficult to determine whether syndromes represent primary disease or secondary drug reactions. Seizures and encephalopathy may be the presenting symptoms of CNS SLE, and the subsequent initiation of anticonvulsants may be wrongfully implicated in the emergence of the disease. To avoid potential confusion in high-risk patients, it may be beneficial to avoid those drugs with the highest incidence of such reactions.

Phenytoin has been implicated in the highest incidence of SLE-like reactions among the anticonvulsants (52). As mentioned, symptoms usually spare the kidneys and CNS (51), although they can be variable.

Carbamazepine may induce SLE, usually after 6–12 mo of therapy (53). Antinuclear antibody titers are highly positive and may persist after discontinuation of the drug. It is not known if oxcarbazepine carries similar risks.

Miscellaneous

Hyponatremia can be a significant dose-related side effect of carbamazepine (54,55). Preliminary studies have shown a similar effect with oxcarbazepine (56,57), usually occurring in the first 3 mo of therapy. Both drugs should be avoided in patients with sodium regulation disorders.

Renal calculi, as mentioned previously, have been associated with topiramate and zonisamide. All patients, especially those with prior stones or known renal dysfunction, should be encouraged to maintain adequate water intake while taking either drug. Screening renal ultrasounds may be of use in clinical follow-up.

Pancreatitis, both subacute and acute hemorrhagic, with pseudocyst formation, have been reported as infrequent complications of valproate therapy (58–60). Early symptoms of abdominal pain may progress to include pericardial effusion and coagulopathy. Reexposure to valproate after normalization of enzymes carries a high risk of recurrence. Amylase levels should be followed in patients on valproate who complain of abdominal pain or excessive nausea.

Chronic phenobarbital therapy has been associated with a variety of connective tissue symptoms, such as contractures with palmar nodules, frozen shoulder, Dupuytren's contractures, and diffuse joint pains (43,61,62). Although it is not clear that the drug exacerbates preexisting arthritic or rheumatic conditions, alternate therapy should be considered for patients who develop isolated symptoms while taking the drug.

Anticonvulsants in Pregnancy

Anticonvulsant use during pregnancy poses a variety of risks to mother and fetus. For pregnant women who require anticonvulsants, or those who may become pregnant while on therapy, certain precautions may limit potential complications.

Folate Supplementation

Maternal treatment with carbamazepine or valproate during pregnancy has been associated with increased rates of neural tube defects in fetuses (1% and 2%, respectively). Inhibition of folate metabolism is believed to have a key role in this process *(63,64)*. As neural tube formation occurs during the third and fourth weeks of fetal development, many women are not yet aware that they are pregnant when they are most at risk. Folate supplementation (1–4 mg/d) is recommended for women receiving either of these drugs, from 3 mo prior to conception through the end of the first trimester *(65,66)*. It is wise to administer folate to all women of childbearing age who receive AEDs. Antenatal ultrasounds and measurements of maternal α-fetoprotein levels can be used to monitor for neural tube defects in the fetus prior to delivery.

Vitamin K

Phytomenadione deficiency occurs in newborns exposed prenatally to the enzyme-inducing anticonvulsants phenobarbital, carbamazepine, and phenytoin. These infants can develop profound hemorrhagic diatheses within 24 h of delivery, with frequently fatal outcomes. Also, women may experience an increased risk of peripartum bleeding as a result of vitamin K deficiency. Pregnant women receiving these anticonvulsants should be supplemented orally with 10 mg/d vitamin K for the last 4 wk of pregnancy. In addition, the neonate should receive a parenteral dose of 1 mg at birth *(65,67)*.

Seizures During Pregnancy

Seizure activity during pregnancy can be escalated by hormonal and pharmacokinetic changes in the mother, as well as by changes in sleep and dietary habits. Although generalized tonic-clonic seizures pose a risk to the fetus, anticonvulsant therapy in the pregnant mother should be conservative. Seizure control should be sought using the lowest therapeutic doses required. Monotherapy is preferred to minimize the cumulative risks of teratogenicity *(65,67)*.

Although initiation of therapy after the first trimester limits the risks of neural tube defects, various other fetal malformations have been associated with anticonvulsant use. Ten to 30% of fetuses exposed to phenytoin develop a complex of multisystem physical anomalies, postnatal growth retardation, and cognitive delay (fetal hydantoin syndrome) *(68)*. Other malformations, including cleft lip/palate, as well as genitourinary and cardiac defects, have been reported in small percentages of those exposed to intrauterine valproate *(69)*, carbamazepine *(70)*, and phenobarbital *(71)*.

Less is known about the fetal effects of the newer anticonvulsants *(67)*. Little clinical data on human fetal exposure have been gathered, and most clinicians continue to recommend early folate supplementation and close monitoring of all such pregnancies.

Seizures occurring later in pregnancy (third trimester) may be attributable to decreasing maternal albumin levels. With a decrease in protein-bound anticonvulsant, there is increased metabolism and clearance of the free drug *(67)*. Patients receiving highly protein-bound anticonvulsants such as phenytoin, valproate, carbamazepine, and tiagabine may require close clinical monitoring, with small incremental increases in dosing as indicated. It is important to remember that measured total drug levels may not fall, although the unbound fractions may decrease to subtherapeutic concentrations. In addition, increased drug metabolism may lead to higher levels of potentially toxic metabolites (i.e., the carbamazepine 10–11-epoxide).

Seizures During Labor and Delivery

Tonic-clonic seizures can occur during labor and delivery in up to 2% of women with epilepsy *(72)*. This is frequently, but not always, the result of subtherapeutic concentrations of anticonvulsants. Additional acute medications may be required. IV loading with phenytoin or fosphenytoin, as well as with benzodiazepines such as lorazepam, is usually an effective intervention. Infants should receive vitamin K supplementation upon delivery and should be observed for signs of withdrawal when mothers have received benzodiazepines or barbiturates.

Breast-Feeding

Anticonvulsants that are highly protein bound are the least likely to be passed into breast milk *(73)*. Phenytoin and valproate are consequently present in very small concentrations. Conversely, larger fractions of carbamazepine and phenobarbital are passed to the breast-feeding infant. This is particularly troublesome because of the long half-life of phenobarbital, which can have a cumulative sedative effect in the infant.

Among the newer agents, most have low binding fractions. Lamotrigine, topiramate, and gabapentin are all passed in significant concentrations into breast milk. Tiagabine, although highly protein bound, is still passed in large concentrations.

The recommendation of the American Academy of Pediatrics is that women taking phenytoin, valproate, or carbamazepine can breast-feed *(73)*. Breast-feeding is not recommended for those receiving lamotrigine or phenobarbital. In all other cases, mothers should proceed with caution and breast-feed only if the benefits clearly outweigh the risks *(65,73)*.

Alternate Routes
of Anticonvulsant Administration

Patients, especially those acutely ill, often have barriers to easy drug administration. Oral dosing can be limited by altered levels of consciousness, especially in the postictal or encephalopathic patient. IV access can be tenuous in
many patients, particularly in those with peripheral vascular disease. Medication interactions within IV lines may limit windows of opportunity for drug
administration in patients with busy schedules of multiple medications.

Alternatives to oral or IV drug administration exist for many anticonvulsants. These are useful in the setting of acute seizure management where
access cannot be gained, as well as in patients with temporary loss of access
in whom initiation or continuation of a specific anticonvulsant is desired. Rectal administration of oral or parenteral formulations of several drugs may be
substituted when other routes are not available. Dilution of oral solutions with
equal volumes of water may help to minimize the cathartic effects of this
route. Intramuscular administration, although frequently effective, is almost
invariably associated with local necrosis and should be avoided if possible,
especially for repeated doses.

Phenytoin

Phenytoin can be absorbed poorly when given with enteral feedings
(74,75). This can usually be avoided if enteral tubes are flushed and clamped
for 2 h pre- and postdosing. Fosphenytoin (IV solution) can also be given
enterally when phenytoin absorption is poor. Phenytoin doses are converted to
equal amounts of "phenytoin equivalents" of fosphenytoin and given in qd or
divided bid doses *(74)*. Serum monitoring of phenytoin levels should be followed to establish continued therapeutic levels if switching from IV therapy.

Intramuscular (IM) fosphenytoin is also well tolerated. Using equivalent
doses, local irritation and muscle and tissue necrosis caused by crystallization
of phenytoin are greatly reduced *(10)*.

Rectal phenytoin, using the IV preparation or the oral solution, has been
effectively used for loading and maintenance therapy *(76,77)*. Fosphenytoin
has not been studied for rectal administration.

Phenobarbital

Phenobarbital is well absorbed and moderately well tolerated when equivalent doses are given IM *(78)*. Rectal administration of the IV solution is 90%
absorbed, although somewhat less quickly than IM injections (4.4 h vs 2.2 h)
(79). The long half-life of the drug makes this less significant.

Valproic Acid

Various problems have been described, both with absorption and tube leakage in patients receiving divalproex sodium via gastrostomy tubes *(80)*. Whether similar problems (presumably with adherence of drug to the tubes) exist for nasogastric tubes is unclear. In patients with feeding tubes, oral valproate sodium should be replaced with equal IV doses until oral feeding can resume. Divalproex sprinkle capsules are notorious for adhering to tubes and should be avoided altogether when oral feeding is not possible.

Valproate is well absorbed rectally. Oral solution can be administered rectally mixed 1:1 with water in equivalent oral doses, with excellent bioavailability (96.7%) *(81,82)*.

IM dosing of parenteral sodium valproate has shown somewhat decreased bioavailability (70%), as well as toxic muscle necrosis, even at low doses *(83)*. Repetitive IM dosing is discouraged.

Carbamazepine

Although no IV or IM form of carbamazepine has been developed, rectal administration has been well described *(77,84)*. Absorption and bioavailability are similar to oral dosing. Equivalent doses of oral solution are used, mixed 1:1 with water *(84)*. A suppository can also be made by dissolving carbamazepine powder in a standard suppository base *(85)*.

Zonisamide

Zonisamide can be absorbed rectally. A suppository using a polyethylene glycol base is absorbed rapidly and yields higher peak plasma concentrations than oral dosing with near 100% bioavailability *(86)*.

Benzodiazepines

Rectal diazepam is very well absorbed, given its high lipid solubility, and has been used extensively for acute seizure control and status epilepticus *(87)*. The parenteral solution may be given rectally without alteration. A rectal gel is also available in premeasured syringes at standard doses. Dosing for acute seizure management is 0.2 mg/kg in adults *(1)*. The medication is effective within 2–10 min, with peak concentrations achieved in 2–30 min. Respiratory depression is the main side effect of concern, as with all benzodiazepines.

Lorazepam tablets can be given sublingually with absorption equivalent to regular oral doses *(88)*. Rectal administration of the parenteral solution is also effective at equivalent doses *(89)*.

Midazolam solution can be given intranasally *(90)* or in the buccal cavity *(91)*, where it is rapidly absorbed through the mucosa. Therapeutic serum

Table 3
Effects of Commonly Used Medications on Serum Levels of Anticonvulsants *(2,3,93)*

	Phenytoin (DPH)	Valproate (VPA)	Carbamazepine (CBZ)	
Amiodarone	⇑		⇑	150–300% increase in plasma DPH
Antifungals	⇑⇑		⇑	Fluconazole causes 200–400% increase of DPH. Monitoring recommended for mico/keto/itraconazole. Ketoconazole may increase CBZ via CYP3A4 inhibition. No effect on either by ampho B, flucytosine.
Calcium channel blockers			⇑	Verapamil, diltiazem can increase CBZ by 40–60%. No effect with ranitidine, famotidine
Cimetidine	⇑⇑		⇑	Increased DPH, CBZ via CYP 2C19 inhibition. No effect with ranitidine, famotidine.
Macrolides			⇑⇑	Erythro/clarithro/troleandomycin inhibit CYP 3A4. No effect with azithromycin.
Omeprazole	⇑			Via inhibition of CYP 2C19. No data on Lansoprazole.
Propoxyphene	⇑		⇑⇑	Increases serum CBZ by CYP 3A4 inhibition, DPH via CYP 2C9.
Salicylates		⇑		Displace protein binding and inhibit B-oxidation of VPA.
SSRI[a]	⇑			Few reports with fluoxetine. No effect from paroxetine, sertraline, fluvoxamine.

⇑, increased serum levels.
⇓, decreased serum levels.
[a]Serotonin-specific re-uptake inhibitor.

levels can be achieved quickly via these routes, and buccal delivery has been favorably compared to rectal diazepam for acute seizure control *(92)*. Rectal administration of midazolam is also well-absorbed *(89)*.

No routes of administration other than enteral have been established for lamotrigine, topiramate, gabapentin, oxcarbazepine, tiagabine, or levetiracetam.

Significant Drug–Drug Interactions

Many drugs interact with anticonvulsants, frequently by virtue of enzyme induction or displacement from protein binding sites. The effects of the major anticonvulsants on commonly used classes of medications are outlined in **Table 3,** and the effects of similar medications on levels of anticonvulsants are outlined in **Table 4.**

Table 4
Effects of Anticonvulsants on Serum Levels of Commonly Used Medications (1–3,94)

	Phenytoin (DPH)	Phenobarbital (PB)	Carbamazepine (CBZ)	
Antipsychotics	⇓	⇓	⇓	EIAEDs[a] induce metabolism of chlorpromazine, clozapine, fluphenazine, haloperidol, risperdal, and mesoridazine (active metabolite of thioridazide)
Calcium channel blockers	⇓	⇓	⇓	Nimodipine metabolism significantly increased by EIAEDs.
Corticosteroids	⇓⇓	⇓⇓	⇓⇓	May require twofold increase in steroid dosing.
Cyclosporine	⇓⇓	⇓⇓	⇓⇓	Decreased blood levels by 30–50%. Increased clearance via CYP 3A4 induction.
Narcotics	⇓	⇓	⇓	EIAEDs enhance metabolism of fentanyl, meperidine, methadone, as well as additive effect on neurotoxic status epilepticus.
Neuromuscular blockers	⇓	⇓	⇓	CBZ and DPH decrease duration of blockade by doxacurium, pancuronium, vecuronium, rocuronium, possibly D-tubocurarine. No effect on atacurium, mivacurium.
Oral contraceptives (OCPs)	⇓	⇓	⇓	EIAED's induce metabolism of estrogen and progestin components of OCP's, as well as levonorgestrel from implants, up to 40%. 30% decrease in ethynyl estradiol with topiramate by unclear mechanism.
Tricyclics	⇓	⇓	⇓	EIAED's increase metabolism of amitriptyline, clomipramine, desipramine, doxepin, imipramine, nortriptyline, and proptiptyline.
Theophylline	⇓⇓	⇓⇓	⇓⇓	30–60% reduction in serum levels by EIAEDs.
Warfarin	⇓	⇓⇓	⇓⇓	CBZ, PHT cause increased clearance by 25–50%. DPH initially inhibits metabolism via CYP 2C9, then induces after 1–2 wk. Monitoring of international normalized ratios (INR) for 3–4 wk recommended.

⇓, decreased serum levels.
[a]EIAED = hepatic enzyme-inducing antiepileptic drug.

351

Conclusions

The choice of an anticonvulsant for the medically ill patient can be complex. No drug is truly without potentially dangerous side effects or the risk of drug–drug interactions. Patients with preexisting illness are especially at risk for such complications, and the choice of anticonvulsant can be difficult. Many of the newest agents have promising profiles, offering safe and effective therapy options, even for patients with hepatic and renal dysfunction. As with all medications, especially in this population, initiation of a new drug must be accompanied by careful monitoring for adverse reactions. With proper drug selection, dosing, and monitoring, seizure control can be achieved in patients, even with the most complex medical conditions.

References

1. *Physicians' Desk Reference.* Montvale, NJ: Medical Economics, 2000.
2. Levy RH, Mattson RH, Meldrum BS (eds.), *Antiepileptic Drugs.* New York: Raven, 1995.
3. Wyllie E. *The Treatment of Epilepsy: Principles and Practice.* Baltimore, MD: Williams & Wilkins, 1997.
4. UCB Pharma. *Keppra Prescribing Information.* Smyrna, GA: UCB Pharma, 2000.
5. Novartis. *Trileptal Prescribing Information.* East Hanover, NJ: Novartis Pharmaceuticals, 2000.
6. Pharma E. *Zonegran Prescribing Information.* South San Francisco, CA: Elan Pharmaceuticals, 2000.
7. Donovan PJ, Cline D. Phenytoin administration by constant intravenous infusion: selective rates of administration. *Ann Emerg Med* 1991;20:139–142.
8. Meek PD, Davis SN, Collins DM, et al. Guidelines for nonemergency use of parenteral phenytoin products: proceedings of an expert panel consensus process. Panel on Nonemergency Use of Parenteral Phenytoin Products. *Arch Intern Med* 1999;159:2639–2644.
9. Graves NM, Ramsay RE. Phenytoin and fosphenytoin. In: Wyllie E (ed.), *The Treatment of Epilepsy.* Baltimore, MD: Williams & Wilkins, 1997, pp 833–844.
10. Wilder BJ, Campbell K, Ramsay RE, et al. Safety and tolerance of multiple doses of intramuscular fosphenytoin substituted for oral phenytoin in epilepsy or neurosurgery. *Arch Neurol* 1996;53:764–768.
11. Jones AL, Proudfoot AT. Features and management of poisoning with modern drugs used to treat epilepsy. *Q J Med* 1998;91:325–332.
12. Boesen F, Andersen EB, Jensen EK, Ladefoged SD. Cardiac conduction disturbances during carbamazepine therapy. *Acta Neurol Scand* 1983;68:49–52.
13. Kasarskis EJ, Kuo CS, Berger R, Nelson KR. Carbamazepine-induced cardiac dysfunction. Characterization of two distinct clinical syndromes. *Arch Internal Med* 1992;152:186–191.
14. Terrence CF, Fromm G. Congestive heart failure during carbamazepine therapy. *Ann Neurol* 1980;8:200–201.
15. Herzberg L. Carbamazepine and bradycardia. *Lancet* 1978;1:1097–1098.
16. Beerman B, Edhag O, Vallin H. Advanced heart block aggravated by carbamazepine. *Br Heart J* 1975;37:668–671.

17. Sillanpaa M. Carbamazepine. In: Wyllie E (ed.), *The Treatment of Epilepsy*. Baltimore, MD: Williams & Wilkins, 1997, pp 808–823.
18. Sudhop T, Bauer J, Elger CE, von Bergmann K. Increased high-density lipoprotein cholesterol in patients with epilepsy treated with carbamazepine: a gender-related study. *Epilepsia* 1999;40:480–484.
19. Dam M, Ekberg R, Loyning Y, Waltimo O, Jakobsen K. A double-blind study comparing oxcarbazepine and carbamazepine in patients with newly diagnosed, previously untreated epilepsy. *Epilepsy Res* 1989;3:70–76.
20. Bourgeois BFD. Phenobarbital and primidone. In: Wyllie E (ed.), *The Treatment of Epilepsy*. Baltimore, MD: Williams & Wilkins, 1997, pp 845–855.
21. Boggs J, Waterhouse E, DeLorenzo RJ. The use of antiepileptic medications in renal and liver disease. In: Wyllie E (ed.), *The Treatment of Epilepsy*. Baltimore, MD: Williams & Wilkins, 1997, pp 753–762.
22. Howard PA, Engen PL, Dunn MI. Phenytoin hypersensitivity syndrome: a case report. *DICP* 1991;25:929–932.
23. Ratnaike RN, Schapel GJ, Purdie G, Rischbieth RH, Hoffmann S. Hyperammonaemia and hepatotoxicity during chronic valproate therapy: enhancement by combination with other antiepileptic drugs. *Br J Clin Pharmacol* 1986;22:100–103.
24. Bryant AE III, Dreifuss FE. Valproic acid hepatic fatalities. III. U.S. experience since 1986. *Neurology* 1996;46:465–469.
25. Konig SA, Schenk M, Sick C, et al. Fatal liver failure associated with valproate therapy in a patient with Friedreich's disease: review of valproate hepatotoxicity in adults. *Epilepsia* 1999;40:1036–1040.
26. Horowitz S, Patwardhan R, Marcus E. Hepatotoxic reactions associated with carbamazepine therapy. *Epilepsia* 1988;29:149–154.
27. Porto I, John EG, Heilliczer J. Removal of phenobarbital during continuous cycling peritoneal dialysis in a child. *Pharmacotherapy* 1997;17:832–835.
28. Askmark H, Wiholm BE. Epidemiology of adverse reactions to carbamazepine as seen in a spontaneous reporting system. *Acta Neurol Scand* 1990;81:131–140.
29. Hogg RJ, Sawyer M, Hecox K, Eigenbrodt E. Carbamazepine-induced acute tubulointerstitial nephritis. *J Pediatr* 1981;98:830–832.
30. Dasgupta A, Jacques M, Malhotra D. Diminished protein binding capacity of uremic sera for valproate following hemodialysis: role of free fatty acids and uremic compounds. *Am J Nephrol* 1996;16:327–333.
31. Moreiras Plaza M, Rodriguez Goyanes G, Cuina L, Alonso R. On the toxicity of valproic-acid. *Clin Nephrol* 1999;51:187–189.
32. Wong MO, Eldon MA, Keane WF, et al. Disposition of gabapentin in anuric subjects on hemodialysis. *J Clin Pharmacol* 1995;35:622–626.
33. Gilmore RL. Seizures and antiepileptic drug use in transplant patients. *Neurol Clin* 1988;6:279–296.
34. Sylvester RK, Lewis FB, Caldwell KC, Lobell M, Perri R, Sawchuk RA. Impaired phenytoin bioavailability secondary to cisplatinum, vinblastine, and bleomycin. *Ther Drug Monit* 1984;6:302–305.
35. Sobotka JL, Alexander B, Cook BL. A review of carbamazepine's hematologic reactions and monitoring recommendations. *DICP* 1990;24:1214–1219.
36. Holmes GL. Carbamazepine: toxicity. In: Levy RH, Mattson RH, Meldrum BS, (eds.), *Antiepileptic Drugs*. New York: Raven, 1995, pp 567–580.
37. Rapeport WG, Connell JC, Thompson GG, Moore MR, Brodie MJ. Effect of carbamazepine on haem biosynthesis in man. *Eur J Clin Invest* 1984;14:107–110.

38. Yeung Laiwah AA, Rapeport WG, Thompson GG, et al. Carbamazepine-induced non-hereditary acute porphyria. *Lancet* 1983;1:790–792.

39. Gidal B, Spencer N, Maly M, et al. Valproate-mediated disturbances of hemostasis: relationship to dose and plasma concentration. *Neurology* 1994;44:1418–1422.

40. Kis B, Szupera Z, Mezei Z, Gecse A, Telegdy G, Vecsei L. Valproate treatment and platelet function: the role of arachidonate metabolites. *Epilepsia* 1999;40:307–310.

41. MacDougall LG. Pure red cell aplasia associated with sodium valproate therapy. *JAMA* 1982;247:53–54.

42. Dreifuss FE. Valproic acid: toxicity. In: Levy RH, Mattson RH, Meldrum BS, (eds.), *Antiepileptic Drugs.* New York: Raven, 1995, pp 641–648.

43. Iivanainen M, Savolainen H. Side effects of phenobarbital and phenytoin during long-term treatment of epilepsy. *Acta Neurol Scand Suppl* 1983;97:49–67.

44. Bruni J. Phenytoin: toxicity. In: Levy RH, Mattson RH, Meldrum BS, (eds.), *Antiepileptic Drugs.* New York: Raven, 1995, pp 345–350.

45. Bardana EJ, Jr., Gabourel JD, Davies GH, Craig S. Effects of phenytoin on man's immunity. Evaluation of changes in serum immunoglobulins, complement, and antinuclear antibody. *Am J Med* 1983;74:289–296.

46. Rosenthal CJ, Noguera CA, Coppola A, Kapelner SN. Pseudolymphoma with mycosis fungoides manifestations, hyperresponsiveness to diphenylhydantoin, and lymphocyte disregulation. *Cancer* 1982;49:2305–2314.

47. Mattson RH, Cramer JA, Collins JF, et al. Comparison of carbamazepine, phenobarbital, phenytoin, and primidone in partial and secondarily generalized tonic-clonic seizures. *N Engl J Med* 1985;313:145–151.

48. Baciewicz AM. Carbamazepine drug interactions. *Ther Drug Monit* 1986; 8:305–317.

49. Kutt H. Phenobarbital: interactions with other drugs. In: Levy RH, Mattson RH, Meldrum BS (eds.), *Antiepileptic Drugs.* New York: Raven, 1995, pp 389–400.

50. Kutt H. Phenytoin: interactions with other drugs. Part 1: clinical aspects. In: Levy RH, Mattson RH, Meldrum BS (eds.), *Antiepileptic Drugs.* New York: Raven, 1995, pp 315–328.

51. Hess E. Drug-related lupus. *N Engl J Med* 1988;318:1460–1462.

52. Drory VE, Korczyn AD. Hypersensitivity vasculitis and systemic lupus erythematosis induced by anticonvulsants. *Clin Neuropharmacol* 1993;16:19–29.

53. Drory VE, Yust I, Korczyn AD. Carbamazepine-induced systemic lupus erythematosis. *Clin Neuropharmacol* 1989;12:115–118.

54. Kalff R, Houtkooper MA, Meyer JW, Goedhart DM, Augusteijn R, Meinardi H. Carbamazepine and serum sodium levels. *Epilepsia* 1984;25:390–397.

55. Lahr MB. Hyponatremia during carbamazepine therapy. *Clin Pharmacol Ther* 1985;37:693–696.

56. Schachter SC, Vazquez B, Fisher RS, et al. Oxcarbazepine: double-blind, randomized, placebo-control, monotherapy trial for partial seizures. *Neurology* 1999; 52:732–737.

57. Van Amelsvoort T, Bakshi R, Devaux CB, Schwabe S. Hyponatremia associated with carbamazepine and oxcarbazepine therapy: a review. *Epilepsia* 1994;35:181–188.

58. Camfield PR, Bagnell P, Camfield CS, Tibbles JA. Pancreatitis due to valproic acid. *Lancet* 1979;1:1198–1199.

59. Williams LH, Reynolds RP, Emery JL. Pancreatitis during sodium valproate treatment. *Arch Dis Child* 1983;58:543–544.

60. Asconape JJ, Penry JK, Dreifuss FE, Riela A, Mirza W. Valproate-associated pancreatitis. *Epilepsia* 1993;34:177–183.
61. Arafa M, Noble J, Royle SG, Trail IA, Allen J. Dupuytren's and epilepsy revisited. *J Hand Surg* 1992;17:221–224.
62. Critchley EM, Vakil SD, Hayward HW, Owen VM. Dupuytren's disease in epilepsy: result of prolonged administration of anticonvulsants. *J Neurol Neurosurg Psychiatry* 1976;39:498–503.
63. Dansky LV, Andermann E, Rosenblatt D, Sherwin AL, Andermann F. Anticonvulsants, folate levels, and pregnancy outcome: a prospective study. *Ann Neurol* 1987;21:176–182.
64. Dansky LV, Rosenblatt DS, Andermann E. Mechanisms of teratogenesis: folic acid and antiepileptic therapy. *Neurology* 1992;42:32–42.
65. Morrell MJ. Guidelines for the care of women with epilepsy. *Neurology* 1998;51:S21–S27.
66. Lewis DP, Van Dyke DC, Stumbo PJ, Berg MJ. Drug and environmental factors associated with adverse pregnancy outcomes. Part I: Antiepileptic drugs, contraceptives, smoking, and folate. *Ann Pharmacother* 1998;32:802–817.
67. Nulman I, Laslo D, Koren G. Treatment of epilepsy in pregnancy. *Drugs* 1999;57:535–544.
68. Gelineau-van Waes J, Bennett GD, Finnell RH. Phenytoin-induced alterations in craniofacial gene expression. *Teratology* 1999;59:23–34.
69. DiLiberti JH, Farndon PA, Dennis NR, Curry CJ. The fetal valproate syndrome. *Am J Med Genet* 1984;19:473–481.
70. Jones KL, Lacro RV, Johnson KA, Adams J. Pattern of malformations in the children of women treated with carbamazepine during pregnancy. *N Engl J Med* 1989;320:1661–1666.
71. Seip M. Growth retardation, dysmorphic facies, and minor malformations following massive exposure to phenobarbitone in utero. *Acta Paediat Scand* 1976;65:617–621.
72. Malone FD, D'Alton ME. Drugs in pregnancy: anticonvulsants. *Semin Perinatol* 1997;21:114–123.
73. American Academy of Pediatrics Committee on Drugs: The transfer of drugs and other chemicals into human milk. *Pediatrics* 1994;93:137–150.
74. Bauer LA. Interference of oral phenytoin absorption by continuous nasogastric feedings. *Neurology* 1982;32:570–572.
75. Doak KK, Haas CE, Dunnigan KJ, et al. Bioavailability of phenytoin acid and phenytoin sodium with enteral feedings. *Pharmacotherapy* 1998;18:637–645.
76. Bialer M, Cloyd JC. Drug formulations and routes of administration. In: Levy RH (ed.), *Antiepileptic Drugs*. New York: Raven, 1995, pp 161–178.
77. Van Hoogdalem EJ, De Boer AG, Briemer DD. Pharmacokinetics of rectal drug administration, part 1. *Clin Pharmacokinet* 1991;21:11–26.
78. Kuile F, Nosten F, Chongsuphajaisiddhi T, Holloway P, Maelankirri L, White NJ. Absorption of intramuscular phenobarbitone in children with severe falciparum malaria. *Eur J Clin Pharmacol* 1992;42:107–110.
79. Graves NM, Holmes GB, Kriel RL, Jones-Saete C, Ong B, Ehresman DJ. Relative bioavailability of rectally administered phenobarbital sodium parenteral solution. *DICP* 1989;23:565–568.
80. Jones-Saete C, Kriel RL, Cloyd JC. External leakage from feeding gastrostomies in patients receiving valproate sprinkle. *Epilepsia* 1992;33:692–695.

81. Margarit MV, Rodriguez IC, Cerezo A. Rectal bioavailability of water-soluble drugs: sodium valproate. *J Pharm Pharmacol* 1991;43:721–725.
82. Holmes GB, Rosenfeld WE, Graves NM, Remmel RP, Carlson GH, Kriel RD. Absorption of valproic acid suppositories in human volunteers. *Arch Neurol* 1989;46:906–909.
83. Gallo BV, Slater JD, Toledo C, DeToledo J, Ramsay RE. Pharmacokinetics and muscle histopathology of intramuscular valproate. *Epilepsy Res* 1997;28:11–15.
84. Graves NM, Kriel RL, Jones-Saete C, Cloyd JC. Relative bioavailability of rectally administered carbamazepine suspension in humans. *Epilepsia* 1985;26:429 433.
85. Olson WL. Carbamazepine suppository. *Neurology* 1990;40:1472–1473.
86. Nagatomi A, Mishima M, Tsuzuki O, Ohdo S, Higuchi S. Utility of a rectal suppository containing the antiepileptic drug zonisamide. *Biol Pharm Bull* 1997;20:892–896.
87. Dreifuss FE, Rosman NP, Cloyd JC, et al. A comparison of rectal diazepam gel and placebo for acute repetitive seizures. *N Engl J Med* 1998;338:1869–1875.
88. Gram-Hansen P, Schultz A. Plasma concentrations following oral and sublingual administration of lorazepam. *Int J Clin Pharmacol Ther Toxicol* 1988;26:323–324.
89. Rey E, Treluyer JM, Pons G. Pharmacokinetic optimization of benzodiazepine therapy for acute seizures. Focus on delivery routes. *Clin Pharmacokinet* 1999;36:409–424.
90. Scheepers M, Scheepers B, Clough P. Midazolam via the intranasal route: an effective rescue medication for severe epilepsy in adults with learning disability. *Seizure* 1998;7:509–512.
91. Scott RC, Besag FM, Boyd SG, Berry D, Neville BG. Buccal absorption of midazolam: pharmacokinetics and EEG pharmacodynamics. *Epilepsia* 1998;39:290–294.
92. Scott RC, Besag FM, Neville BG. Buccal midazolam and rectal diazepam for treatment of prolonged seizures in childhood and adolescence: a randomised trial. *Lancet* 1999;353:623–626.
93. Fischer JH. *Drug Interactions with Antiepileptic Drugs.* New York: McMahon Publishing Group, 1999.
94. Spina E, Pisani F, Perucca E. Clinically significant pharmacokinetic drug interactions with carbamazepine. An update. *Clin Pharmacokinet* 1996;31:198–214.

Index

Edema
  neuronal, 322
  pulmonary, 323
Electrocardiograms (EKGs)
  in syncope, 274, 275–277
Electroencephalograms (EEGs)
  acute neurological disturbances
    and, 39–41
  acute stroke and, 40
  with ARSs, 175
  brain trauma and, 41
  CNS infection and, 40–41
  critically ill patients and, 324
  with HIE, 236–237
  ICH and, 40
  with organ transplantation, 261
  in SE, 315
  with SE, 324
  in syncope, 274, 277–278
  syncope and, 279
Electrolyte balance, 14, 85–100
Emboli, 31, 217, *see also* Cerebral
    embolism
Enalapril, 257
Encephalitis
  Japanese, 296–297
Encephalopathy
  acute, 219
  bilirubinemic, 298
  diffuse, 217
  Hashimoto's, 113–114
  hepatic, 15
  hypertensive, 252–257
  hyponatremic, 90
  hypothyroid, 78
  hypoxic-ischemic (HIE), 236–238
  mitochondrial, *see* Mitochondrial
    encephalopathy, lactic acidosis,
    and stroke-like episodes (MELAS)
  rejection, 264–265
  uremic, 74–75
Endocarditis, 183
  bacterial, 242
Endocrine disorders, 107–115
Endocrine failure, 77–80
Enflurane, 160
Entamoeba histolytica, 294
Environmental toxins, 193–203
Eosinophilia, 289

Epilepsy
  acute stroke and, 26
  alcohol-related seizures (ARSs) and, 171
  classification, 309–310
  defined, 3
  drug-associated seizures and, 149
  OCIs and, 299–300
  permanent, and SE, 329
  temporal lobe, 275
  in tropics, 285, 286
Epileptogenesis, 34–36
Escherichia coli, 126
Essential thrombocythemia, 77
Ethanol, *see* Alcohol
Ethanol-related hypoglycemia, 170
Etomidate, 160
  •
Fat embolism syndrome, 62–63
Febrile convulsions (FCs), 127
  assessment, 132
  clinical features, 132
  EEG and, 132
  epidemiology, 127–128
  etiology, 128
  genetic analysis and, 15–16
  in malaria, 294
  management, 132–133
  MRI in, 130–131
  MTS and, 130–132
  pathology, 129
  prognosis, 129–130
  treatment, 132–133
  in the tropics, 298
Felbamate, 267
Fever, 121–123, *see also* Hyperthermia
  brain injury and, 124–126
FK506, 155
Flumazenil, 160
Fluoroquinolones, 152–153
Focal motor seizures
  with cerebrovascular disease, 26
Focal necrotizing meningoencephalitis, 266
Focal seizures, 3
Foscarnet, 154
Fosfamide therapy, 219
Fosphenytoin, 312, 313, 326, 336, 341,
    342, 348
Free radical scavengers, 238
Fungal infections, 297